Essentials of Operative Cardiac Surgery

Prakash P. Punjabi
Panagiotis G. Kyriazis
Editors

Essentials of Operative Cardiac Surgery

Second Edition

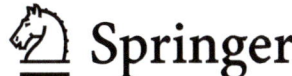 Springer

Editors
Prakash P. Punjabi
National Heart and Lung Institute
Faculty of Medicine, Imperial College
London
London, England, UK

Department of Cardiothoracic
Surgery
Hammersmith Hospital
Imperial College Healthcare NHS Trust
London, UK

Panagiotis G. Kyriazis
National Heart and Lung Institute
Faculty of Medicine, Imperial College
London
London, England, UK

Department of Cardiothoracic
Surgery
Hammersmith Hospital
Imperial College Healthcare NHS Trust
London, UK

ISBN 978-3-031-14556-8   ISBN 978-3-031-14557-5   (eBook)
https://doi.org/10.1007/978-3-031-14557-5

This Springer imprint is published by the registered company Springer Nature Switzerland AG
The registered company address is: Gewerbestrasse 11, 6330 Cham, Switzerland

Preface

"The life so short, the craft so long to learn."—Hippocrates of Kos (460–370 BC) aka Father of Medicine was a Greek physician, one of the most outstanding figures in the history of Medicine

According to the World Health Organization, around 7.2 million men and women die every year from coronary heart disease (CHD), which is the leading cause of cardiovascular death worldwide [1, 2]. In Europe, CHD accounts to approximately 1.95 million deaths yearly of which over 66,000 are in the UK and over 53,000 of those are in England alone [1–3]. It has also been estimated that 2.3 million people live with CHD in the UK of which 1.9 million people are in England [1, 3]. Considering the UK has a population of approximately 67 million, it has been deduced that 3.7% of the UK population is suffering from CHD.

The number of heart disease cases accelerated in early 2000, thereafter recent advances in primary prevention coupled with percutaneous intervention for acute myocardial infarction which stabilised and gradually declined the morbidity rate [3]. Associated with this decline, a rise in valvular heart disease has compensated in maintaining the total number of cardiac surgery procedures in adults. Multiple studies and guidelines have recommended ongoing improvement of techniques minimising risks to maintain and enhance safety. Currently, it is estimated that more than one million cardiac operations are performed each year worldwide with the use of the heart-lung machine, more specifically in the UK 35,158 cardiac surgeries were performed in 2015 [4]. In most cases, the operative mortality is quite low, approaching 1% for some operations [5].

Inspired by cardiac surgery and driven to simplify the charm of surgical principles, the goal of this book is to provide surgeons the necessary tools with review of techniques along with tips and tricks to finetune and excel their skills in an ever-expanding field of adult cardiac surgery. The second edition offers the readership an opportunity to widen their repertoire by reading each chapter and introductory literature review, major technical essentials and conclude with the results and long-term outcomes. The Philosophy of Essentials of Operative Cardiac Surgery remains the same 'keep simple cases simple and turn complex cases into simple cases'.

"The important thing in science is not so much to obtain new facts as to discover new ways of thinking about them."—Sir William Bragg (1862–1942), Physics Nobel Laureate 1915, was a British physicist, chemist, and mathematician

References

1. British Heart Foundation. England factsheet; April 2019.
2. Mackay J, Mensah G, eds. The atlas of heart disease and stroke. World Health Organization, Geneva; 2004.
3. British Heart Foundation. UK Factsheet; April 2019.
4. The Society for Cardiothoracic Surgery in Great Britain & Ireland, Blue Book Online.
5. Punjabi PP, Taylor KM. The science and practice of cardiopulmonary bypass: from cross circulation to ECMO and SIRS. Global Cardiol Sci Pract. 2013:32.

London, UK   Prakash P. Punjabi
London, UK   Panagiotis G. Kyriazis

Contents

Echocardiography in Adult Cardiac Surgery

Rasa Ordiene, Karan P. Punjabi,
and Egle Ereminiene

Learning Objectives

- Understand the principles of echocardiography in cardiac surgery as an essential guiding tool
- Understand the role of each different technique based on its sophistication and sensitivity
- Understand the process of assessing the information gathered from each technique
- Understand how each technology can assist and support the decision making process of a surgeon
- Understand its necessity as a diagnostic tool in adult cardiac surgery

R. Ordiene (✉) · K. P. Punjabi
Department of Cardiology, Medical Academy,
Lithuanian University of Health Sciences,
Kaunas, Lithuania
e-mail: rasa.ordiene@lsmuni.lt

K. P. Punjabi
School of Medicine, St. George's University of
London, London, UK

E. Ereminiene
Department of Cardiology, Medical Academy,
Lithuanian University of Health Sciences,
Kaunas, Lithuania

Institute of Cardiology, Lithuanian University of
Health Sciences, Kaunas, Lithuania

Introduction

Echocardiography has become the major imaging and diagnostic modality of cardiac diseases, so all cardiac specialists, cardiologists and cardiac surgeons, need to know basic principles of this investigation in order to make the right decisions in the management of the patients.

A complete transthoracic echocardiogram (TTE) is routinely performed before any cardiac surgical procedure. It consists of two-dimensional (2D) anatomic imaging, M-mode, and three Doppler techniques: pulsed-wave (PW), continuous-wave (CW), and color-flow imaging and provides a surgeon with information on the dimensions, areas, and volumes of cardiac chambers, biventricular function, cardiac valve anatomy and function, and pericardium. Currently available new techniques—Doppler tissue imaging and speckle-tracking echocardiography add very important data about early changes of regional and global myocardial dysfunction in surgery patients.

2D and 3D transesophageal echocardiography (TOE) examination provides additional information in patients who are not optimally imaged by the transthoracic approach. In addition, structures that are not well visualized by TTE (left atrial appendage, thoracic aorta, prosthetic valves) can be assessed by the transesophageal approach. A third indication is to guide intraoperative management during cardiac surgery. Class I indications for perioperative TOE are listed in Table 1.1.

© Springer Nature Switzerland AG 2022
P. P. Punjabi, P. G. Kyriazis (eds.), *Essentials of Operative Cardiac Surgery*,
https://doi.org/10.1007/978-3-031-14557-5_1

Table 1.1 Class I Indications for perioperative TEE

- Acute and life-threatening hemodynamic instability
- Valve repair or complex valve replacements
- Hypertrophic obstructive cardiomyopathy
- Aortic dissection with possible aortic valve involvement
- Endocarditis (perivalvular involvement)
- Congenital heart surgery
- Pericardial windows (posterior or located effusions)
- Placement of intracardiac devices

TOE also may be useful in surgical procedures in patients at risk of myocardial ischemia or hemodynamic instability, minimally invasive surgery, or intracardiac mass resection, detecting intracardiac air or aortic atheromatous disease. According to the guidelines, TOE should be used in all open heart and thoracic aortic surgical procedures to confirm the preoperative diagnosis, detect new or unsuspected pathology, and to assess the results of surgical intervention [1, 2].

In this chapter, we will highlight the applications of echocardiography on the following topics, most relevant for cardiac surgeons: assessment of biventricular geometry and function, mitral, tricuspidal, and aortic valve morphology and function, evaluation of aorta, valve repair and replacement results.

Assessment of Biventricular Geometry and Function

LV Geometry, Global and Regional Function

Evaluation of LV dimensions and function is essential for the **preoperative** assessment of the patient. LV dilatation and systolic dysfunction, as well as increased LV end-systolic dimension and volume are important parameters in valvular surgery timing. Internal dimensions can be obtained with a 2DE guided M-mode approach, although linear measurements obtained from 2D echocardiographic images are preferred. LV volumes are measured using 2DE or 3DE. One of the advantages of 3D echocardiographic volume measurements is that they do not rely on geometric assumptions, are accurate and reproducible, closer to those obtained by cardiac magnetic resonance (CMR) and should therefore be used when available and feasible. LV size and volume measurements should be indexed to BSA. 2D echocardiographic LV end diastolic volume index of 74 ml/m2 for men and 61 ml/m2 for women and LV end systolic volume index of 31 ml/m2 for men and 24 ml/m2 for women are used as the upper limits of the corresponding normal range. LV systolic function is assessed using 2DE or 3DE by calculating ejection fraction (EF). LV EF of <52% for men and < 54% for women are markers of abnormal LV systolic function [3]. Detailed assessment of LV systolic function is of great importance in patients with severe valve regurgitation for surgery timing and prediction of cardiac events. Surgery in patients with asymptomatic severe MR is recommended when LV dysfunction occurs (LVEF≤60% and/or LV ESD ≥ 40 mm). However, assessment of LV dysfunction by LVEF is often overestimated in MR patients. New 2DE modalities, such as speckle tracking echocardiography enables calculation of global longitudinal LV strain (GLS). Reduced GLS with > − 18.1% showed higher risk of composite events in asymptomatic severe MR patients, and diagnostic value in predicting a reduction in LVEF of >10% with a resulting postoperative LVEF of <50% (area under the curve, 0.93; P < .001 [4–6] and patients with GLS > −19.5% were more likely to have a shorter survival in asymptomatic patients with aortic regurgitation patients who did not undergo aortic valve replacement [7]. This indicates the important value of myocardial longitudinal deformation indices for surgery timing in severe aortic and mitral regurgitation patients (Fig. 1.1).

Determination of regional and global LV systolic function is one of the most common indications of **perioperative** TOE examination. Quick 'eyeballing' of the overall LV systolic function by an experienced observer in the operating room correlate to quantitative measurements of LV ejection fraction. Assessment of LV regional wall motion abnormalities (RWMA) allows detection of areas of myocardial asynergy and identifies coronary territories in compromise. Regional wall motion analysis can be performed using the ME four and two chamber and ME LAX views. However, the TG midpapillary SAX view is of great importance, as the myocardium in these segments is supplied by the LAD, LCX and RCA coronary arteries simultaneously (Fig. 1.2). New

RWMA in the perioperative setting may indicate native coronary artery (accidental ligation) or early graft failure, inadequate myocardial preservation during cardioplegia or off-pump surgery. This is particularly important in the right coronary artery territory as, due to its anterior and superior location, air embolism may occur. Occasionally, the left circumflex artery (supplying blood to the lateral wall) may become compromised as there is a risk of accidental ligation of the artery in the atrioventricular groove while applying sutures in the posterior mitral annular area. TOE assists the surgeon while weaning-off the patient from cardiopulmonary bypass (CPB) and helps ensure complete de-airing of the car-

diac chambers by providing visualisation of residual air bubbles in the LV cavity, thus, reducing the risk of coronary air embolism and subsequent biventricular dysfunction. Perioperative LV dimensions help to assess systemic volume status, mainly in TG midpapillary SAX view. While assessing LV function in the operating room, it is useful to remember that: CPB unloads both ventricles and LV function may appear better than it really is. Systemic volume underfilling status may falsely 'shrink' the LV; at a slow heart rate, the LV appears 'sluggish' and the increase in heart rate may improve the systolic function in such case. Paradoxical motion of the interventricular septum is a common finding after pericardiotomy and, when observed in isolation, does not indicate new myocardial ischemia. To avoid possible pitfalls in LV assessment, its volumes and function should be assessed, not only while coming off bypass, but also at the very end of the surgery (fully off-bypass).

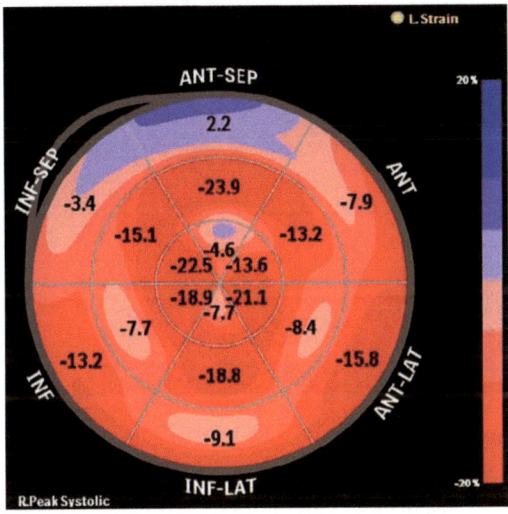

Fig. 1.1 Reduced LV global longitudinal strain (−12.2%) in severe MR with preserved LV ejection fraction

RV Geometry and Function

Right ventricular (RV) function in the context of cardiac surgery confers a high perioperative mortality rate. The reported incidence of refractory RV failure varies from 0.1% (post-cardiotomy) to 30% (post-LV assist device insertion). Perioperative factors that increase the risk of RV dysfunction/failure include: long cardiopulmonary bypass time (>150 min) and acute pulmonary hypertension, suboptimal intraoperative

Fig. 1.2 Regional wall motion analysis using TOE mid esophageal four (**a**) and two chambers (**b**), long axis (**c**) and transgastric midpapillary short axis views (**d**). *RCA* right coronary artery, *LAD* left anterior descending artery, *CX* circumflex artery

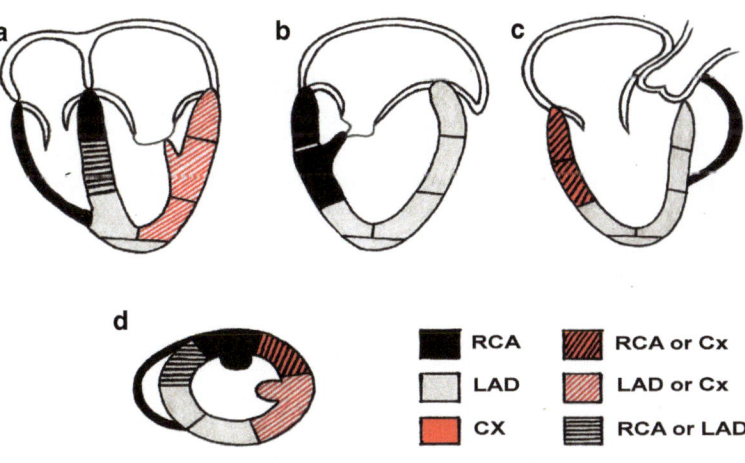

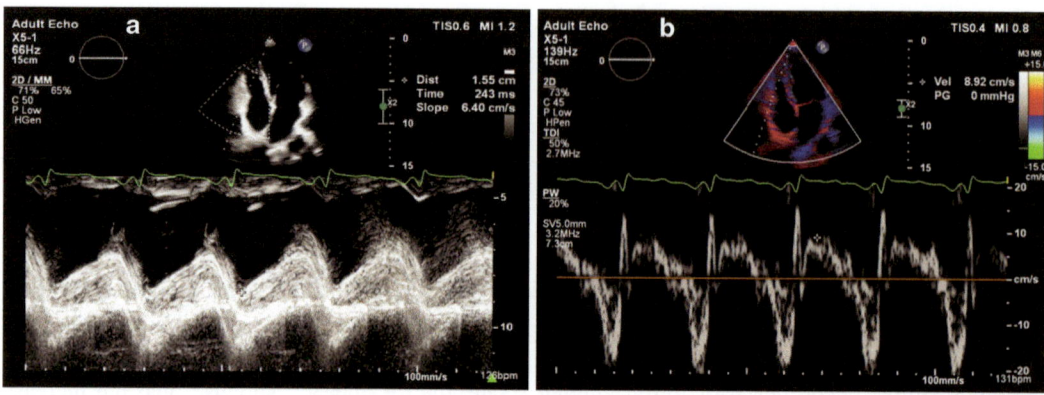

Fig. 1.3 Assessment of RV function: tricuspid annular plane systolic excursion (**a**) and longitudinal myocardial velocity (s') (**b**), showing slightly reduced longitudinal RV function

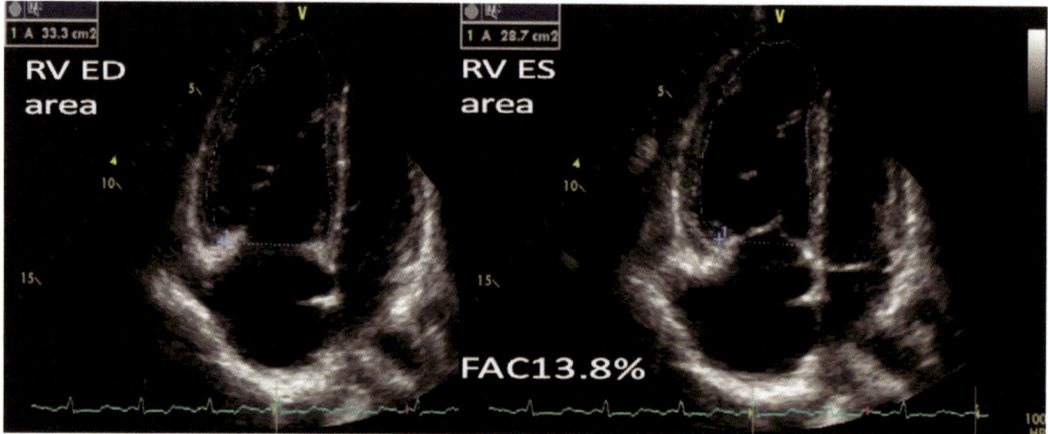

Fig. 1.4 RV fractional area change shows severely reduced RV function

myocardial protection (stunning), coronary embolism or graft occlusion causing RV ischemia, pre-existing pulmonary vascular dysfunction, injurious perioperative mechanical ventilation leading to lung injury and acute respiratory distress syndrome [8].

Patients with clinically suspected RV dysfunction assessed by 2D and 3D TTE and perioperative TEE may have RV dilatation (volume overload) and/or septal dyskinesia during end-systole (pressure overload). Due to its complex geometry, measurements by 2DE can be challenging. In the RV-focused view, RV diameter > 41 mm at the base and > 35 mm at the midlevel indicates RV dilatation. Multi, not single echocardiographic parameters have been proven in diagnosis of perioperative RV dysfunc-

tion: tricuspidal annular plane systolic excursion (TAPSE) <17 mm, pulsed-Doppler systolic myocardial velocity (s') <9.5 cm/s, RV fractional area change (RVFAC) <35%, RV 3D ejection fraction <45% [3, 8, 9] (Figs. 1.3, 1.4, and 1.5). The assessment of RV function goes hand in hand with pulmonary artery (PA) pressure estimation. Systolic PA pressure is obtained if there is a sufficient degree of tricuspid regurgitation (TR).

2DE allows to diagnose elevated right atrial pressure by dilatation of inferior vena cava (>21 mm) and absence of inspiratory variation.

These echocardiographic parameters together with invasive hemodynamic monitoring are crucial to diagnose RV failure and to guide therapy in operative room or intensive care unit and reduce mortality in cardiac surgical patients.

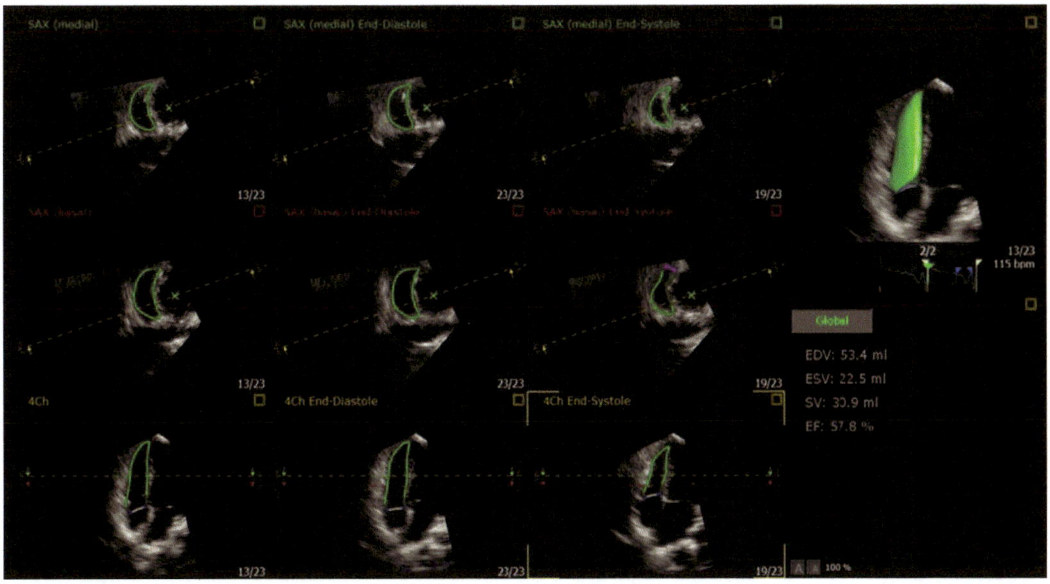

Fig. 1.5 Measurement of RV systolic function: ejection fraction, measured by 3D TEE

Intraoperative echocardiography for valve Surgery

As the repair techniques for heart valves evolved, there is the need for detailed and accurate intraoperative imaging of the valves before and after cardiopulmonary bypass. Multiplane 2D and/or 3D TOE are recommended for all valve repair procedures in order to better define the mechanism of valve dysfunction, severity of valve stenosis or regurgitation and provide comparison images for postoperative evaluation. The alterations in loading conditions from general anesthesia and positive pressure ventilation have effects on valve dysfunction severity—reduce valvular regurgitation in comparison to preoperative data. Reduced systemic blood pressure causes reflective tachycardia and general anaesthetics may provoke atrial fibrillation, consequently, the estimation of valvular lesions may be difficult. Once the surgical procedure commences, electrocautery is used, which creates reduced quality of 2DE, also creates stitching artifacts during multiple beat acquisitions on 3D TOE.

MV Assessment

Anatomic Backgound

The mitral valve (MV) complex is composed from mitral annulus, anterior and posterior leaflets, the subvalvular apparatus (chordae tendinea and two papillary muscles), and the LV. An imperfection in any one of these components can cause the valve to leak.

The mitral annulus is a frequent surgical target in cardiac surgery and its unique saddle-shaped anatomy was first understood by the help of 3DE (Fig. 1.6). This shape facilitates valve closure and minimize leaflet stress. The annulus is not a static structure, the dynamic motion includes systolic antero-posterior shortening as well as alteration of the height to facilitate filling and minimize regurgitation. The mitral leaflets become confluent at the lateral and medial commissures. According to Carpentier classification the posterior leaflet has three scallops: P1, or lateral, P2, central and P3, medial with the central scallop usually the largest. The anterior leaflet, though

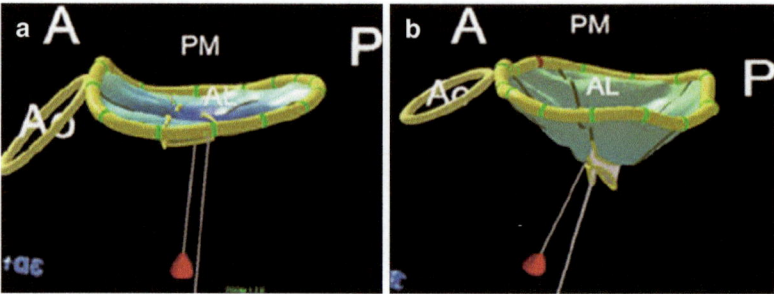

Fig. 1.6 (**a**) Normal MV with a saddle shape of the annulus, with anterior and posterior points being higher than the posteromedial and anterolateral; (**b**) MV leaflet coaptation defect as a result of ischaemic heart disease. Note the annular distortion, loss of saddle shape, significant tenting and ventricular displacement of mitral valve leaflets. *A* anterior, *P* posterior, *Ao* aorta, *AL* anterolateral, *PM* posteromedial

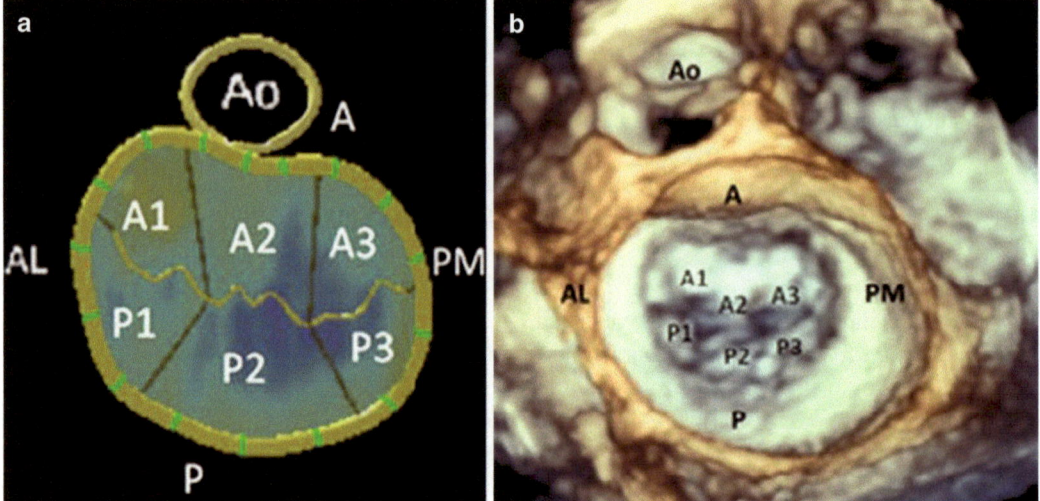

Fig. 1.7 Carpentier's MV and scallop nomenclature in (**a**) reconstructed 3D MV model and (**b**) real-time 3D TEE 'surgical' view of MV. *A* anterior, *P* posterior, *Ao* aorta, *AL* anterolateral, *PM* posteromedial, P1, P2, P3 posterior mitral leaflet scallops with the corresponding segments of the anterior leaflet (A1, A2, A3)

longer, covers one third of the annular circumference. Although the anterior leaflet lacks scallops, the corresponding posterior segments are named A1, A2 and A3, (Fig. 1.7). This classification enables better communication among the cardiac anaesthetists, cardiologists and cardiothoracic surgeons while addressing the underlying MV pathology. 3D TOE imaging of MV provides 'surgical view' of the valve, which is a good match of what the surgeon expects to see in theatre. The images can be rotated by 360° to visualize the valve from either left atrial or LV sides. The proper coaptation of the leaflets is approximately 1 cm and is subtended by primary and secondary chordae. Strut chords attach to the rough zone of the anterior leaflet and maintain direct continuity among the valve, the papillary muscles, and the LV myocardium. LV shape and function are also of great importance in normal MV function. Alteration in LV geometry and function may lead to valvular tethering and mitral insufficiency.

Mitral Valve Regurgitation (MR)

The role of 2D/3D TOE in MR is to determine aetiology, lesion, mechanism, localization of regurgitant orifice, quantification of MR severity, assessment of suitability for repair, estimation of risk of SAM, evaluation of surgical results.

Aetiology and Mechanisms of MR

According to aetiology, MR can be classified as primary (organic/structural) or secondary (functional) (Table 1.2).

Evaluation of leaflet morphology and mobility is crucial in mitral valve surgery. Carpentier's classification of leaflet lesion type and motion disturbances distinguishes three major types of leaflet motion:

Type I: normal leaflet motion, MR is derived from a dilated mitral annulus, mitral cleft or leaflet perforation due to trauma or endocarditis and the jet tends to be central. Annular dilatation is identified when the ratio annulus/anterior leaflet is >1.3 (in diastole) or when

Table 1.2 Aetiology of mitral regurgitation

• Organic (primary) mitral regurgitation
• Degenerative disease (Barlow, fibroelastic deficiency (FED), Marfan, Ehler-Danlos, annular calcification)
• Infective endocarditis;
• Rheumatic heart disease;
• Congenital structural abnormalities (prominent leaflet cleft, parachute mitral valve);
• Toxic valvulopathy
• Ruptured papillary muscle secondary to myocardial infarction
Secondary (functional) MR
• Dilated cardiomyopathy
• Ischaemic heart disease,
• Systolic LV dysfunction, conduction disturbances (dyssynchronous contraction);
• Severe LA dilatation

the annulus diameter is >35 mm. 3D TOE method has been shown to be superior in diagnosis of indentation and clefts—with sensitivity 93% and specificity of 92%. This type also includes patients with dilated cardiomyopathy and functional MR in cases when the motion of the mitral valve leaflets is not restricted (Fig. 1.8).

Type II: MV is structurally abnormal with one or more prolapsing segments. It is characterised by excessive leaflet motion often secondary to Barlow disease, fibroelastic deficiency, ruptured or elongated chordae or papillary muscles and the regurgitant jet is directed away from the diseased leaflet (Fig. 1.9).

Type III: the responsible mechanism in this type is restrictive motion of the leaflets and the regurgitant jet can be directed towards the affected leaflet, or it can be central if both leaflets are equally affected. There are 2 subtypes—III A: systolic/diastolic—when MV apparatus is damaged by rheumatic heart disease and III B: systolic—when LV dilatation/ischaemia results in systolic leaflet restriction (tenting of the leaflets), or regional wall motion abnormalities, areas of thinning and ventricular aneurysms that result in asymmetric tenting patterns of the MV apparatus and functional (ischemic) MR. LV dilatation causes displacement of papillary muscles, annular dilatation and increased systolic and diastolic tension of the valve, thus, impeding normal valve closure [10, 11] (Fig. 1.10).

Quantitation of MR

The assessment of MR includes integration of data from 2D/3D imaging of the valve and the evaluation LV as well. The severity of MR can be quantified by various echocardiographic techniques: colour flow jet area, vena contracta

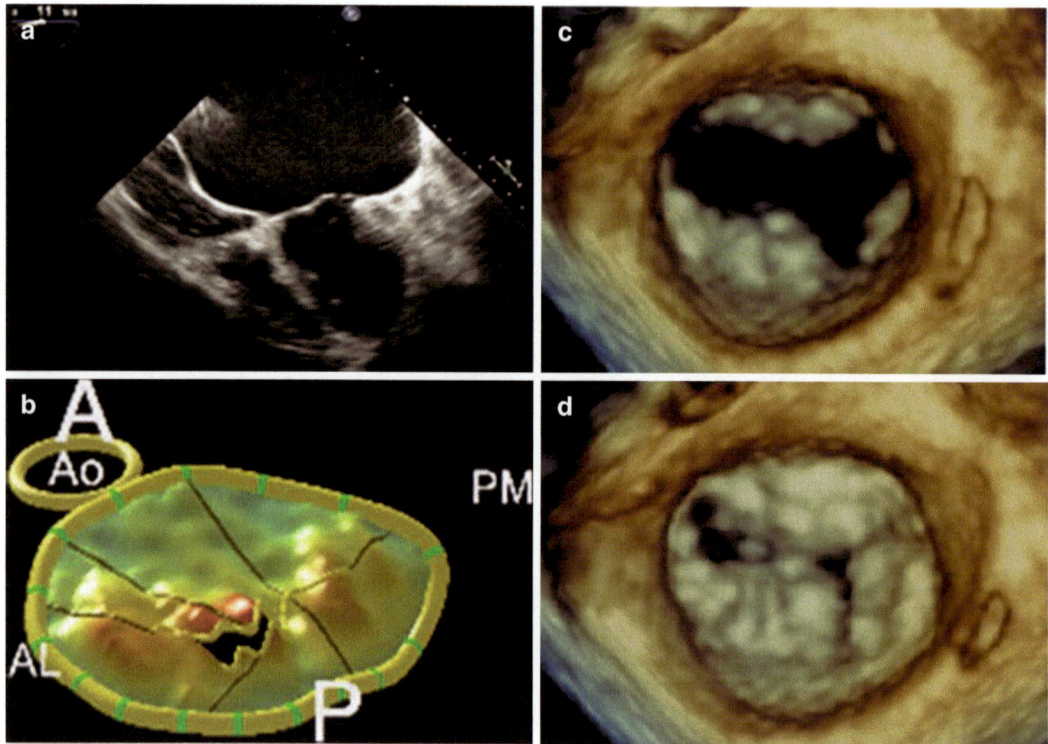

Fig. 1.8 Type I (Carpentier's) MR: (**a**) Significant mitral annular dilatation secondary to severe LA enlargement resulting in significant leaflet malcoaptation most appreciated on 3D TEE reconstructed mitral annular model (**b**). Note, a flattened annular shape and secondary prolapse of A2 segment. (**c, d**) show mitral valve cleft at 5 o'clock and another coaptation defect at the posteromedial commissure (10 o'clock) in diastole and systole respectively. *A* anterior, *Ao* aorta, *AL* anterolateral, *PM* posteromedial, *P* posterior

width, proximal isovelocity surface area (PISA) and detection of flow reversal in the pulmonary veins (Table 1.3). Both the VC width and the regurgitant orifice area (EROA) by the PISA method are recommended for MR estimation. VC > 7 mm and an EROA ≥40 mm2 or an regurgitant volume (R Vol) ≥ 60 ml indicates severe organic MR. In functional ischaemic MR, an EROA ≥20 mm2 or an R Vol ≥ 30 ml identifies patients with severe functional MR [12–14]. 3D echocardiography allows overcoming many limitations of conventional 2D echocardiographic assessment. 3D TOE provides direct planimetry of regurgitant orifices in an en face projection. This also illustrates that often ROA is not circular, which is an erroneous assumption that the PISA method is based upon and there may be multiple regurgitant orifices and jets present (Figs. 1.11 and 1.12). It's important to remember that the alteration in loading conditions from general anesthesia and positive pressure ventilation have dramatic effect on indices of MR severity that's why the severity of MR must be preciously assessed preoperatively [11].

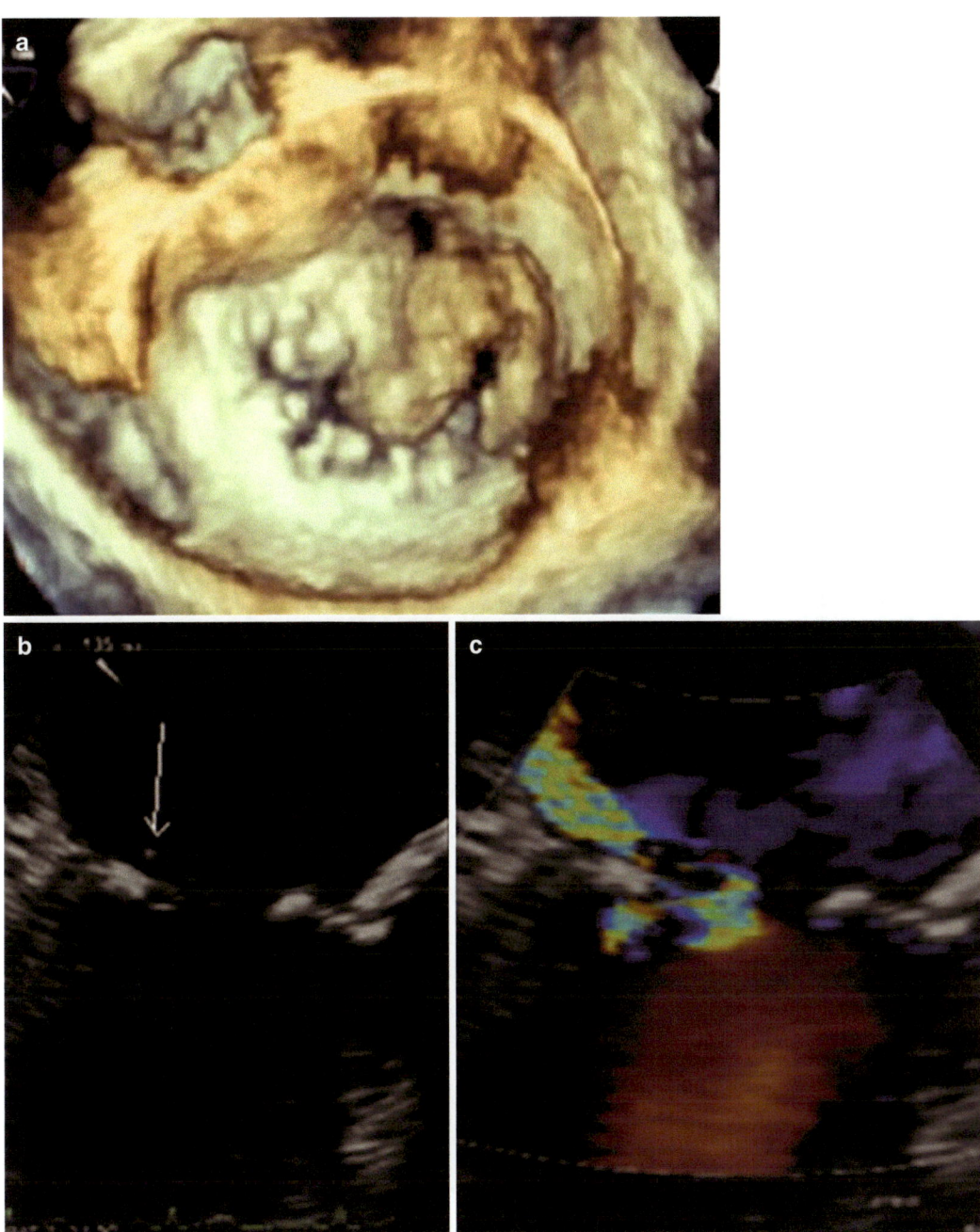

Fig. 1.9 Type II (Carpentier's) MR. (**a**) show 3D TEE images of extensive myxomatous valve disease, prolapse of A2 segment, A3/P3 segments, and posteromedial com-missure, (**b, c**): degenerative MV disease with a flail A2 segment secondary to a ruptured chord (*arrow*). Severe MR directed posteriorly

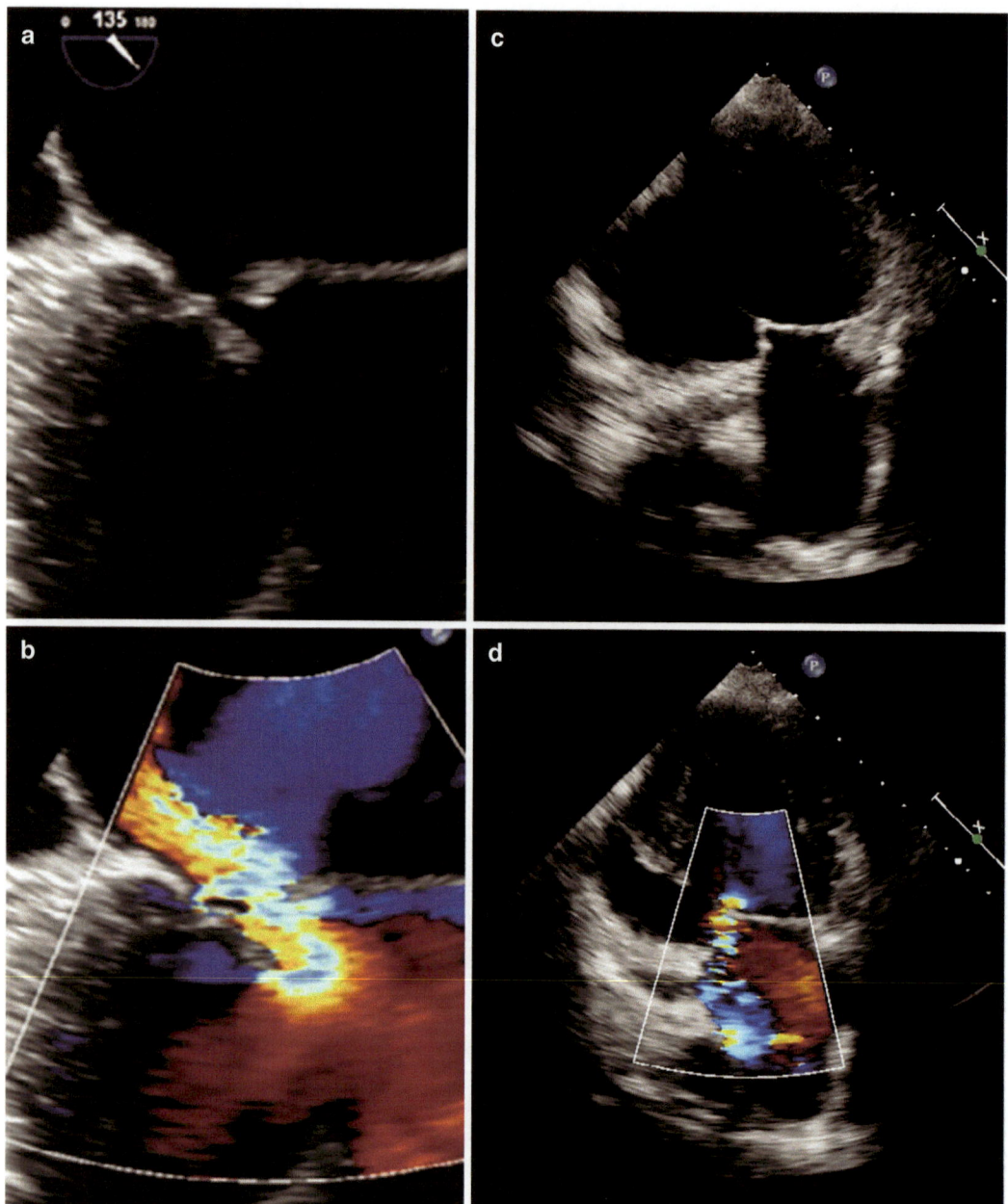

Fig. 1.10 Type III (Carpentier's) MR. (**a, b**): Type IIIa. Rheumatic mitral valve with severely restricted posterior mitral valve leaflet (PML). The anterior leaflet is mobile and overrides the PML in systole, leading to a very eccentric and severe posteriorly directed MR jet. Both leaflets are thickened at the tips. (**c, d**) Type IIIb. Inferior LV myocardial infarction, aneurysm of inferior wall, restriction of the MV posterior leaflet, resulting in functional severe MR

Table 1.3 Criteria for severe primary MR

Quantitative Measures	Specific Criteria[a]
EROA ≥40 mm2	Flail leaflet
Reg volume ≥ 60 ml	VC width ≥ 0.7 mm
Regurgitant fraction ≥50%	PISA radius ≥ 1.0 cm at Nyquist of 30–40 cm/s
	Central large jet >50% of LA area
	Pulmonary vein systolic flow reversal
	Dilated with normal function LV

[a] Definitely severe if ≥4 specific criteria

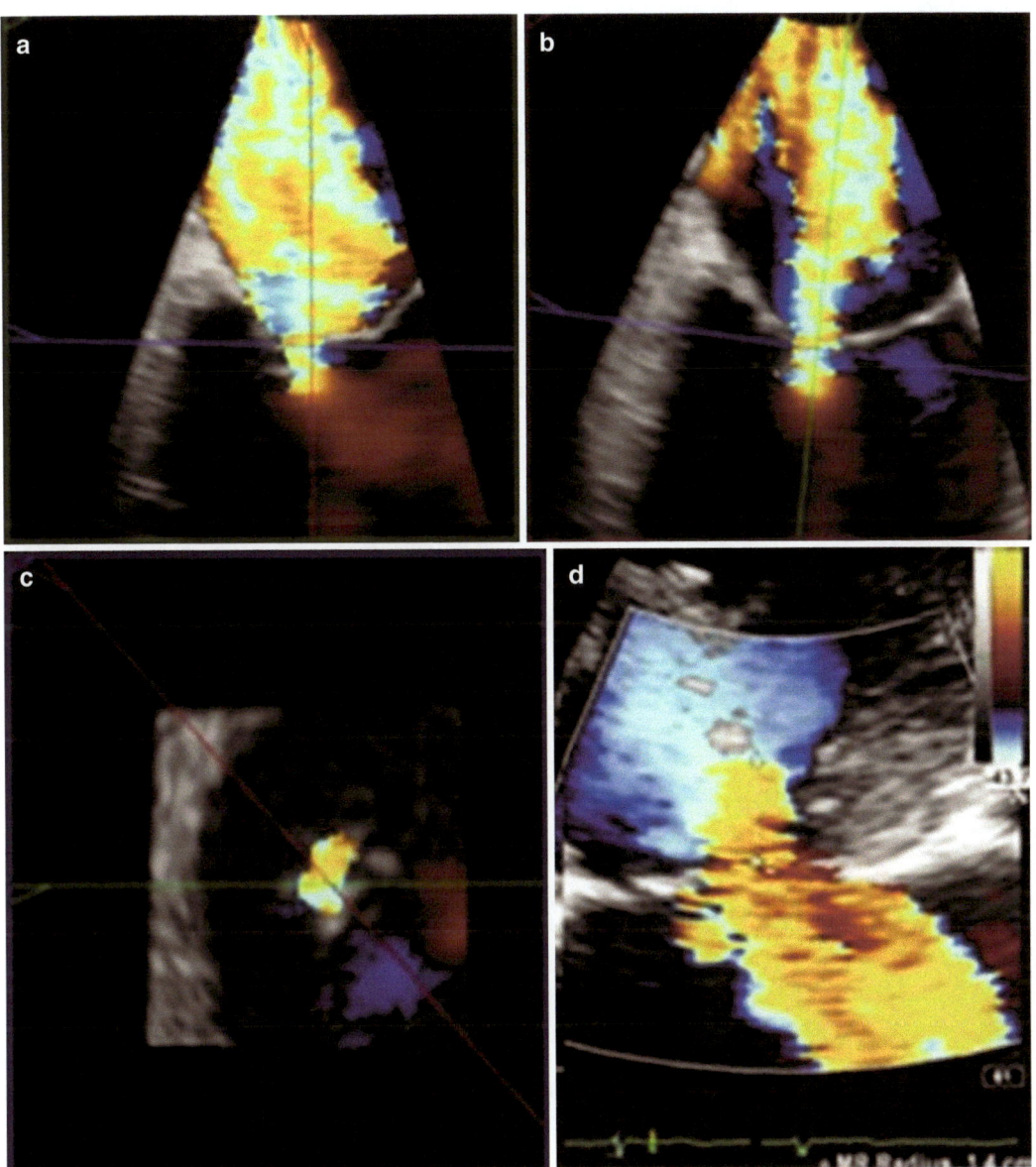

Fig. 1.11 3D-guided 2D reconstruction of severe MR colour flow Doppler images (**a–c**). The cursors are placed at the tips of mitral valve leaflets and the neck (VC) of the regurgitant MV jet. Off-line reconstruction allows appre-ciation of elliptical VC and regurgitant orifice shape in functional MR. (**d**) PISA measurement on TOE color flow Doppler image. (**e**) Systolic flow reversal in the pulmo-nary veins is in keeping with severe MR

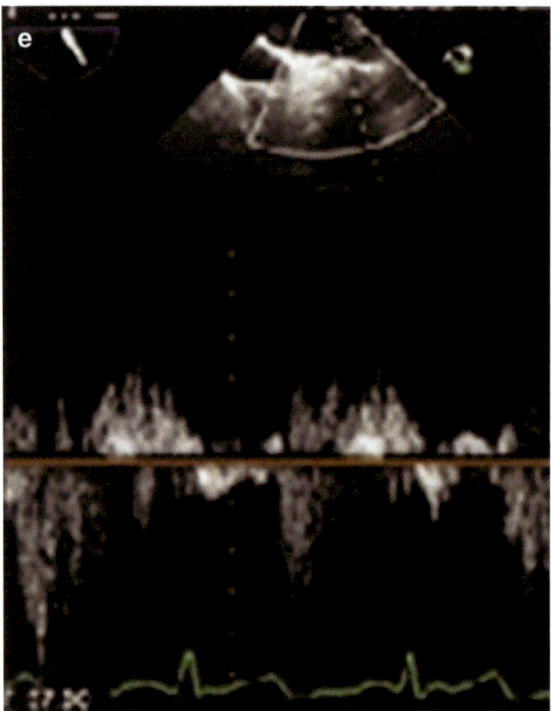

Fig. 1.11 (continued)

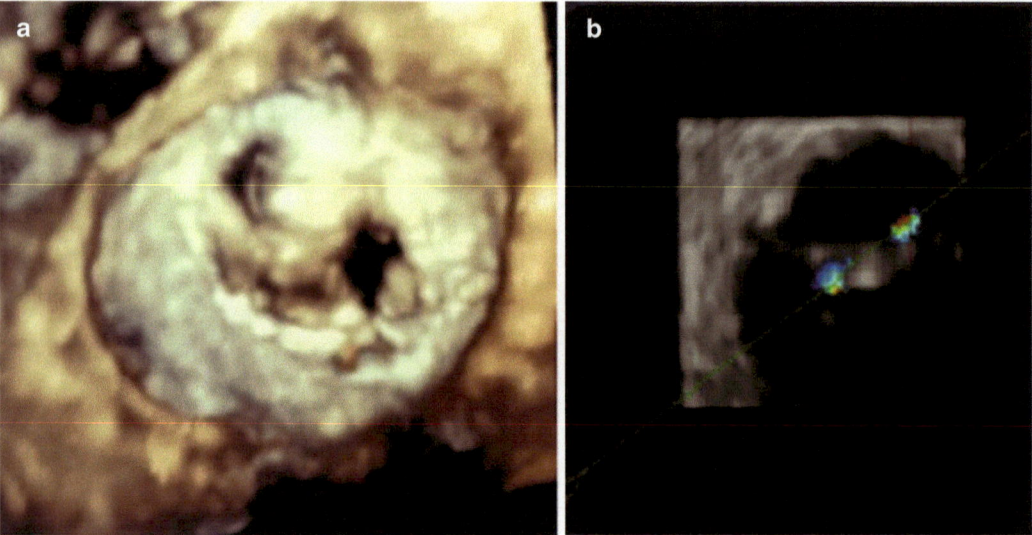

Fig. 1.12 (**a, b**) 3D TOE imaging allows direct visualization of multiple regurgitant orifices (**b**) Assessment of MR severity, by calculation of two regurgitant orifice areas

The Role of Echo in Guiding MV Repair

Preoperative 2D and 3D TOE allows the estimation of MV reparability and its use in the perioperative setting has contributed greatly to increase the success of MV repair. Different 3D TOE appearances of the mitral valve are depicted in Fig. 1.13.

In *primary MR*, type I lesions or posterior MV (PMV) leaflet prolapse, valve reconstruction has excellent results. With contemporary surgery techniques, the results of anterior MV leaflet (AML) prolapse repair are improving. The complexity of the repair increases with the increasing number of prolapsing scallops, commissural involvement and superimposed leaflet or annular calcification. Determination of the morphology

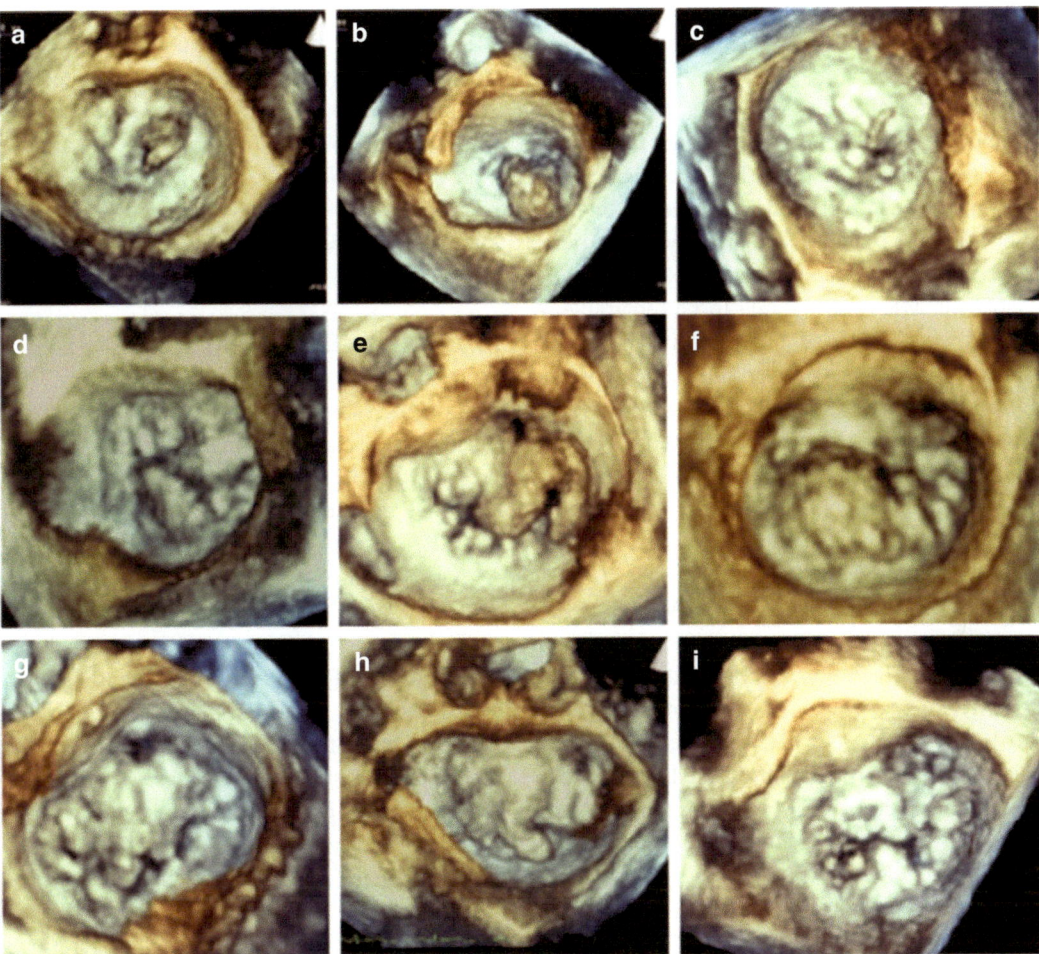

Fig. 1.13 *Row 1*: Type 1 repairable MV lesions. (**a**, **b**) Large mobile echogenic mass with mobile elements attached to LA surface of P2 and posterior MV annulus visible on 3D MV views. (**c**) *Row 2*: Lesions, requiring more complex surgical approach to MV repair. (**d**) Degenerative mitral valve disease with P2 prolapse, extending to P1. (**e**) Extensive myxomatous mitral valve disease and dilated annulus. Thickening of the anterior leaflet affecting all 3 segments, but A2 and A3 are more markedly affected. Prolapse of A2 segment and flail A3/ P3 segments and posteromedial commissure. Flail chords seen attached to A3 and P3. (**f**) Degenerative/myxomatous mitral valve disease with extensive posterior leaflet prolapse mainly affecting the middle and lateral (P2 and P1) scallops. *Row 3*: Difficult to repair MV lesions: (**g**) degenerative mitral valve disease with bileaflet prolapse and loss of coaptation; (**h**) Elongated AML with a vegetation at the tip. There is prolapse of A2 and a flail A1 segment with a ruptured chord; (**i**) flail P1, prolapse of P3, degenerative MV disease

of complex prolapse (commissural, bileaflet) requires more complex surgical techniques, e. g. commissural plication, Alfieri technique (stitching together the tips of A2 and P2, and converting MV into a double orifice valve). Identification of chordal rupture or elongation directs to chordal transfer/shortening or replacement techniques. Rheumatic MV disease is usually advanced and complex at the time of referral for surgery. A combination of thickened, calcified and deformed leaflets with commissural fusion, as well as subvalvular involvement, is generally unsuitable for MV repair.

Chronic ischaemic MR is a result of LV remodelling: ischaemic injury and myocardial scarring leads to LV dilatation, increased papillary muscle separation and symmetric or assymetric tenting of the valve leaflets, with restricted systolic motion and consequential MR. Generally, ischaemic MR is considered to be repairable. A careful assessment of the mechanism of MR allow the surgeon to better select the type and extent of ischaemic MR repair. Still, some authors present the proportion of patients with recurrent moderate or severe MR during the 2-year period more than 50% [15]. Several preoperative parameters can help to identify patients at risk of treatment failure Table 1.4 [12].

One more complication of MV reconstructive surgery—LV outflow tract obstruction with or without MR due to systolic anterior motion (SAM) range between 1–16% of MV repair [16]. This number can be minimized by identification of high-risk patients based on echocardiographic factors. SAM can be predicted by a small LV diameter, acute aortic-mitral angle,

Table 1.4 Preoperative 2DE parameters associated with reccurent MR after ischaemic MV repair

• MV deformation indices:
Coaptation distance ≥1 cm, tenting area > 2.5–3 cm2, complex jets, posterolateral angle >45°;
• Local LV remodelling:
Interpapillary muscle distance >20 mm, posterior papillar–fibrosa distance >40 mm, lateral wall motion abnormality;
• Indices of global LV remodelling
LV EDD > 65 mm, ESD > 51 mm (ESV > 140 ml), systolic sphericity index >0.7.

increased posterior and anterior mitral valve leaflets length, hight of prolapse >15 mm, coaptation point to interventricular septum distance less than 2.5 cm and the ratio of AML length to PML length of 1.3 cm or less [17]. 3D TOE provides dynamic measurements of the mitral annulus on a beating heart in systole and diastole while sizing the mitral annuloplasty ring. Larger ring sizes are suggested for cases of higher likelihood of postoperative SAM, while smaller rings are used in correcting ischaemic MR. Limited triangular or quadrangular resection is sufficient to resolve MR in isolated one scallop prolapse. However, in the presence of predictors of post-repair SAM, a sliding annuloplasty technique in addition to quadrangular resection of the PML to reduce its length is known to be advantageous.

Post-Bypass Evaluation

Before assessing the results of a mitral valve repair, it is essential to bring up the systolic blood pressure (SBP) to just above 90–100 mmHg. Low SBP may seriously underestimate any residual MR.

Assessment of MV repair is comprised of the following key elements:

- **Residual MR**. Detection and quantification of residual MR is of paramount importance. If more than mild residual MR is present, the mechanism should be clarified (residual prolapse, excessive restriction, inadequate downsizing of the annulus, paravalvular leak, leaflet perforation). Patients with greater than mild residual MR should be returned on CPB for further correction as the risk of re-operation is high if more than mild MR is present after MV repair.
- Evaluation of **coaptation of the leaflets**. Each scallop and segment should be thoroughly evaluated for the adequacy of coaptation in mid systole. However, there are no uniform standards for the value of the coaptation height because of the difficulty in exact measurements in clinical practice. Still, leaflet coapta-

tion height should be at least 5 mm by intraoperative TOE for a satisfactory repair to ensure valve competence and long-term durability of repair.

- Assessment of **leaflet motion**. Residual or new restriction or prolapse may cause residual MR. It should be noted, that fixed and immobile PML, acting as a doorstop, and moving AML are normal echocardiographic findings following MV repair.
- **SAM** is featured in degenerative MV repairs with small LV diameter and lengthy PML. Following MV repair, the leaflet coaptation point is shifted towards the LVOT, resulting in systolic flow obstruction and posteriorly directed MR jet. The condition is worsened by volume depletion and hypercontractile LV. In mild forms of SAM, adequate LV filling and reduction of inotropic support may help. Significant SAM unamenable to conservative treatment requires return on CPB and surgical correction (sliding annuloplasty, larger annuloplasty ring or MV replacement).
- **Assessing the transvalvular gradient**. Mean transmitral gradient helps to exclude mitral stenosis following MV repair. It should be noted that the pressure half time method is unreliable postoperatively due to varying compliance of the LV and LA. A mean gradient of >5 mmHg is unacceptable and warrants correction or valve replace- ment, if further repair is not feasible.
- **Aortic regurgitation** must be looked for, keeping in mind the proximity of aortic and mitral valves. Surgical manoeuvers in the anterior MV annulus area and AML region may distort the aortic valve anatomy, resulting in new or worsened aortic regurgitation after MV surgery.
- **Biventricular function** should be carefully assessed. Postoperative global and regional LV function must be assessed to identify potentially correctable myocardial ischaemia during the operation (e. g. surgical treatment in the anterolateral commissural region may result in accidental suturing or kinking of the left circumflex artery, which is found adja-

cently). RV dysfunction may be the result of the persistent severe MR, intracoronary air emboli, or inadequate ventricular protection during the period of aortic cross-clamping. Any ancillary procedures, such as tricuspidal annuloplasty, must be evaluated.

If MR is surgically managed by MV replacement, the motion of occluders must be visualised. Pressure gradients should be assessed. It's important, that increased post-bypass cardiac output and anemia, pressure recovery may increase gradients. Later in follow up, the presence of high gradients may demonstrate pathological valve obstruction or patient-prothesis mismatch. With a tissue prosthesis, as well as with a bileaflet mechanical prosthesis, there is a small central intravalvular MR. Paravalvular jets are always abnormal. Small paravalvular leaks often disappear after heparin reversal, but larger leaks should be corrected surgicaly [18].

Mitral Valve Stenosis

Despite the decrease in the incidence of rheumatic heart disease, mitral valve stenosis (MS) remains prevalent, even in industrialized countries. As in other valvular lesions, 2D and 3D echocardiography plays a major role in decision-making for MS, allowing for analysis of valve anatomy, assessing MS cause (rheumatic, calcific, congenital), the severity of this lesion and hemodynamic consequences (Table 1.5).

Impairment of mitral anatomy is expressed in scores (Wilkins, Cormier scores) combining different components of mitral apparatus and it is important in planning type of MV correction (choosing between percutaneous balloon mitral valvotomy (PBMV) and surgery). In symptomatic patients with favourable characteristics, such as young age with pliable valves and moderate subvalvular disease (echo score ≤ 8), results of PBMV are generally excellent. This procedure can be done in critically ill patients. However, surgical correction of MS is indicated in symptomatic moderate and severe MS if there are con-

Table 1.5 Echocardiographic factors in the evaluation of MS

• Valve anatomy
Leaflet thickening and mobility;
Diastolic doming of the anterior mitral valve leaflet;
Reduced valve opening;
Commissural fusion;
Subvalvular involvement (chordal thickening, thickening and fusion);
Secondary calcification;
• Severity of MS
MS is considered significant when valve area is less than 1.5 cm^2 and severe, when it is ≤1 cm^2, mean gradient >10 mmHg and systolic pulmonary artery pressure > 50 mmHg.
• Associated findings
Associated other valve lesions (aortic valve involvement in rheumatic disease, MR, tricuspidal valve organic changes or functional TR due to pulmonary hypertension);
Left atrial enlargement (increased index of LA volume);
Left atrium thrombus, spontaneous contrast in LA (recommended TOE evaluation) (Fig. 1.16);

traindications for balloon mitral valvotomy: LA thrombus, moderate/severe MR, severe or bicommissural calcification, severe concomitant aortic or combined tricuspidal stenosis and regurgitation, concomitant coronary artery disease, requiring bypass surgery [19]. Current surgical techniques often allow the repair of even severely regurgitant and stenosed valves; if the stenosed MV cannot be repaired, MV replacement can be chosen (for post- operative assessment refer to assessment of MV repair) (Fig. 1.14).

Intervention should be performed in patients with significant MS (valve area < 1.5 cm2). Planimetry is one of the most accurate mitral valve area (MVA) estimation method. Real-time 3D echocardiography provides the precise measurement of the valve area contained by the open leaflet tips. However, planimetry may be difficult in the case of an irregular and heavily calcified orifice [20]. In severe asymptomatic patients or when symptoms do not correlate with MV area—stress testing enables to assess mean mitral gradient and systolic pulmonary artery pressure changes for increased workload and to guide surgery timing (Figs. 1.15 and 1.16).

Aortic valve and Aortic Root

The aortic valve is a part of the aortic root complex, which is composed of the sinuses of Valsalva, the fibrous interleaflet triangles, and the three valvular leaflets themselves [21]. The non-coronary cusp is superior, next to the interatrial septum; the right coronary cusp lies inferiorly and the left coronary cusp is on the right and associated with the offset of the left main coronary artery seen at 3 o'clock (Fig. 1.17). The localized apical thickening of the free edge of each cusp (nodules of Arantius) is a normal finding. Some small fibrous strands may also be seen on TOE, their significance, however, is not always clear. These normal structures do not interfere with valve function and should not be confused with vegetations or fibroelastomas.

Assessment of normal anatomy should always be followed by confirmation of normal physiology. Continuous flow (CW) Doppler in the aortic valve area and pulsed wave Doppler in the left ventricular outflow tract area should confirm normal transvalvular gradients with laminar flow. These parameters can be used for calculation of AVA by the volumetric method. 2D or 3D en face TOE views are particularly useful while assessing aortic valve area (AVA) by planimetry and colour flow Doppler with colour flow compare mode may help to identify the site of the leak or cusp coaptation defects. In long axis aortic valve views, one may identify diastolic prolapse or reduced cusp opening in stenotic disease.

The thoracic aorta is divided into 4 parts: the aortic root (which includes the aortic valve annulus, the aortic valve cusps, the sinuses of Valsalva and sinotubular junction), the ascending aorta (which includes the tubular portion of the ascending aorta, the aortic arch and the descending aorta.

LVOT is a region of the LV that is located between the anterior cusp of the MV insertion to the interventricular septum and the aortic annulus. Measurements of the LVOT are important in calculating the aortic valve area and selecting the diameter for the aortic valve prosthesis. True (anatomical) *aortic annulus* is a complex three-

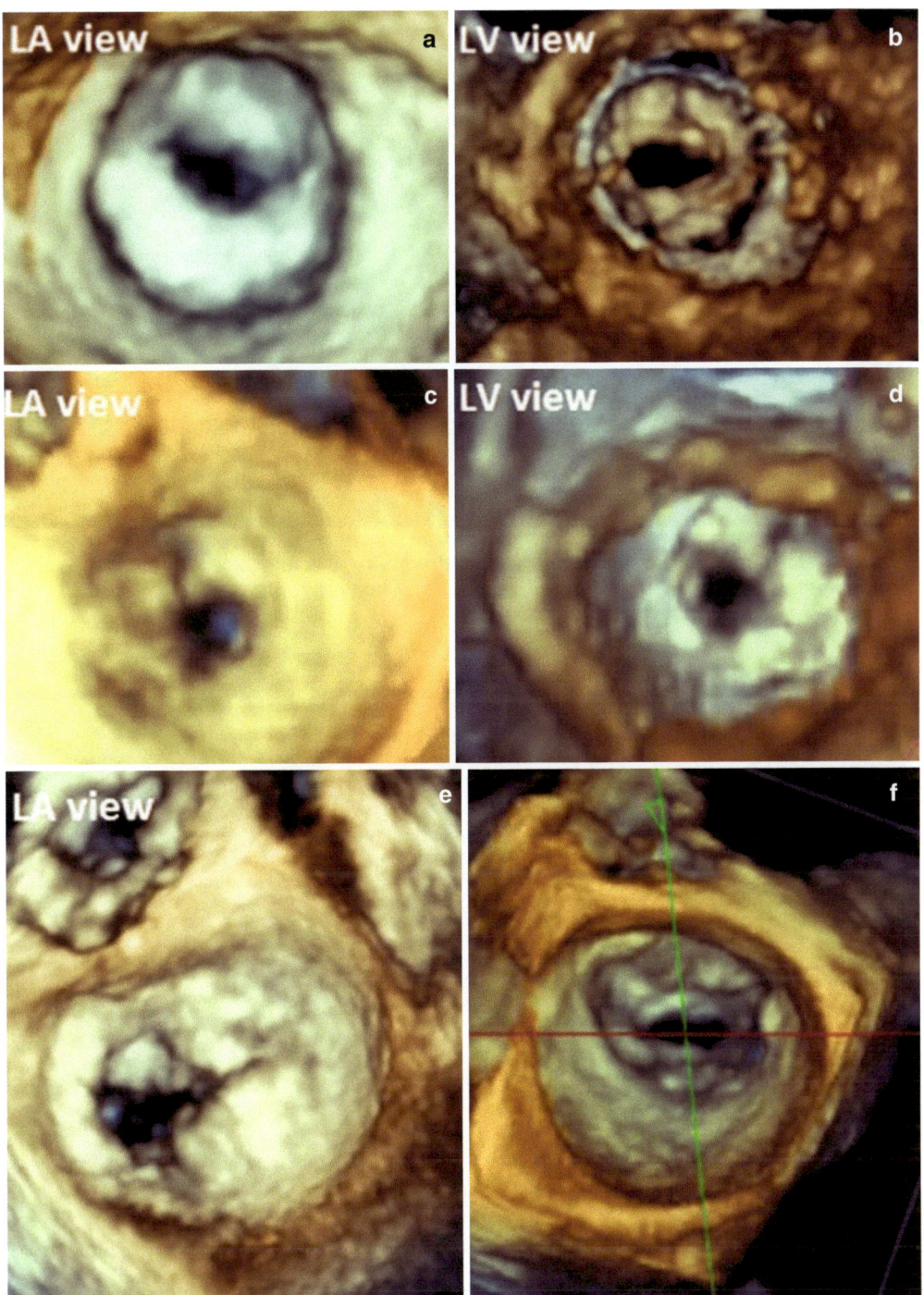

Fig. 1.14 (**a**, **b**) Rheumatic mitral stenosis (MS) with visible, but identifiable, commissural fusion; favourable for balloon valvuloplasty. (**c**, **d**) Severe rheumatic mitral stenosis (MS) with symmetrically fused unidentifiable commissures; anatomy highly unfavourable for balloon valvuloplasty. (**e**, **f**) Calcific mitral stenosis. Posterior mitral annular calcification extends below the valve into the myocardium (**f** LV view). The calcium is more severe medially, leading to fusion of the PM commissure and immobile A3 and P3 scallops which appear fused. The A2 and P2 scallops are also affected with restricted mobility. Visible triangular valve opening only between A1 and P1 scallops

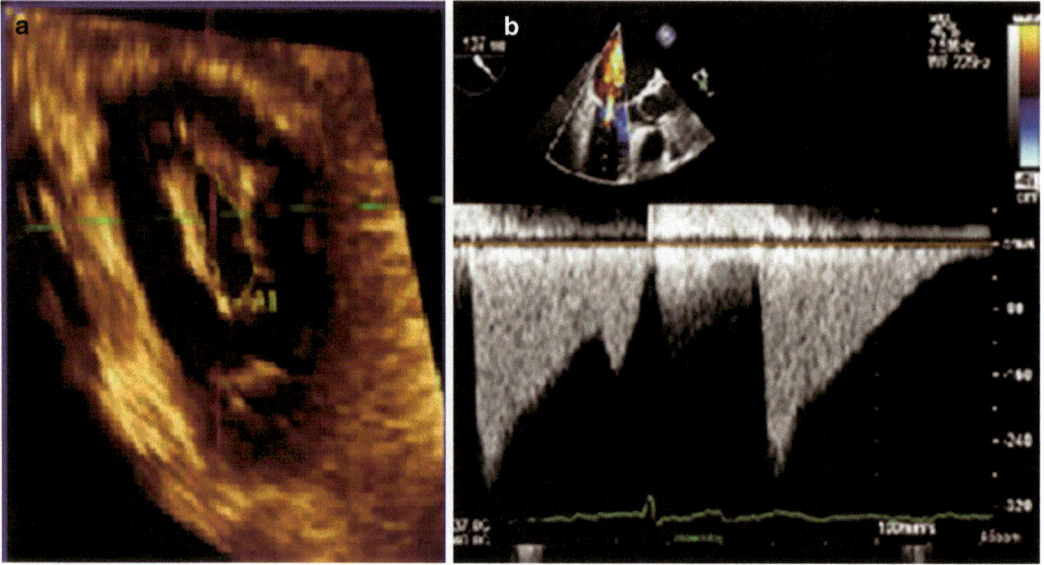

Fig. 1.15 Assessment of severe mitral stenosis. (**a**) 3D imaging allows visualization of mitral valve opening and orifice area contained by mitral leaflets in rheumatic MS. (**b**) Severe mitral stenosis with mean gradient of 13.3 mmHg and moderate MR

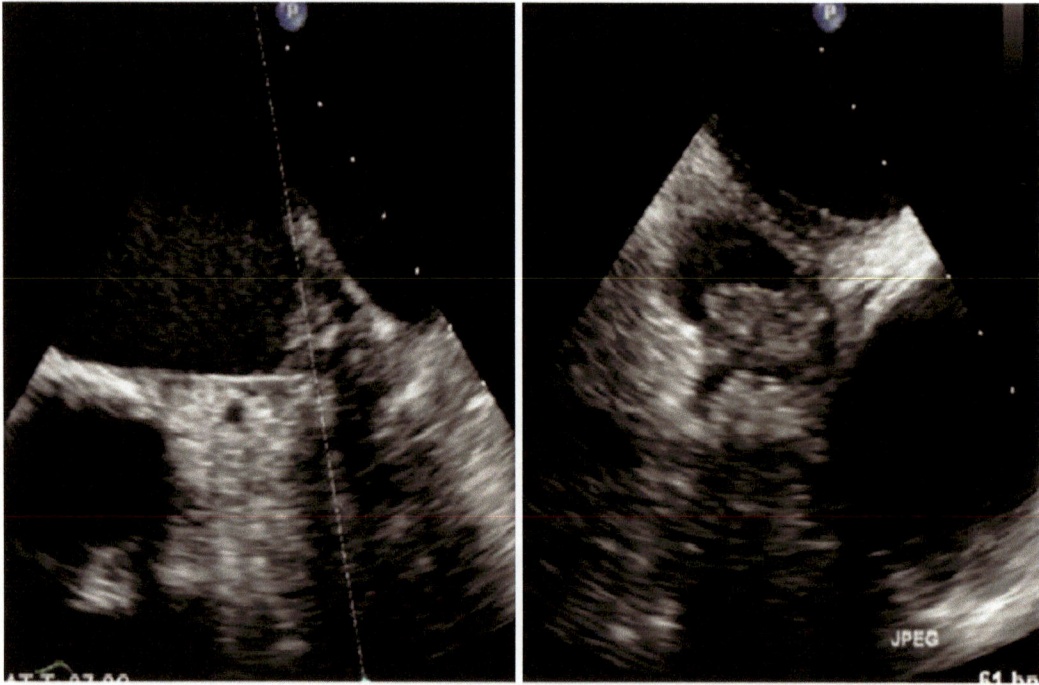

Fig. 1.16 Thrombus in left atrial appendage, visualized from TOE cross-sectional view. Note spontaneous contrast in LA cavity

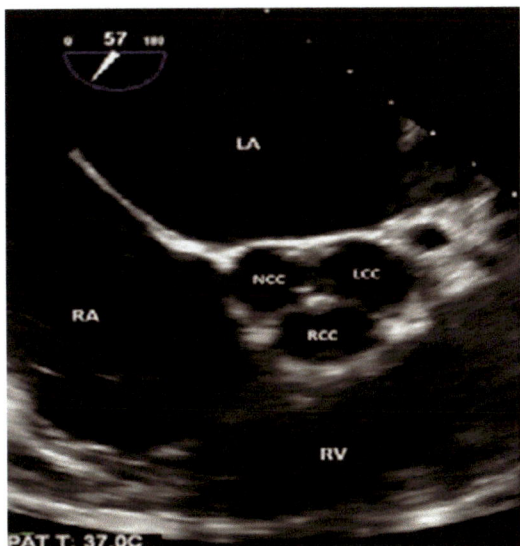
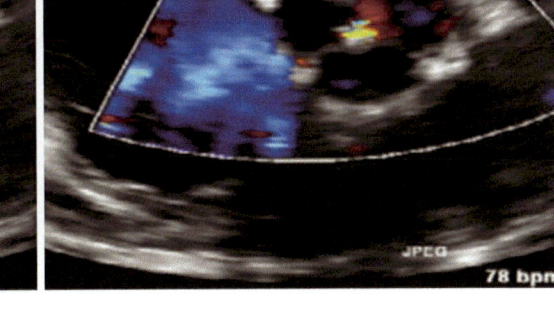

Fig. 1.17 Mildly thickened aortic valve leaflets in diastole (*left*) with mild central aortic regurgitation, arising from the coaptation point of the cusps. *LA* left atrium, *RA* right atrium, *RV* right ventricle, *NCC* non-coronary cusp, *LCC* left coronary cusp, *RCC* right coronary cusp. Left coronary artery stem arises at 3 o'clock

dimensional crown-shaped structure formed by the anchoring of the aortic cusps to the walls of the aortic sinuses. It can be recognized by visual inspection by of the surgeon and the aid of 3D echocardiography. However, visualisation of this structure by either means is imperfect. Echocardiography often provides a simplified aortic annular measurement, taken at the base of aortic valve cusps. This virtual basal ring is often non-circular (may be oval or elliptical) and may be even more irregular due to superimposed calcification. It is important to keep in mind that a surgically implanted aortic valve prosthesis is sewn at the level of the anatomic aortic annulus (between the base of the leaflets and sinotubular junction) and even most advanced echocardiographic modalities (3D TOE) may underestimate the true aortic annular dimensions.

Aortic sinuses are anatomic recesses of proximal ascending aorta just above the aortic valve. There are generally three aortic sinuses, named after the valve cusps and coronary arteries that they are associated with: the left, the right and the non-coronary (or posterior).

Sinotubular junction is defined by the sinotubular ridge demarcating the junction of the aortic sinuses and proximal ascending aorta.

Ascending aorta continues its course as a tubular structure after the sinotubular junction and turns into the aortic arch at the upper sternal level. There is a 'blind spot' for echocardiographic imaging in the distal ascending aorta, just before the take-off of the innominate artery, attributable to interposition of the right bronchus and trachea. Aortic dimensions are strongly related to body surface area (BSA) and age, thus, these factors have to be taken into consideration while assessing aortic dilatation. TOE is superior to other imaging modalities in assessing aortic atheromas, as it provides information on size and mobility of the plaques in real time. Atheromas typically get worse proceeding distally, therefore, large mobile atheromas are unlikely to be found in the ascending aorta in the absence of distal aortic plaques.

TTE allows the assessment of aortic root and proximal ascending aorta; however, visualisation of the ascending aorta may be difficult, and measurements are known to significantly underestimate the true dimensions. In operating theatre, TOE is helpful in providing high-quality imaging of nearly all of the ascending and descending thoracic aorta. Measurements of aortic diameter should be taken at reproducible anatomic landmarks, perpendicular to the axis of blood flow (Fig. 1.18). TOE is valuable in assessing aortic dilatation, atherosclerosis, dissection and monitoring surgical treatment (Fig. 1.19). TOE incorporates all the functionality of TTE, including 3D imaging, which can reliably interrogate cardiovascular anatomy, function, hemodynamics, and blood flow, still it often fails to adequately visualize the distal ascending aorta, aortic arch and its branches, because of interposition of the trachea [22]. With advances in imaging technology, CTA, MRA, aortography can be preferred in different clinical situations.

Aortic Regurgitation (AR)

Aortic regurgitation has multiple causes involving abnormalities of aortic valve leaflets, aortic root, or both. 2D TTE commonly does not allow a complete assessment of the anatomy and causes of AR. 3D echo provides better delineation of the aortic valve morphology. However, in many cases

of AR, TOE is needed for assessing the causes and mechanisms of AR together with the measurements of the aortic root dimensions and morphology, determining the feasibility of valve repair.

Aetiology and Mechanisms of AR

In the case of AR, the echo report provides information about aetiology, the lesion process and the type of dysfunction. The most frequent causes of leaflet abnormalities are calcification, congenital abnormalities (bicuspid, unicuspid, quadricuspid valves), infective endocarditis, rheumatic disease, myxomatous degeneration, fenestrations. Aortic root abnormalities include annuloaortic ectasia, Marfan's syndrome, aortic dissection, atherosclerotic aneurysm, syphilitic aortitis, collagen vascular diseases, other systemic inflammatory disorders. The Carpentier' classification is used to describe the mechanism of AR [12, 23].

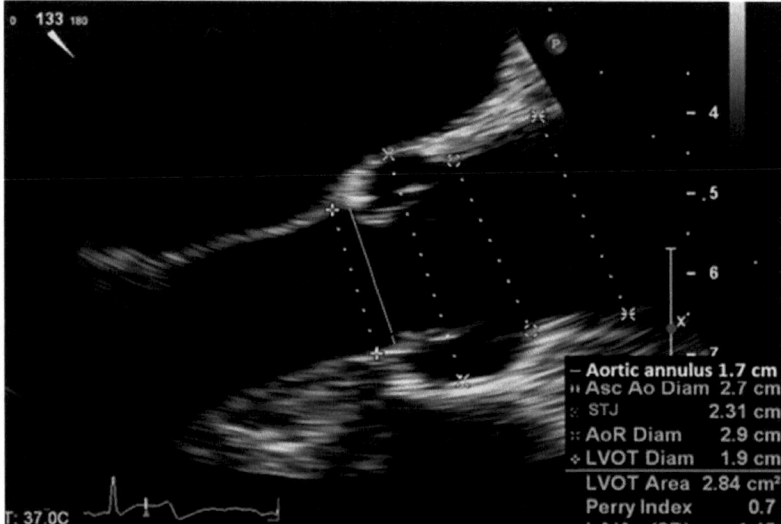

Fig. 1.18 Sites for measurements of the aortic root and ascending aorta. From left to right: LV outflow tract, aortic annulus, aortic sinuses, sinotubular junction and proximal ascending aorta

Fig. 1.19 Aortic pathology. (**a**) Dilated aortic sinuses. (**b**) Dilated ascending aorta. (**c**) Dilated ascending aorta with visible dissection flap (arrow). (**d**) Aortic dissection intimal flap visible in the aortic arch. (**e**) Thoracic aorta with atherosclerotic plaques. (**f**) Longitudinal view of the thoracic aorta, allowing estimation of atheromatous plaque extent. *LV* left ventricle, *Ao* ascending aorta, *ThA* thoracic aorta

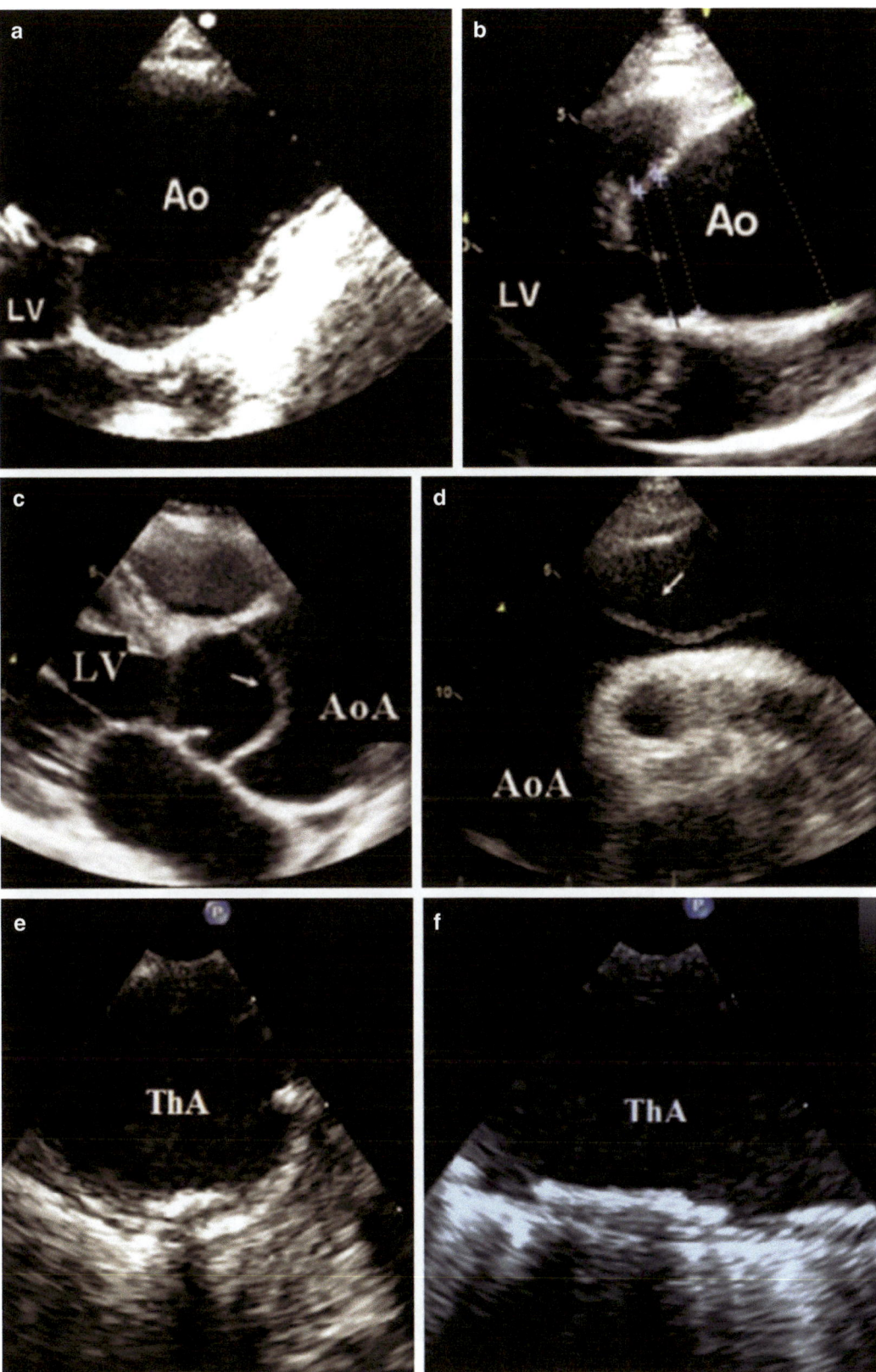

Type I: Aortic valve cusps structurally are normal with dilatation of any segment of the aortic root (aortic annulus, sinuses of Valsalva, sinotubular junction). The regurgitant jet usually is central, because of the reduction of leaflets coaptation.

Type II: The responsible AR mechanisms are—aortic valve prolapse (IIA): partial or whole cusp prolapse/flail, or free edge fenestration (IIB) with eccentric AR jet, directed away from the diseased leaflet.

Type III: This type of AR is induced by poor leaflet quality, thickened cusps, reduced motion, different degree of calcification, or tissue destruction because of infective endocarditis. The regurgitant jet can be directed towards the affected leaflet, or it can be central if both leaflets are equaly affected (Figs. 1.20, 1.21, and 1.22).

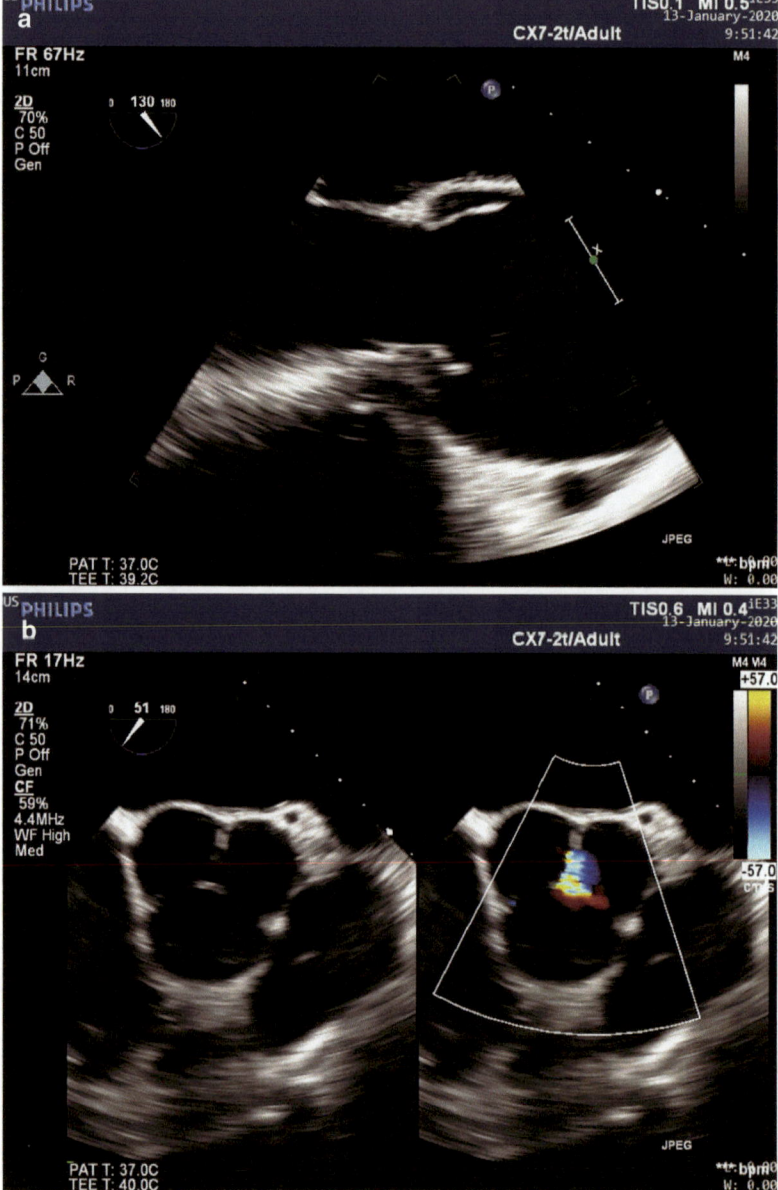

Fig. 1.20 Type I AR with dilated aortic root, reduction of leaflet coaptation and central AR jet (**a**—long axis view, **b**—short axis view)

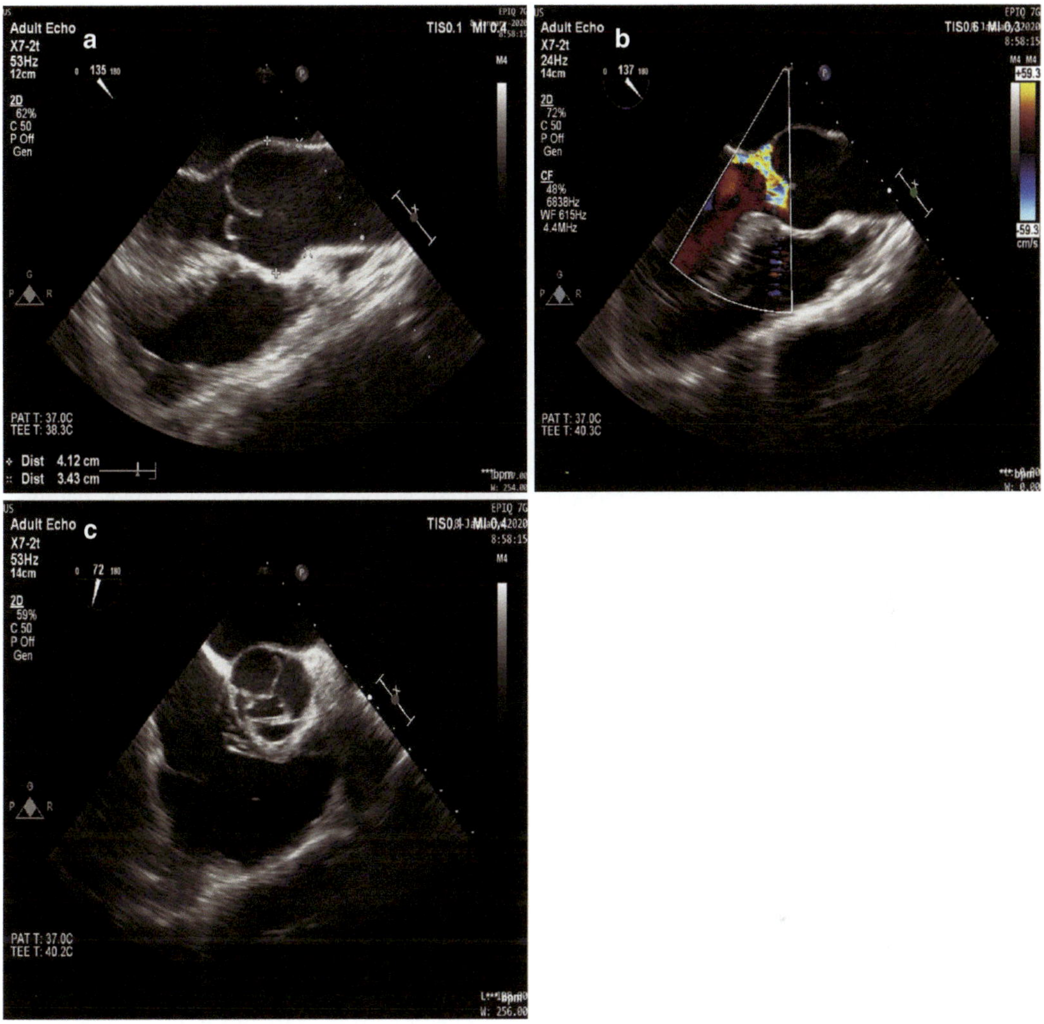

Fig. 1.21 Type II AR with (**a**, **c**) slightly dilated Ao sinuses, flail of right coronary cusp and (**b**) eccentric regurgitant jet directed from prolapsing cusp

In majority of type I or type II cases, valve repair may be considered and often may be successfully performed, though AV repair is still underused. However, if cusp tissue quality is poor (type III AR) or there is mixed stenotic and regurgitant valve disease, the valve is generally considered unrepairable and replacement strategy should be chosen if surgical treatment is indicated [24].

Quantitation of AR

No single measurement or Doppler parameter is precise enough to quantify AR in individual patients. Integration of multiple parameters is required. Criteria for the definition of severe AR is presented in Table 1.6 [13].

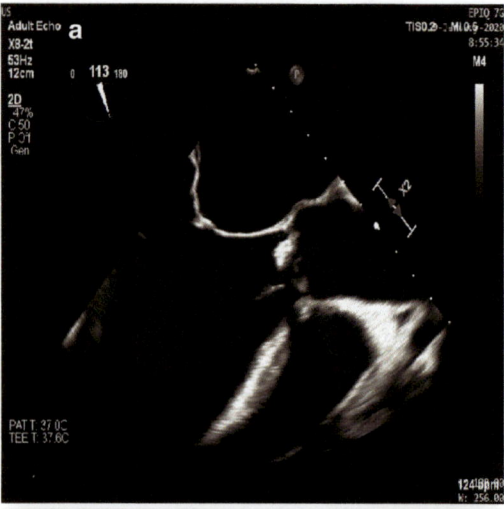

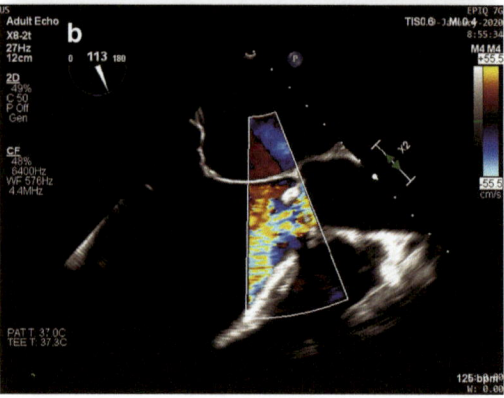

Fig. 1.22 Type III AR—aortic valve tissue destruction because of infective endocarditis causing severe aortic regurgitation (**a, b**)

Table 1.6 Echocardiographic criteria for severe AR

Quantitative Measures	Specific Criteria[a]
EROA ≥30 mm2 Regurgitant volume ≥ 60 ml Regurgitant fraction ≥50%	Flail leaflet VC width > 0.6 cm Central jet, width ≥ 65% of LVOT Large flow convergence PHT < 200 ms Prominent holodiastolic flow reversal in the descending aorta Dilated with normal function LV

[a]Definitely severe if ≥4 specific criteria

Consequences of AR on LV Size and Function and Timing for Surgery

LV remodelling is a consequence of chronic severe AR and may be a specific marker of regurgitation severity. The timing for surgery is based on symptoms, severity of AR and changes of LV systolic function, as well as dimensions. Surgery is indicated in symptomatic patients with severe AR, or in asymptomatic patients with severe AR and LV dysfunction at rest (LVEF≤50%). In asymptomatic severe AR without LV dysfunction, LV enlargement with LV EDD >70 mm or LVESD >50 mm or > 25 mm2/m2, guide for surgical AR correction. Echocardiographic parameters obtained by three-dimensional (3D) echocardiography, tissue Doppler and strain rate imaging may be useful, particularly in patients with borderline left ventricular ejection fraction (LVEF), where they may help in the decision for surgery [19]. Recently a study focused on prognosis demonstrated that asymptomatic severe AR patients with dilated LV and GLS > −19.5% were more likely to have a shorter survival without aortic valve replacement [13]. In patients with dilated aorta, the rationale for surgery has been defined by aetiology and extent of aortic dilatation. Surgery should be considered in patients with maximal ascending aortic diameter ≥ 45 mm in the presence of Marfan syndrome and additional risk factors, ≥50 mm in the presence of a bicuspidal valve, and ≥ 55 mm for all other patients. When surgery is indicated for the aortic valve, replacement of the aortic root or ascending part is considered when aortic diameter is ≥45 mm, particularly in bicuspid valve [19].

The Role of Echo in Guiding AV Repair

Intra-operative TOE provides a road map and predicts techniques to be used for an effective and durable repair. Pre-pump intra-operative echocardiography protocol includes the main objectives to be assessed:

- Valve type and geometry. Valve type is defined by number of cusps, which is based on the number of functional commissures (a tricuspidal valve with three fully developed commissures, a bicuspid valve (BAV) with two developed commissures and 0 or one raphe on the fused cusp, a unicuspid AV with one fully developed commissure and two raphes and quadricuspid valve with four commissures). Commissure orientation, which varies between 120° (tricuspid) and 180° (bicuspidal symmetrical configuration) and the aortic annulus must be assessed. Additional measurements are of great importance in planning valve reconstruction: the effective height (eH)—the distance from the annulus to the middle of the free margin of the cusp (normal value is close to 9 mm), the geometric height (gH) (also called cusp height)—the distance between the cusp nadir and the middle of the free margin (cusp retraction when gH is 16 mm or less), the coaptation height (cH) or coaptation length—the distance of cusp apposition in diastole with normal range 4–5 mm. (Fig. 1.23). The motion of the cusps and the jet direction must be evaluated [25]. 3D has several advantages in individualizing each cusp and in detail measurement of eH and gH. Restriction per se is not considered an absolute contraindication for valve repair, however combination with valve retraction is a predictor of poor repair result. Another lesion with surgical implications is the presence of fenestrations, seen as filament—like structures on the free margins of the leaflets. The complexity of repair increases if these fenestrations are multiple, big size and fragile.

- Aortic diameters, that enables to diagnose aortic phenotype: normal root with aortic diameters <40 mm, aortic root dilatation, aorta at the sinuses of Valsalva >45 mm, ascending aortic aneurysm—aortic root < 40 mm, ascending aorta > 45 mm.

- LV diameters and function, as well as evaluation of other valves.

After AV repair postoperative TOE including 3D imaging is mandatory to evaluate the surgery result. It is ideal when the valve is competent without any or trace residual AR, without cusp restriction and mean transvalvular gradient <10 mmHg, with coaptation length ≥ 4 mm, with individual cusps eH ≥ 9 mm (by 3DE), with aortic annulus <25 mm. These measurements are important determinants of good long term postoperative results [25, 26].

Aortic valve Stenosis (AS) [19, 27]

AS is one of the most common valvular disorders leading to valve replacement procedure. Despite the chosen technique—TAVI (transcatheter aortic valve implantation) or surgical aortic valve replacement, detailed information is required. By the time the patient arrives to the cardiac theatre, the diagnosis usually has been made according to clinical symptoms, signs and by TTE as it's the first line diagnostic method in aortic stenosis. Additional information (e.g. invasive hemodynamics, low dose dobutamine stress echocardiography, computed tomography) can be important for decision making. 2D and 3D TOE should be considered for: better ana-

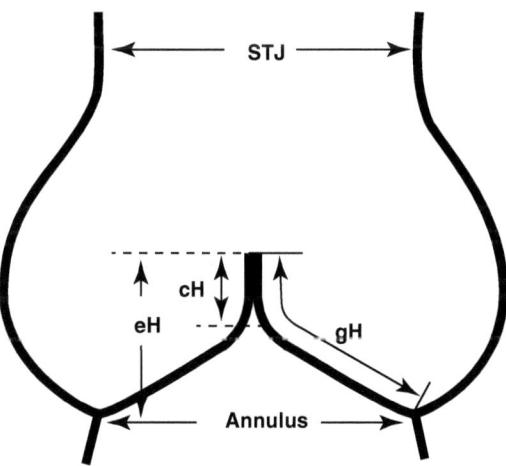

Fig. 1.23 Definitions used in aortic valve repair: *STJ* sinotubular junction, *eH* effective height, *cH* coaptation height, *gH* geometric height

tomic assessment, underlying morphology (bicuspid vs tricuspid), extent and distribution of calcification, assessment of annulus dimension in discording grading of stenosis severity, measurement of aortic valve area planimetry in cases of coexisting subvalvular stenosis, in severe valve calcification and "low gradient, low flow" patients with LV dysfunction.

Echocardiographic Factors in the Evaluation of AS

- *Assessment of valve anatomy and morphology.*
- Confirmation of aetiology of aortic stenosis is mandatory. Calcific degenerative aortic stenosis is the commonest valve lesion in the ageing Western world population. It is identifiable as trileaflet and calcified, with reduced cusp opening and mobility. Bicuspid aortic valve is another cause of isolated aortic stenosis in the younger age group with or without echocardiographic signs of aortopathy. Rheumatic aortic stenosis can be recognized by commissural fusion and thickening, reduced leaflet motion. Mitral valve can also be affected (Fig. 1.24).
- *Severity of AS*
- AS is considered **severe** when peak jet velocity is >4 m/s, transvalvular mean pressure gradient >40 mmHg, valve area is less than 1 cm2 (or < 0.6 cm2/m2) by continuity equation, LV outflow tract/AV velocity/VTI ratio ≤ 0.25 (Fig. 1.25). Discording of grading is common in clinical practice (20–30%). 3D guided 2D planimetry of the aortic valve in systole may be used to evaluate the precise AV area, also in perioperative setting this method is preferred over the gradients, as the severity of AS may not necessarily follow a high gradient (Fig. 1.26). AV calcium scoring is a quantitative and flow independent method of assessing AS severity. Severe AS is likely when calcium score by CT is more than 2.000 in men and more than 1.200 in woman [27].
- Current evidence suggests that a low gradient cannot exclude the presence of severe AS.

"Low flow, low gradient" severe AS with decreased LV systolic function is diagnosed when AVA < 1 cm2, mean pressure < 40 mmHg, LVEF <50% and systolic volume index SVi < 35 ml/m2. In these cases low dose dobutamine stress echo provides info on contractile response and helps to differentiate severe AS, causing LV dysfunction and moderate AS with another cause of LV dysfunction. Paradoxical "low gradient, low flow" AS with preserved LV systolic function is a challenging situation when AVA <1 cm2, mean pressure < 40 mmHg, a peak velocity < 4 m/s with maintained LV EF and SVi < 35%. This refers to patients with hypertrophied, small ventricles. Technical mistakes in AVA calculation have to be excluded. AV replacement might improve outcome of this group of patients [27, 28].

- Intervention (AV replacement or TAVI) is recommended is symptomatic patients with proven severe AS. Prognostic markers to impact decision for surgery in asymptomatic severe AS is velocity > 5,5 m/s, severe valve calcification with rapid increase in transvalvular velocity (>0,3 m/s/y) and increase transvalvular gradient with exercise more than 20 mmHg [27].
- *Associated Findings*
  - Changes of LV geometry and function. LV hypertrophy is the consequence of pressure overload and can lead to severe diastolic dysfunction and pulmonary hypertension in AS patients with poor outcomes of the surgical treatment. Global longitudinal strain (GLS) in severe AS may detect impairment of LV systolic function when ejection fraction is still normal and may predict prognosis in this group of patients.
  - Changes of aortic root and ascending aorta—echocardiography may provide information on the extent of aortic dilatation, severe calcification and the presence of mobile atheromas, indicative of increased risk of embolism or aortic cannulation. Extensive aortic calcification

Fig. 1.24 3D image of congenitally bicuspid aortic valve with moderate stenosis and continuous flow Doppler through the valve

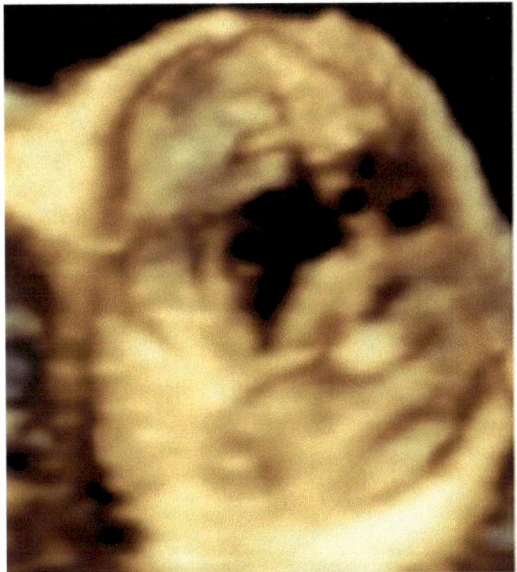

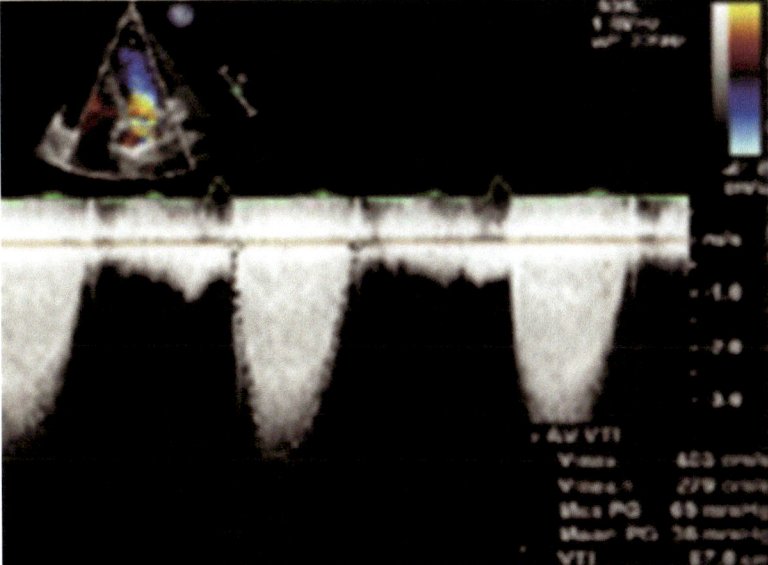

(porcelain aorta)—is a considerable contraindication to AV replacement.

- Evaluation of other valves and unexpected lesions.

During surgery for AS some notes for pre- and postoperative echocardiographic examination are important—.

Selection of the prosthetic valve type and size preoperatively. Echocardiographically derived small aortic annular dimensions may lead towards the selection of a stentless bioprothesis or aortic root enlargement to prevent the patient-prothesis mismatch.

Postoperative evaluation includes the assessment of transvalvular gradients, intra- and/or paravalvular regurgitation, LV function and integrity of the aortic wall.

Tricuspid Valve

The tricuspid valve (TV) is often called the 'forgotten' valve as it is relatively understudied in

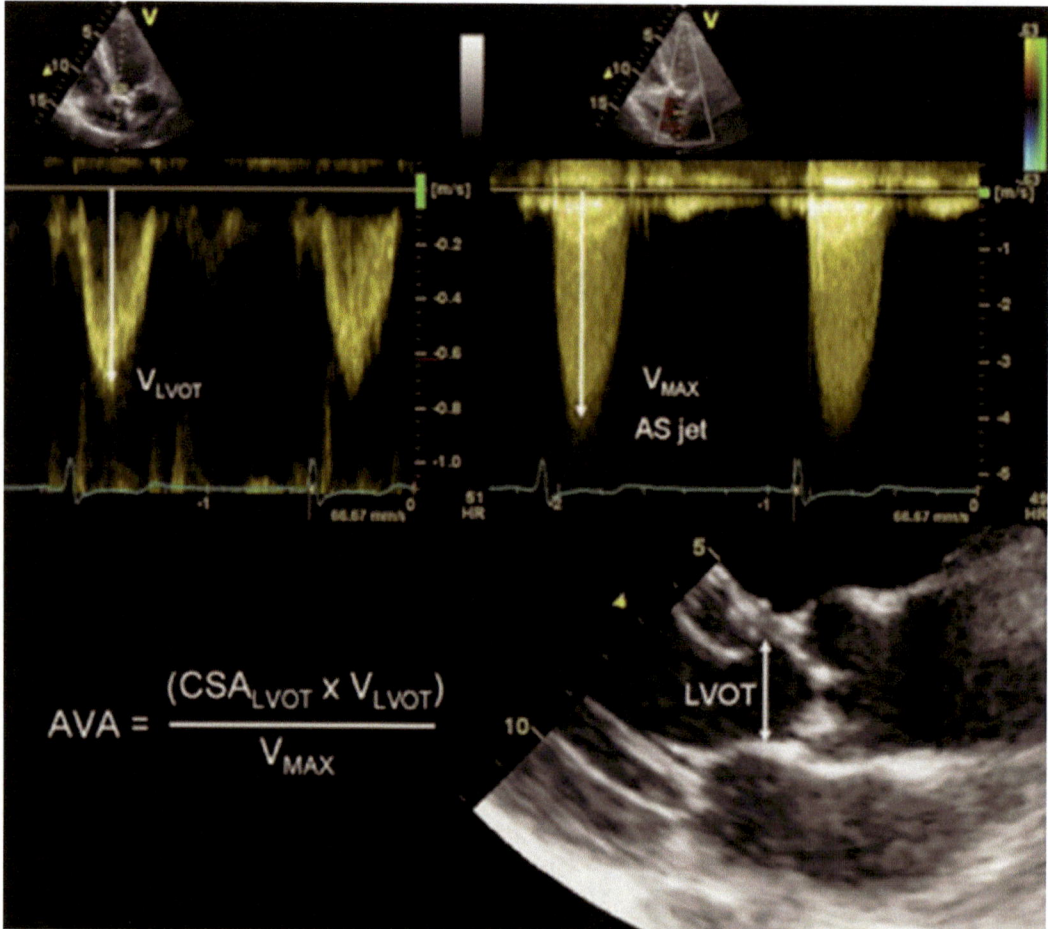

Fig. 1.25 Illustration of AV area calculation

comparison to the other heart valves and the imaging of this valve is more difficult by TTE and TOE due to the inability to visualize its structures in one cross-sectional view (e. g. imaging of all three TV leaflets) (Fig. 1.27). However, recent advances in 3D TTE and TOE has enabled to visualize the TV anatomy, define the mechanism of tricuspid regurgitation, measure the size and geometry of the tricuspid annulus, analyze the anatomic relationships between TV apparatus and surrounding cardiac structures, to assess volumes and function of the right atrium and ventricle, and to plan surgical repair or guide and monitor transcatheter interventional procedures [29].

Echocardiography allows differentiation of functional (dilatation of RV and/or tricuspid annulus leading to malcoaptation of the leaflets due to RV dysfunction, pulmonary hypertension, or left heart disease) and organic TR causes (infective endocarditis, congenital anomalies, rheumatic disease, carcinoid syndrome, prolapse, trauma, iatrogenic complications), as well as diagnosing different morphologic types of TR (leaflet damage, annular dilation, and distinct patterns of right—heart remodelling) (Fig. 1.28).

TV repair is indicated when primary and secondary TR is severe in patients undergoing left heart surgery or in pts. with progressing RV dilation/dysfunction [19]. No single Doppler and echocardiographic parameter is precise enough, therefore integration of multiple parameters is required. In poor TTE quality or when parameters are discordant TOE or CMR for quantitation could be used (Table 1.7).

Fig. 1.26 3D guided 2D planimetry of the aortic valve area in systole

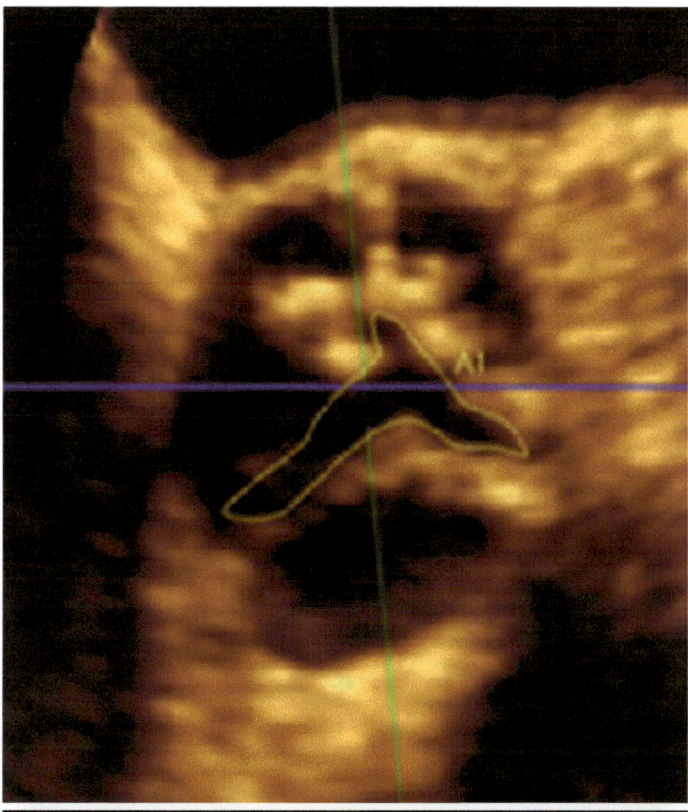

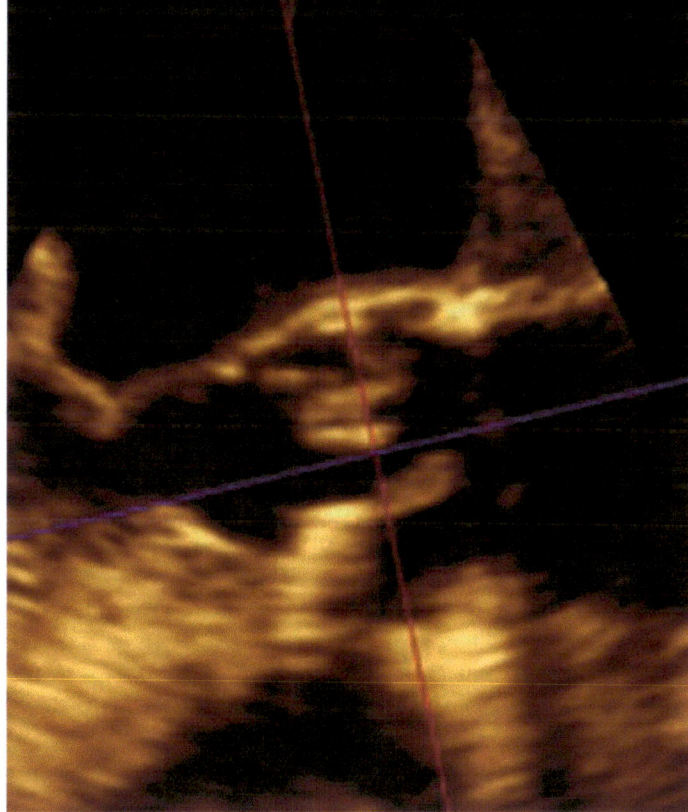

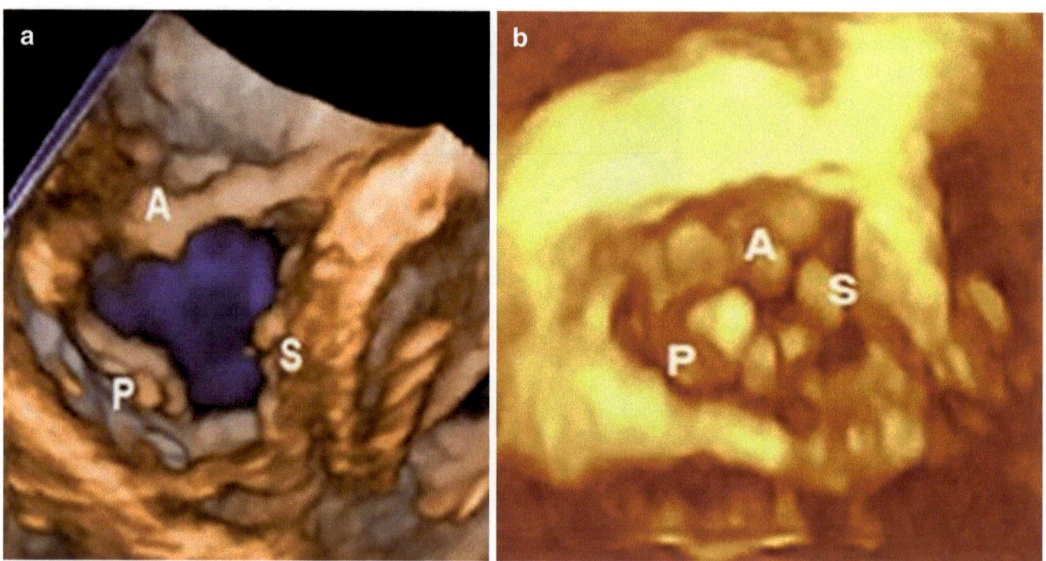

Fig. 1.27 3D image of a tricuspid valve "en face" in diastole (**a**) and in systole (**b**) with visible three cusps: A anterior, P posterior and S septal

Significant annular dilatation is defined by an end-diastolic diameter ≥ 40 mm or > 21 mm/m2 in the four-chamber transthoracic view and it is the indication for secondary TR surgical correction during left sided surgery even in the absence of substantial TR as this demonstrated to provide reverse RV remodelling and to improve functional status of the patients [19]. 3D echocardiography allows more detail evaluation tricuspid annulus size and geometry (Fig. 1.29). Assessment of TV deformation parameters is important as it was shown that marked leaflet tethering (coaptation height > 1 cm) was associated with failed annuloplasty repair. In these patients adjunctive repair techniques or valve replacement maybe required [30].

Evaluation of RV geometry, function and pulmonary systolic pressure should be carried out in TR patients. Parameters of RV systolic function helps to detect the deterioration of RV muscle function. A tricuspidal annular excursion measurement <16 mm and an RV fractional area change <35% are suggestive of RV dysfunction [13]. In severe TR indices of longitudinal RV systolic function can be misleading. CMR or 3D RV volumes and ejection fraction provides more accurate information for quantification of RV

geometry and function. Preoperative pulmonary hypertension has the impact on postoperative outcomes and must be carefully assessed in this group of patients.

Tricuspid stenosis is often combined with tricuspid regurgitation, most frequently of rheumatic origin. Echocardiographic evaluation of the anatomy of the valve and its subvalvular apparatus is important to assess valve repairability. A mean transvalvular gradient ≥5 mmHg at a normal heart rate indicates significant tricuspid stenosis and requires intervention [19].

Artificial Valves

Prior to evaluating the patient with an artificial valve, it is imperative to know the type and size of the valve, as different types of prosthetic valves have different flow characteristics.

Comprehensive echocardiographic assessment of the prosthetic valve function comprises the evaluation of valve leaflet/occluder morphology and mobility, peak and mean transvalvular gradients, effective orifice area (EOA) calculation, assessment of any transvalvular or paravalvular regurgitation and, finally, evaluation of LV dimensions and function and systolic pulmonary artery pressure [31]. These parameters obtained

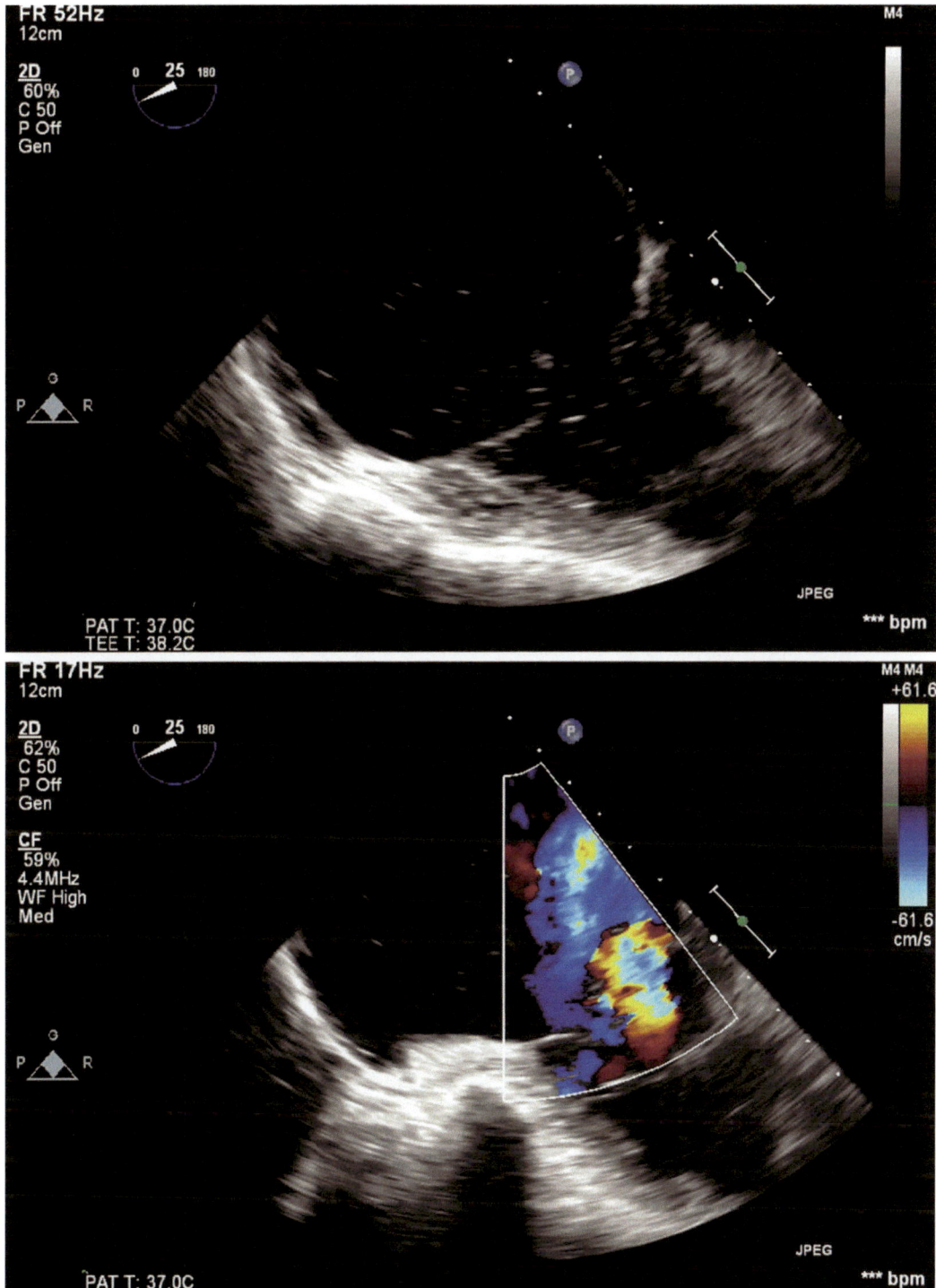

Fig. 1.28 2D TOE images of traumatic TV anterior cusp flail and severe TR

in operating theatre tend to change after the effects of GA wear off and the associated hyperdynamic state resolves. A baseline postoperative TTE assessment of prosthetic valve function is recommended to be performed before hospital discharge or 3–12 weeks after the operation.

Table 1.7 Echocardiographic criteria for severe TR [13]

Quantitative Measures, whenever possible	Specific Criteria
EROA ≥40 mm2 Regurgitant volume ≥ 45 ml VC width ≥ 0.7 cm	Flail leaflet or dilated annulus with no valve coaptation VC width > 0.7 cm Central jet, >50% of right atrium PISA radius > 0.9 cm Dense, triangular CW jet Systolic reversal of hepatic vein flow Dilated RV with preserved function

Normal gradients through artificial valves are slightly higher than the gradients of normal native valves. Doppler echocardiographic parameters are presented for the normal prosthetic valves and suspected stenotic prosthetic valve dysfunction. (From Version 2015) Abnormally high velocities and gradients through a prosthetic valve may be indicative of valve stenosis, patient-prosthesis mismatch (PPM), high flow states, regurgitation or localised high velocity central jet in bileaflet prostheses. TTE imaging is often difficult, especially in mechanical valves, due to reverberation and shadowing artefacts, therefore, TOE has marked superiority in prosthetic valve assessment. Valve type and size should be taken into consideration and effective orifice area (EOA) of the type and size of the implanted valve should be indexed to the patient's body surface area (BSA). In the early postoperative period, stentless bioprostheses, especially if implanted by subcoronary technique, may have higher gra-

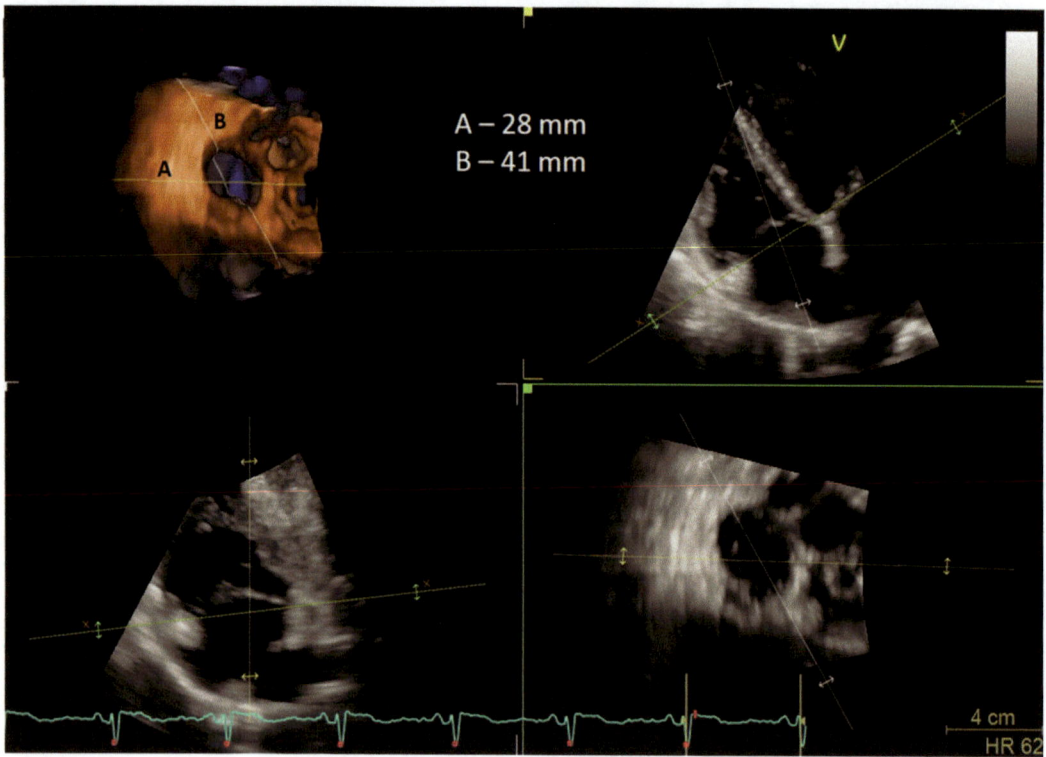

Fig. 1.29 3D TTE evaluation of tricuspid annulus size and geometry

dients, which regress over a few weeks as the aortic wall oedema regresses and LVOT remodels. If the EOA/BSA ratio is <0.85 cm^2/m^2 in the aortic position or < 1.2 cm^2/m^2 in the mitral position, PPM is present and may totally or partially be responsible for high transvalvular gradients. If PPM is excluded or not severe enough to account for transvalvular gradient leaflet/occluder mobility, calcification, additional structures (thrombus, pannus and presence of vegetations) and pathological regurgitation have to be looked for. In the absence of any abnormal findings or hyperdynamic state, the possibility of a technical error should be considered, especially in measuring LVOT dimension.

Normal bioprosthetic valves should have no more than trace regurgitation detectable on echocardiographic assessment through the central leaflet coaptation point. In the meantime, mechanical prostheses have a degree (not more than mild) of 'built-in' regurgitation known as 'washing jets' (minimal back leakage necessary to close the valve occluders), which is detectable and characteristic for each valve model, depending on architecture, number of leaflets and orifices. Normal closing jets are brief, narrow and symmetric (Fig. 1.30). Difficult visualisation of allogeneic structures in the heart and the possibility of complex regurgitant mechanisms (paraprosthetic leaks, eccentric jets) make detection and quantification of pros- thetic valve regurgitation challenging. In the presence of significant regurgitation, it is important to localize the location, determine the mechanism and quantify its severity (Figs. 1.31, and 1.32). It is important to note that methods of regurgitant native valve lesion quantification are applicable in such cases, however, less reliable, especially when multiple jets are present.

Postoperative Complications

Intraoperative TOE provides allows quick evaluation of cardiac haemodynamics and rapid diagnosis in potentially life- threatening complications in the cardiothoracic theatre setting where prompt decision making is of paramount importance. In cases of difficult weaning of patients off-bypass, echocardiography can promptly detect the following postoperative complications:

- Left or right ventricular failure: RV/LV dilatation with decreased systolic function; new regional WMA are findings alerting of myocardial ischemia and its location needs to be identified;
- Mechanical complications (iatrogenic aortic dissection following cross-clamping); valve leaflet perforation, resulting in new or worsened regurgitant lesions (Fig. 1.33);
- Valve/LVOT obstruction: transvalvular/LVOT gradients; leaflet/occluder motion helps to detect these abnormalities. Raising systemic blood pressure may help to unmask latent valve incompetence or worsening LVOT obstruction.
- Persistent or new valvular/paravalvular regurgitation;
- New or residual intracardiac shunts (ASD in MV approach through RA, VSD in surgical myectomy of interventricular septum);
- Pericardial effusion and cardiac tamponade manifesting as cardiac arrest or haemodynamic deterioration when the patient is fully off bypass and the surgical wound is closed (usually in the intensive care unit) (Fig. 1.34).

The role of intraoperative TOE is mostly appreciated when quick and definite information on cardiac function and haemodynamics needs to be obtained in real time. Perioperative echocardiography is a highly reliable imaging tool when being handled and interpreted with sufficient expertise when critical decisions have to be made. It is a cost-effective procedure for patients undergoing cardiac surgery, associated with a decrease in long-term complications including stroke, cardiac complications, and death [32]. Current trends towards the introduction of accreditation in transthoracic, transoesophageal and critical care echocardiography highlights the importance of achieving and maintaining high standards while operating this imaging technique.

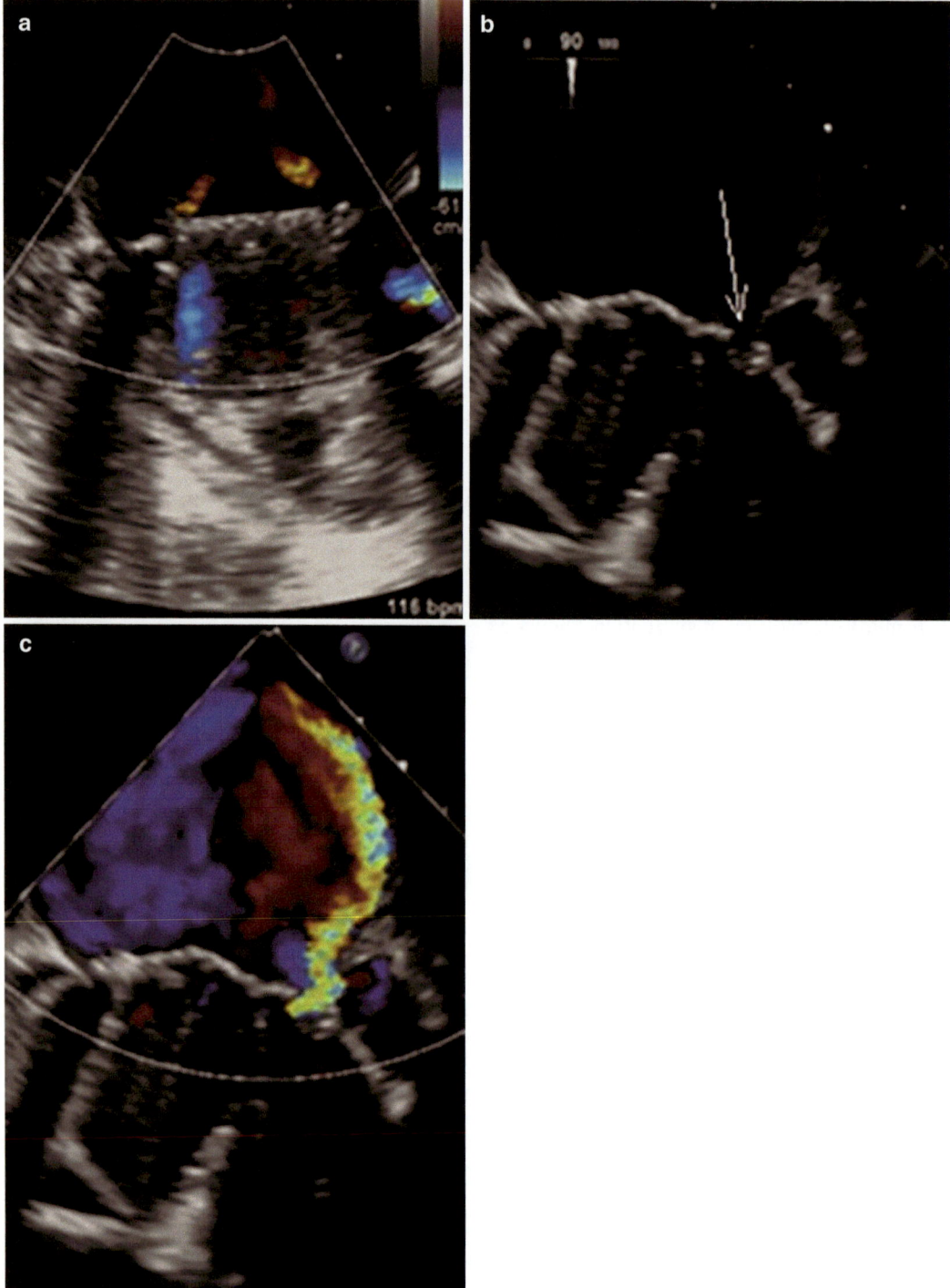

Fig. 1.30 Mechanical bileaflet mitral valve. (**a**) normal washing jets. (**b**) paravalvular defect on 2D TOE images (arrow). (**c**) Paraprosthetic regurgitant jet seen on colour Doppler image

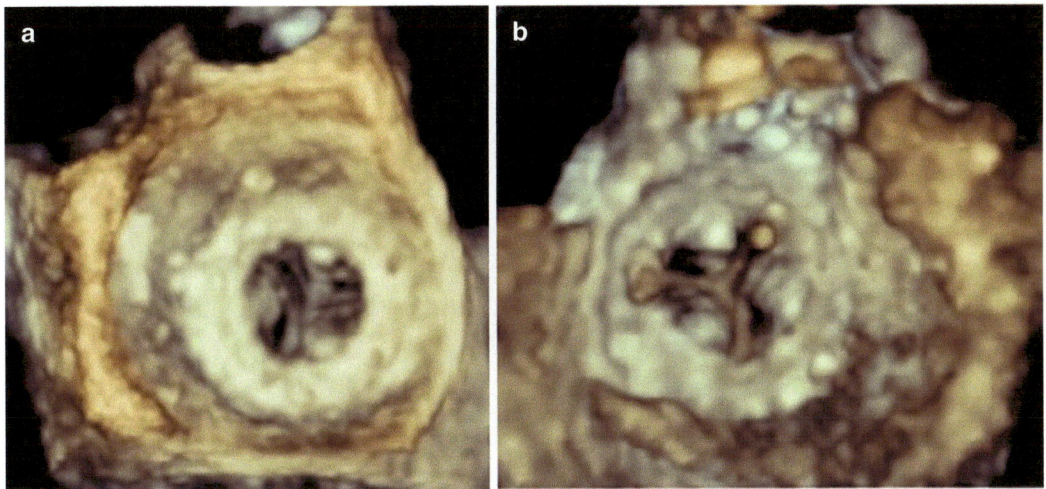

Fig. 1.31 Bioprosthetic valve in the mitral position with normal appearance from the LA side (**a**) and LV side (**b**): 3D TOE images

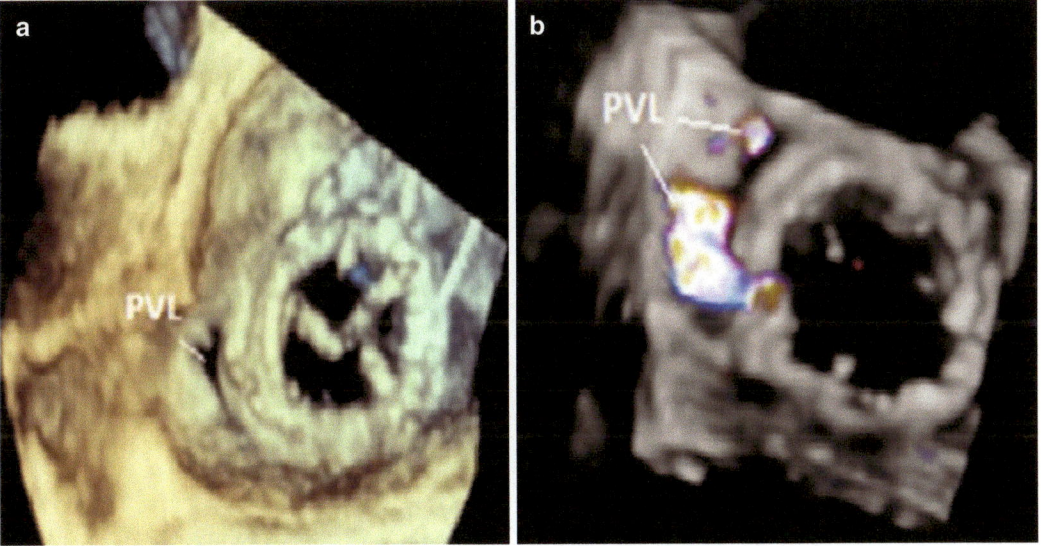

Fig. 1.32 The tissue bioprothesis in the mitral position with paraposthetic defect (**a**) and paravalvular regurgitation with color doppler arising from two holes around the anterolateral portion of the valve (**b**) on plain 3D en face image. No transvalvular MR

Key Pearls & Pitfalls

- A complete transthoracic echocardiogram (TTE) is routinely performed before any cardiac surgical procedure
- 2D and 3D transesophageal echocardiography (TOE) examination provides additional information in patients who may benefit from additional imaging
- LV systolic function is assessed using 2DE or 3DE and calculating ejection fraction (EF). LV EF of <52% for men and < 54% for women are markers of abnormal LV systolic function

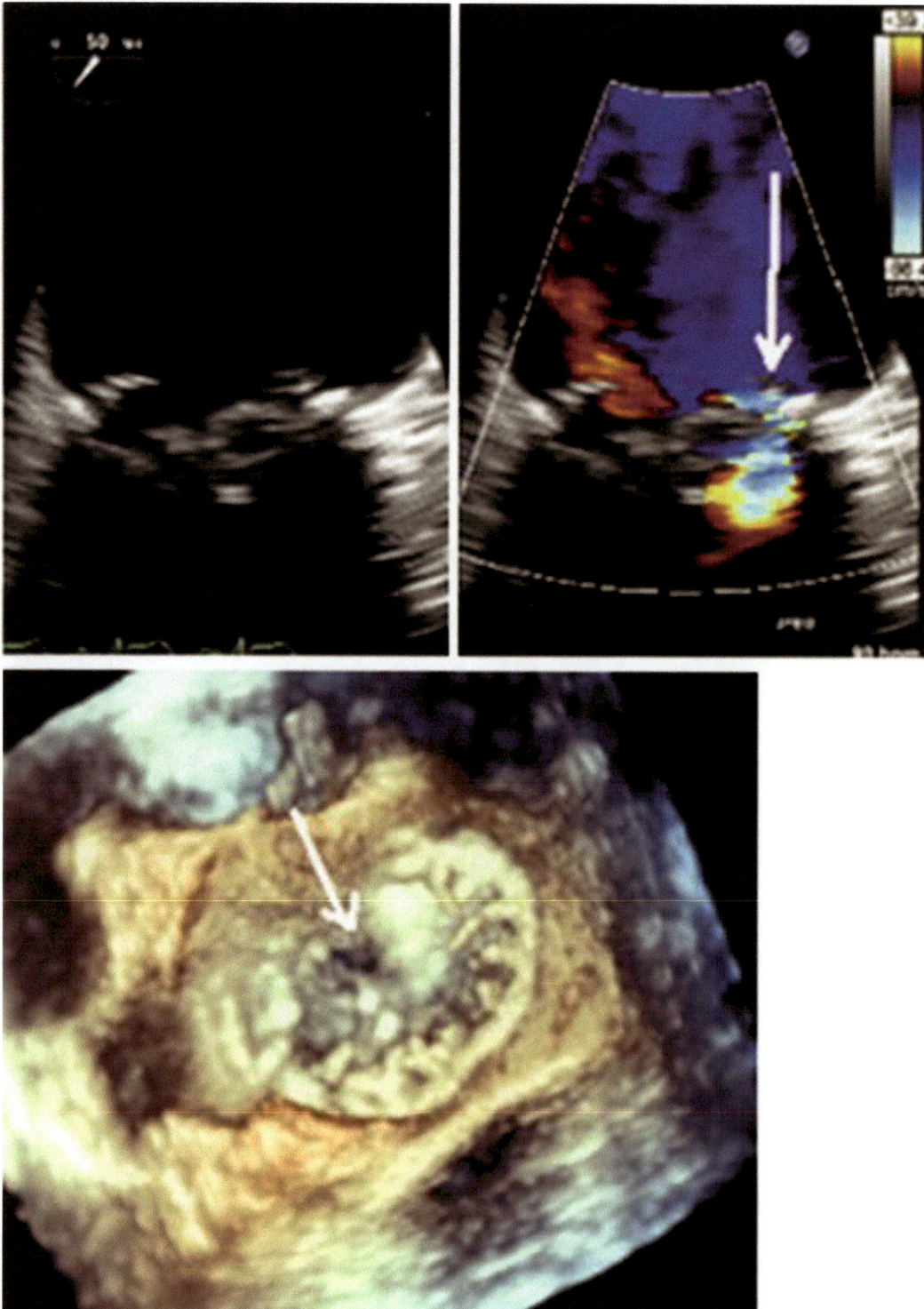

Fig. 1.33 2D and 3D TOE view post MV repair with color flow showing a spot of regurgitation through the defect in the anterior MV leaflet body (arrow)

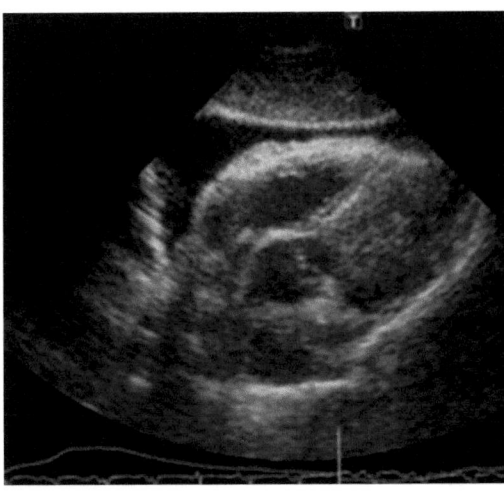 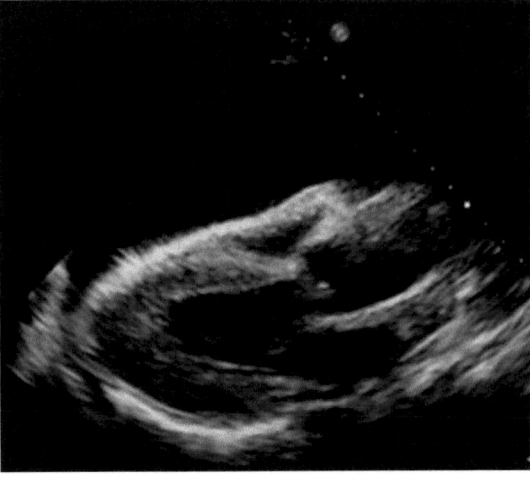

Fig. 1.34 Image on the *left*: small- to medium-sized pericardial effusion. Image on the *right*: large pericardial effusion with evidence of right ventricular diastolic compression indicative of cardiac tamponade

- 3D TOE provides direct view of the mitral valve in an en face projection
- Preoperative 2D and 3D TOE allows assessment of MV reparability and its use in the perioperative setting has contributed greatly to increase in the success of MV repair.

Review QS

1. Abnormal Right Ventricular function in the context of cardiac valve disease may
   a. decrease perioperative mortality rate
   b. have no effect on perioperative mortality rate
   c. **increase perioperative mortality rate**
2. What procedures are recommended to assess valvular pathology?
   (a) 2D TTE
   (b) **2D and/or 3D TOE**
   (c) TOE
3. Alteration in LV geometry and function may lead to
   (a) **Valvular tethering and mitral insufficiency**
   (b) Mitral stenosis
   (c) Aortic stenosis
4. Which of the following best describes the Carpentier's Type III A classification
   (a) Structural abnormal MV characterised by excessive leaflet motion

   (b) **MV apparatus damaged by Rheumatic Heart disease**
   (c) LV dilatation/ischaemia resulting in systolic leaflet restriction
5. Which of the following is difficult to visualise with a TTE?
   (a) Aortic root
   (b) Proximal ascending aorta
   (c) **Arch of aorta**

References

1. Thys DM, Chair MD, Abel MD, et al. Practice guidelines for perioperative transesophageal echocardiography. Anesthesiology. 2010;112:1084–96.
2. Reeves ST, Finley AC, Skubas NJ, et al. Basic perioperative transesophageal echocardiography examination: a consensus statement of the American Society of Echocardiography and the society of cardiovascular anesthesiologists. J Am Soc Echocardiogr. 2013;26:443–56.
3. Lang RM, Badano LP, Mor-Avi V, et al. Recommendations for cardiac chamber quantification by echocardiography in adults: an update from the American Society of Echocardiography and the European Association of Cardiovascular Imaging. J Am Soc Echocardiogr. 2015;28:1–39.
4. Nishimura RA, Otto CM, Bonnow RO, et al. 2017 AHA/ACC focused update of the 2014 AHH/ACC guideline for the management of patients with valvular heart disease. Circulation. 2017;135:e1159–95.

5. Kim HM, Cho GY, Hwang I-C, et al. Myocardial strain in prediction of outcomes after surgery for severe mitral regurgitation. JACC Cardiovasc Imaging. 2018;1:1235–44.

6. Pandis D, Sengupta PP, Castillo JG, et al. Assessment of longitudinal myocardial mechanics in patients with degenerative mitral valve regurgitation predicts postoperative worsening of left ventricular systolic function. J Am Soc Echocardiogr. 2014;27:627–38.

7. Cavalcante JL. Global longitudinal strain in asymptomatic chronic aortic regurgitation. JACC Cardiovasc Imaging. 2018;11:683–5.

8. Zochios V, Protopapas AD, Parhar K, et al. Markers of right ventricular dysfunction in adult cardiac surgical patients. J Cardiothorac Vasc Anesth. 2017;31:1570–4.

9. Rudski LG, Lai WW, Afilalo J, et al. Guidelines for the echocardiographic assessment of the right heart in adults. J Am Soc Echocardiogr. 2010;23:685–713.

10. Quader N, Rigolin VH. Two and three-dimensional echocardiography for pre-operative assessment of mitral valve regurgitation. Cardiovasc Ultrasound. 2014;12(42)

11. Oxorn DC. Intraoperative echocardiography for mitral valve surgery. In: Otto CM, Bonow RO, editors. Valvular heart disease: a companion to Braunwalds' heart disease; 2014. p. 353–75.

12. Lancellotti P, Tribouilloy C, Hagendorff A, et al. Recommendations for the echocardiographic assessment of native valvular regurgitation: an executive summary from the European Association of Cardiovascular Imaging. European Heart Journal–Cardiovascular Imaging. 2013;14:611–44.

13. Zoghbi WA, Adams D, Bonow RO, et al. Recommendations for noninvasive evaluation of native Valvular regurgitation: a report from the American Society of Echocardiography developed in collaboration with the Society for Cardiovascular Magnetic Resonance. J Am Soc Echocardiogr. 2017;30:303–71.

14. Vahanian A, Beyersdorf F, Praz F, et al. 2021 ESC/EACTS guidelines for the management of valvular heart disease: developed by the task force for the management of valvular heart disease of the European Society of Cardiology (ESC) and the European Association for Cardio-Thoracic Surgery (EACTS). Eur Heart J. 2022;43:561–632.

15. Goldstein D, Moskowitz AJ, Gelijus AC, et al. Two years outcomes of surgical treatment of severe ischaemic mitral regurgitation. N Engl J Med. 2016;28:344–53.

16. Ibrahim M, Rao C, Ashrafian H, et al. Modern management of systolic anterior motion of the mitral valve. Eur J Cardiothorac Surg. 2012;41:1260–70.

17. Maslow A, Regan MM, Haering JM, et al. Echocardiographic predictors of left ventricular outflow tract obstruction and systolic anterior motion of the mitral valve after mitral valve reconstruction for myxomatous valve disease. JACC. 1999:342096–104.

18. Lancellotti P, Pibarot P, Chambers J, et al. Recommendations for the imaging assessment of prosthetic heart valves. European Heart J–Cardiovasc Imaging. 2016:2–47.

19. Baumgartner H, Falk V, Bax JJ, et al. 2017 ESC/EACTS guidelines for the management of valvular heart disease. Eur Heart J. 2017;38:2739–91.

20. Iung B, Vahanian A. Rheumatic mitral valve disease. In: Otto CM, Bonow RO, editors. Valvular heart disease: a companion to Braunwalds' heart disease; 2014. p. 255–74.

21. Piazza N, de Jaegere P, Schultz C, et al. Anatomy of the aortic valve complex and its implications for transcatheter implantation of the aortic valve. Circ Cardiovasc Interv. 2008;1:74–81.

22. Goldstein SA, Evangelista A, Abbara S, et al. Multimodality imaging of the diseases of the thoracic aorta in adults. J Am Soc Echocardiogr. 2015;28:119–82.

23. DeWaroux JB, Pouleur AC, Goffinet C, et al. Functional anatomy of aortic regurgitation: accuracy, prediction of surgical repairability, and outcome implications of transesophageal echocardiography. Circulation. 2007;116:I264–9.

24. Boodhwani M, de Kerchove L, Glineur D, et al. Repair-oriented classification of aortic insufficiency: impact on surgical techniques and clinical outcomes. J Thorac Cardiovasc Surg. 2009;137:286–94.

25. Berrebi A, Monin J-L, Lansac E. Systematic echocardiographic assessment of aortic regurgitation–what should the surgeon know for aortic valve repair? Ann Cardiothorac Surg. 2019;8:3.

26. Vanoverschelde JL, van Dyck M, Gerber B, et al. The role of echocardiography in aortic valve repair. Ann Cardiothorac Surg. 2013;2:65–72.

27. Baumgartner H, Hung J, Bermejo J, et al. Recommendations on the echocardiographic assessment of aortic valve stenosis: a focused update from the European Association of Cardiovascular Imaging and the American Society of Echocardiography. Eur Heart J Cardiovasc Imaging. 2017;18(3):254–75.

28. Baumgartner H. Low-flow, low-gradient aortic stenosis with preserved ejection fraction. J Am Coll Cardiol. 2012;60:1268–70.

29. Muraru D, Hahn RT, Soliman OI, et al. 3-dimensional echocardiography in imaging the tricuspid valve. JACC Cardiovasc Imaging. 2019;12:3.

30. Rodes-Cabau J, Taramasso M, O'Gara P. Diagnosis and treatment of tricuspid valve disease: current and future perpectives. Lancet. 2016:1–11.

31. Pibarot P, Dumesnil JG. Doppler echocardiographic evaluation of prosthetic valve function. Heart. 2012;98:69–78.

32. Dieleman JM, Myles PS, Bulfone L, et al. Cost-effectiveness of routine transoesophageal echocardiography during surgery: a discrete-event simulation study. Br J Anaesth. 2020;124(2):136–45.

Cardiac Magnetic Resonance Imaging in Cardiothoracic Surgery

2

Nikita P. Punjabi, Zahra Raisi-Estabragh, and Gajen Sunthar Kanaganayagam

Abbreviations

CMR cardiac magnetic resonance
LGE late gadolinium enhancement
LV left ventricle
LVOT left ventricular outflow tract
RV right ventricle
RVOT right ventricular outflow tract
TOE transoesophageal echo

Chapter Learning Objectives

- Understand the role of CMR in quantification of left and right ventricular structure and function.

- Understand the value of CMR in assessment of ischaemic heart disease, including stress perfusion CMR, and late gadolinium enhancement.
- Understand the role of CMR in assessment of valvular heart disease, including quantification of severity with flow mapping.
- Understand the role of CMR in assessment of aortic disease.
- Understand safety and technical considerations relevant to CMR including for patients with cardiac devices and renal impairment.

Introduction

Cardiovascular magnetic resonance (CMR) imaging technology has advanced exponentially in the last two decades. Volumetric accuracy due to superior endocardial border definition and versatile imaging planes, as well as detailed tissue characterisation have established CMR as the reference modality for assessment of cardiac structure and function. Development of flow sequences has also allowed accurate quantification of regurgitant volumes, and peak velocities. Accordingly, CMR has gained notable presence in international guidelines and its use in clinical practice has become increasingly widespread [1, 2]. In certain clinical scenarios, CMR is the modality of choice, whilst in others, it provides valuable

N. P. Punjabi
Academic Foundation Programme–Imperial College London, London, UK

Z. Raisi-Estabragh
William Harvey Research Institute, NIHR Barts Biomedical Research Centre, Queen Mary University of London, London, UK

Barts Heart Centre, St Bartholomew's Hospital, Barts Health NHS Trust, London, UK

G. S. Kanaganayagam (✉)
Imperial College Healthcare NHS trust, Hammersmith Hospital, London, UK
e-mail: gajenkanaganayagam@nhs.net

© Springer Nature Switzerland AG 2022
P. P. Punjabi, P. G. Kyriazis (eds.), *Essentials of Operative Cardiac Surgery*,
https://doi.org/10.1007/978-3-031-14557-5_2

complementary information or a viable alternative where the first-line modality cannot be used.

The CMR Assessment

The magnetic resonance imaging (MRI) technique is based on the proton spin properties of hydrogen atoms within tissues, and manipulation of their excitation and relaxation properties with magnetic fields and radiowaves. Different sequences are available, with most 'cine' imaging performed via SSFP—steady state free precession imaging. The standard protocol for CMR scans consists of a minimum basic dataset for cardiac chamber quantification and qualitative assessment of valvular structure and function with the remainder of the scan tailored to acquisition of images appropriate to the clinical context (e.g. detailed quantification of a valve lesion (Table 2.1)). Within the same session, gadolinium-based contrast and/or stress agents may be administered if indicated.

Left and Right Ventricular Assessment

CMR allows accurate and reproducible structural assessment and volumetric quantification of the left and right ventricles (LV, RV). The dif-

Table 2.1 Typical image sequences available from CMR assessment

Basic CMR dataset	Additional images based on clinical indication
Localiser	Early and late gadolinium enhancement
Long axis cine images (3, 2, and 4 chamber)	Tissue characterisation with T1 (fat) and T2 (oedema) weighted imaging as well as mapping
Short axis cine stack	Stress imaging
LVOT view	Flow mapping
Short axis view of the aortic valve	3D rendered image of aorta
	Trans-axial stack
	Sagittal RVOT
	Valvular assessment (aortic, mitral, pulmonary, tricuspid)

CMR cardiovascular magnetic resonance, *LVOT* left ventricular outflow tract, *RVOT* right ventricular outflow tract

ferences in magnetic properties of the blood pool and myocardium create intrinsic contrast and high endocardial border definition. CMR is not reliant on acoustic windows, which can limit echocardiography. Further, the long-axis image cut planes can be placed deliberately through the LV apex avoiding foreshortened images, a recognised source of inaccuracy in echocardiography. LV volumes in end-systole/diastole, typically quantified using a series of imaging slices perpendicular to the mitral annulus towards the apex (Fig. 2.1), and an ejection fraction derived from these, are key determinants of many important clinical decisions. Quantification of LV volumes is performed by tracing around the endocardial border, and muscle mass is calculated by tracing around the epicardial border. In cases, where progressive change in LV volumes are important, or for subjects with suboptimal echocardiography windows, CMR may be a better choice for LV assessment. The irregular geometry of the RV and its anterior location in the thorax makes it difficult to image with echo. In cases where visualisation and quantification of the RV is important, CMR is the modality of choice. Quantification is performed by tracing around the endocardium, with increasing use of 'threshold' tools that automatically identify the myocardium and blood pools.

Ischaemic Heart Disease

CMR provides an all-encompassing assessment of ischaemic heart disease (IHD). There are three key features of IHD that may be assessed with CMR: resting LV function, functional significance of coronary artery disease (CAD), and myocardial infarction/viability.

Resting LV Function

The standard cine images allow assessment of global LV function and detection of resting wall motion abnormalities, which may be indicative of infarcted myocardium. Hibernating myocardium may be identified in the presence of hypoki-

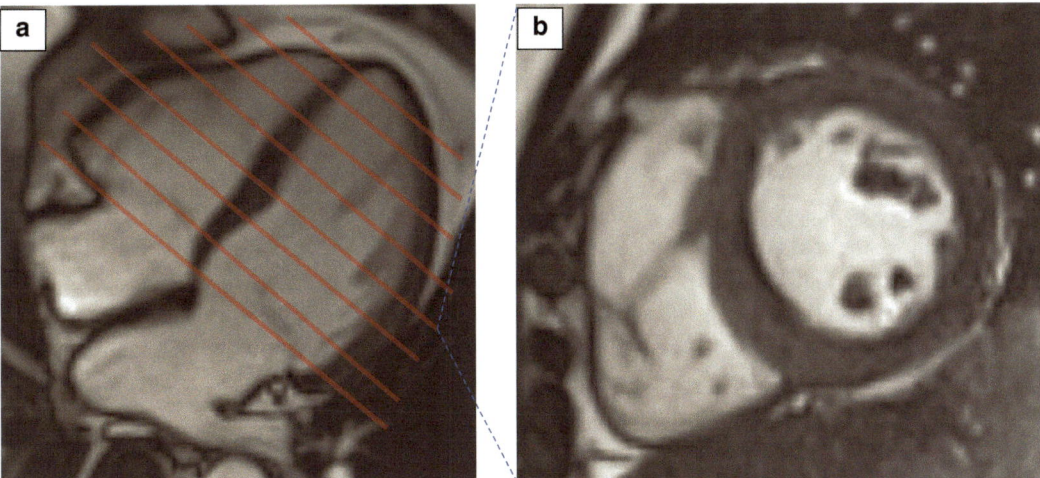

Fig. 2.1 (**a**) 4 chamber view of the heart obtained using SSFP imaging, with further imaging planes (red lines) through the heart to obtain short axis views (**b**). The interval cavities are then traced to obtain volumes

nesia at rest with colocalised ischaemia, and the absence of infarction.

Functional Significance of CAD

Adenosine stress perfusion CMR is an established technique for evaluating the functional significance of CAD with landmark trials demonstrating its utility, with head-to-head comparisons to single photon emission computed tomography (SPECT) [3, 4]. Adenosine administered through an intravenous infusion creates a state of hyperaemia with vasodilatation, and myocardial segments supplied by coronary arteries with flow-limiting disease experience relative hypo-perfusion. Gadolinium is an extracellular, intravascular contrast agent creating a bright signal in the myocardium it enters. Intravenous injection of gadolinium simultaneous to stress with adenosine, and imaging the *first-pass* of contrast to the LV myocardium allows appreciation of differential tissue perfusion patterns. Thus, visual inspection of stress images allows identification of dark areas (i.e. with less contrast entry), which represent areas of hypoperfusion (or perfusion defects) and suggest limitation of blood flow to that segment of myocardium (Fig. 2.2). Other forms of pharmacological stress such as regadenoson and dobutamine are less

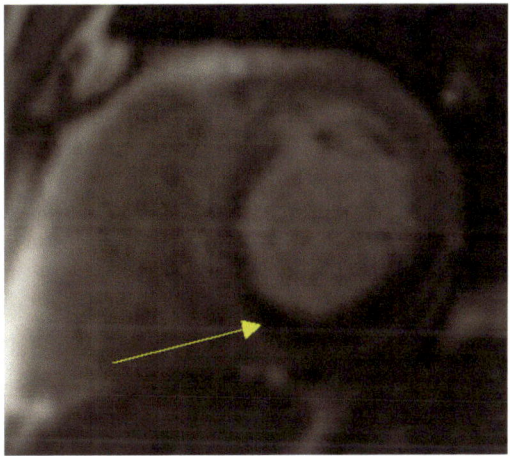

Fig. 2.2 The figure demonstrates a short axis cut of the left ventricle at mid-level taken at time of peak adenosine stress and first pass of gadolinium. The inferior and infero-lateral appear darker than the remaining left ventricular segments, indicating delayed perfusion of these areas. In the absence of corresponding infarction and normal first pass perfusion during rest perfusion imaging, this represents ischaemia

commonly used. Exercise stress CMR is possible but rarely used in clinical settings.

There are recent advances in this field that allow myocardial blood flow quantification, as with PET (positron emission tomography) stress imaging. These absolute values can be colour coded to provide a clearer distinction between areas of ischaemia and normal flow, where a ratio indicates a significant perfusion defect.

Myocardial Infarction and Viability

Due to its larger molecular weight, gadolinium accumulates in the extracellular space and is therefore retained in areas with disrupted myoctes and increased extracellular space for longer than in normal myocardium. This differential wash-out pattern is exploited to identify areas of myocardial infarction, where areas of fibrosis with increased extracellular space can be seen from the subendocardium outwards. The signalling characteristics of gadolinium can be exploited when imaging the heart approximately 10 min after administration, by application of a T1 weighted sequence, that then demonstrates a bright signal in areas of disrupted myocytes and increased extracellular space [late gadolinium enhancement (LGE) due to a shortening of the T1 relaxation time (Fig. 2.3)]. Subendocardial LGE, particularly if in a coronary territory, is suggestive of a myocardial infarction. The transmurality of infarction, quantified as percentage of infarction of the entire myocardial thickness has been shown to be indicative of myocardial viability and to inform decision for revascularisation

based on likelihood of functional recovery. If there are areas of infarction <50% wall thickness, the muscle may be considered viable and should be revascularised if there is ischaemia and the appropriate clinical indications are met. The cut-off of >50% transmurality is commonly quoted to as the threshold for non-viability [5], hence there would be no significant benefit in revascularising an area where the majority of myocardium is non-viable. Reports often provide information on the number of myocardial segments affected based on the American heart association (AHA) 17 segment model.

Valvular Heart Disease

The morphology and function of all heart valves may be assessed with CMR. In addition, CMR incorporates evaluation of the consequences of valve disease on the ventricles and related structures (e.g. aorta). CMR should be seen as a close ally of echocardiography, with the two modalities complementing each other well, with echocardiography the gold standard. When available, CMR adds significant value with difficult to quantify valve lesions. Indeed, it has enjoyed greater attention in the latest European and American Valve guidelines [6, 7].

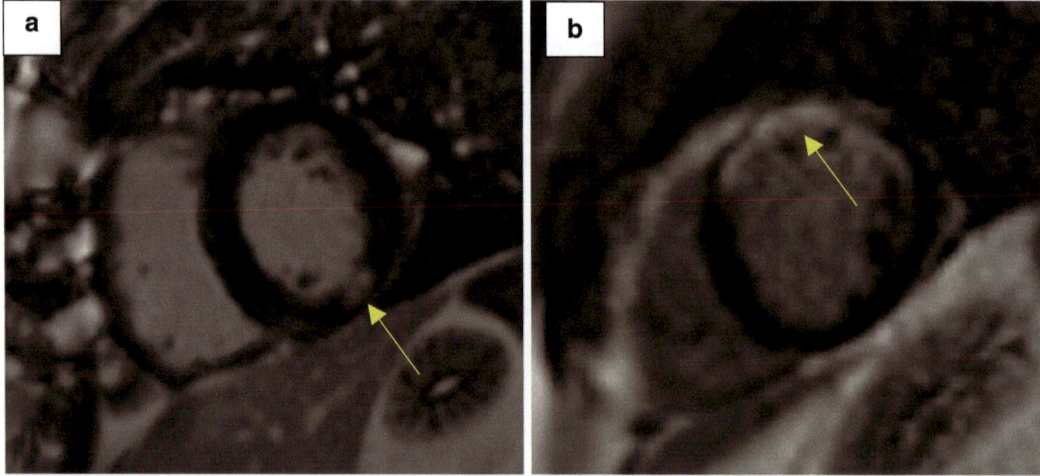

Fig. 2.3 Subendocardial late gadolinium enhancement representing infarction. (**a**) Focal infarct in the inferolateral wall, (**b**) larger infarct in the anterior and anterolateral segments, extending to the anteroseptum

Aortic Stenosis

CMR allows clear visualisation and assessment of the aortic valve, even in the presence of angulated aortic roots or eccentric jets, which can limit evaluation with echo. Valve morphology and function, quantitative grading of stenosis severity by flow mapping, remodelling of the LV (hypertrophy and fibrosis), and aorta dimensions are all readily obtainable.

The aortic valve is routinely imaged in three views (two long axis and one short axis plane). In these views, the mobility of the valve leaflets, flow acceleration, and regurgitation can be qualitatively assessed. Calcification is seen as a signal void. Imaging in short axis allows assessment of valve morphology, leaflet opening, and discrimination of number of leaflets (Fig. 2.4). In this view, the aortic valve area can be directly measured by planimetry.

Through-plane flow mapping allows measurement of mean and peak flow velocities and transvalvular gradients by setting a target velocity encoding peak, with corrections based on aliasing pixels. The long axis images are used to optimally align the through-plan image with the aortic flow jet (Fig. 2.5), in a way that is not possible with echo.

In comparison to echocardiography, there is a tendency to underestimate the peak aortic jet velocity due to partial volume averaging and lower temporal resolution, as well as non-perpendicular slice orientation. Therefore an echocardiogram demonstrating greater severity of stenosis, would take precedence over lower CMR values.

CMR allows excellent haemodynamic differentiation between valvular, sub-valvular, and supra-valvular stenosis. Notably, although larger membranes maybe visualised, very thin, mobile sub-aortic membranes may not be appreciated on CMR. If there is high suspicion for such pathology, trans-oesophageal echo (TOE) would be the

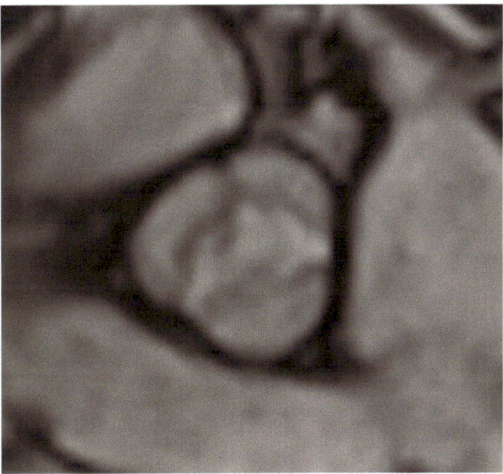

Fig. 2.4 Short axis of the aortic valve showing a bicuspid aortic valve with fusion of the right coronary cusp and left coronary cusp

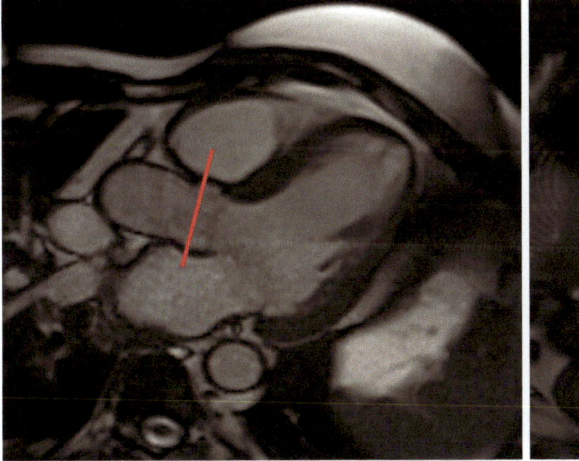
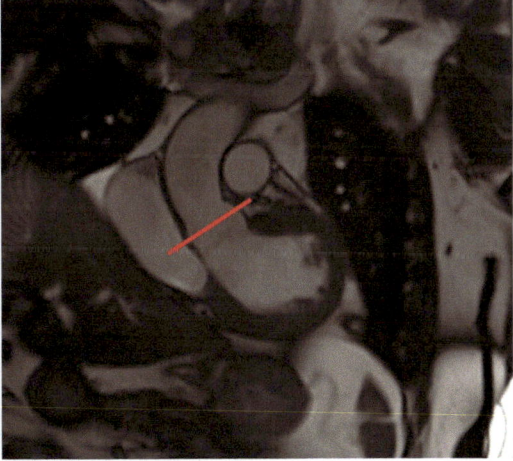

Fig. 2.5 Long axis images used to plan flow mapping plane of the aortic valve (red plane)

optimal modality. The entire length of the aorta may be assessed with CMR, both with and without contrast. Supra-valvular stenosis in the ascending aorta and aortic coarctation are readily identified. Three-dimensional (3D) rendered images of the aorta allow accurate measurement of vessel diameter with proper alignment of measurement planes (double-oblique) with the centre point of the vessel avoiding over/under estimation by incorrect plane measurement.

Aortic pathology related to bicuspid valves, together with eccentric regurgitation patterns and combination of both stenosis with regurgitation make CMR a very useful tool for serial assessment. This is especially the case as the majority of follow up can be performed by a non-contrast and non-radiation based study.

The impact of aortic stenosis on the left ventricle can be assessed with accurate quantification of LV volumes, ejection fraction, and mass. There is increasing suggestion that intervention in asymptomatic severe/very severe aortic stenosis with objective evidence of LV decompensation has outcome benefits. The presence of non-ischaemic LGE and other CMR markers of adverse myocardial remodelling (elevated extracellular volume fraction (ECV), elevated native T1) have been shown to predict outcomes in a variety of settings and may become increasingly important as we move towards consideration of intervention in a broader population of patients [8]. There are ongoing clinical trials assessing outcomes of early valve replacement in asymptomatic severe aortic stenosis guided by CMR LV biomarkers such as LGE (clinicaltrials.gov NCT03094143) [9].

Aortic Regurgitation

As with aortic stenosis, assessment of valvular morphology, the LV, and aorta are of high importance in the assessment of aortic regurgitation. In addition, CMR has unique value in enabling true quantification of regurgitant volume. Through-plane flow mapping above the aortic valve allows accurate measurement of regurgitant volume and fraction, as can LV/RV stroke volume differ-ences. Aortic regurgitation volume = LV stroke volume—RV stroke volume, in the absence of further significant valve disease.

The accurate assessment of cavity dimensions with echocardiography can be challenging, with potentially small changes achievable with small tilts of an echocardiography probe leading to clinically important change in indices. Hence volumetric assessment where changes can be mapped objectively in a linear fashion is immensely appealing. Flow in the descending aorta can also be assessed, with holodiastolic retrograde flow reversal (an indicator of severe aortic regurgitation) easily identified.

The reproducibility of the aortic regurgitant volume with CMR is superior to echocardiography with good evidence that CMR measured regurgitant fraction is a reliable predictor of outcomes [10, 11]. A recent paper used CMR to reclassify patients with previous echocardiography quantification of aortic regurgitation; in this study, CMR (but not echocardiography) quantifiers of aortic regurgitation were significantly associated with outcomes [12].

Mitral Regurgitation

The mitral valve is anatomically complex and its function reliant on the correct working of multiple inter-related components (leaflets, annulus, chordae, papillary muscles, LV). TOE is the preferred modality for assessment of the mitral valve, allowing detailed visualisation of all the fine components of the valve structure. However, CMR provides excellent assessment and may be preferred in patients who are not tolerant of TOE [13]. Limitations include the lower spatial resolution when compared to echocardiography.

The standard long axis cine views allow good qualitative assessment of mitral valve function with visualisation of almost all valve segments. The entire valve and all the scallops may be viewed en-face in the short axis cine view. If systematic evaluation of scallops and papillary muscles is desired, a dedicated stack of images may be planned from the short axis view, comprising a series of cuts perpendicular to the commissure

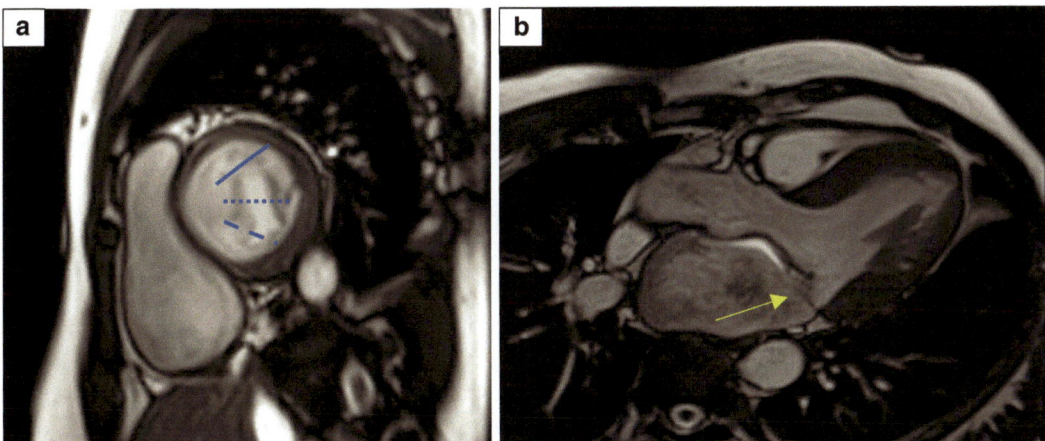

Fig. 2.6 (**a**) Planes through the mitral valve. Solid represents A1/P1, dotted represents A2/P2, dashed represents A3/P3. (**b**) prolapse of P2 with anteriorly directed mitral regurgitation (bright area under anterior leaflet)

and parallel to the LVOT covering the entire valve (Fig. 2.6).

The volume of mitral regurgitation may be quantified by subtracting aortic forward flow (measured on flow mapping) from LV stroke volume, and by stroke volume differences between the LV and RV. In patients with atrial fibrillation, the accuracy of flow measurement may be diminished and quantification of regurgitant volume by subtracting RV from LV stroke volume may be preferred. Quantification with CMR is unaffected by the lack of the perfect hemisphere mandated by PISA (proximal isovolumic surface area) based calculations, jet eccentricity or the presence of multiple jets which can cause problems with quantification by echocardiography. There is a growing body of evidence demonstrating the prognostic value of regurgitant volume measured by CMR and the discrepancies found with echocardiography based assessment [14, 15].

The consequences of mitral regurgitation for the LV may also be assessed through accurate quantification of volume, mass, and ejection fraction. LV dilatation is an early sign of decompensation with reduction of ejection fraction occurring in later stages. Assessment of regional myocardial thickening and papillary muscle function is important for ascertaining mechanism of regurgitation. Papillary muscle fibrosis is also an area of research interest when looking at mitral valve disease, especially with mitral valve

prolapse where fibrosis at the point of insertion may represent a nidus for arrhythmias [16]. In secondary mitral regurgitation, assessment for viability and functionally significant CAD may also be possible within the same study. The left atrium may also be assessed with dilatation indicative of chronic mitral regurgitation or predisposition to atrial fibrillation.

Mitral Stenosis

Thickening and restriction of valve leaflets associated with mitral stenosis can be qualitatively assessed with CMR. The most useful measure on CMR is mitral valve area by direct planimetry. Diastolic flow gradients can be calculated but may not be as accurate, due to difficulty in selecting the appropriate plane, and the likelihood of atrial fibrillation with significant mitral stenosis. Assessment of thickening and calcification of valve leaflets and the sub-valvular apparatus is limited by CMR and echo may be more appropriate. Further, the Wilkins score used for guiding suitability for balloon valvuloplasty is not validated with CMR measures [17]. Left atrial appendage thrombus may be seen on early gadolinium imaging, however, TOE is required to definitively exclude thrombus. For assessment of mitral stenosis, CMR may have value in cases where echocardiography is inadequate or providing conflicting data, with most value from measurement of mitral valve area on planimetry.

Pulmonary Regurgitation

CMR is the modality of choice for assessment of pulmonary regurgitation, allowing clear visualisation of the pulmonary valve, right ventricular outflow tract (RVOT), pulmonary arteries, and the RV.

There is good visualisation of the valve with capability for accurate quantification of the regurgitant volume using flow mapping. The RVOT size and anatomy is clearly visualised and can be considered when planning interventions. The main pulmonary artery and its branches are visualised and may be measured. In pulmonary regurgitation, assessment of the RV is of utmost importance. The irregular geometry of the right ventricle and its anterior position in the thorax limits visualisation and reproducible quantification with echo. CMR allows accurate and reproducible quantification of RV volume, function, and wall thickness. Dilatation of the RV suggests significant regurgitation (in absence of other pathology). Impairment of RV systolic function indicates decompensation and is an important factor in timing intervention.

Pulmonary Stenosis

The pulmonary valve morphology and leaflet motion can be readily visualised with CMR. The outflow tract anatomy is clearly seen, which is of particular importance when balloon valvotomy or valve replacement are being considered. The degree of stenosis can be quantified using through-plane flow mapping (peak velocity, transvalvular gradient) and direct planimetry of the valve area on short axis images. The consequences for the RV can be assessed through accurate measurement of RV volume, wall thickness, and systolic function. The pulmonary arteries can also be measured, with reliable identification of

main or branch pulmonary artery dilatation. Further, co-existent congenital abnormalities (e.g. Tetralogy of Fallot) may be assessed at the same time.

Tricuspid Regurgitation

The tricuspid valve is a large and anatomically complex valve. Most commonly, tricuspid regurgitation occurs secondary to a dilated RV or annulus. The tricuspid valve leaflet motion and morphology can be visualised on routine long axis cine images. Dedicated short axis images can be acquired to obtain en-face view of the valve leaflets, which may reveal areas of non/mal-coaptation and allow identification of the valve segment through which regurgitation is occurring. Whilst such views may be produced with 3D echo or TOE, they are difficult to achieve with 2D echo alone. The degree of regurgitation may be graded by quantification of regurgitant volume using through-plane flow mapping to measure the forward pulmonary flow, which is then subtracted from the RV stroke volume. Alternatively, if flow measurement is not available, LV stroke volume may be subtracted from the RV stroke volume to give the regurgitant volume. Regurgitant fraction is calculated in the normal way. Assessment of the RV is highly important. CMR allows accurate quantification of RV volume, ejection fraction, and wall thickness and therefore remains the gold-standard assessment modality. The right atrial size may also be measured, with dilatation suggestive of chronic tricuspid regurgitation or atrial fibrillation.

Tricuspid Stenosis

Tricuspid stenosis is extremely rare. CMR has value in allowing direct planimetry of the valve area, and accurate assessment of the RV and right atrium.

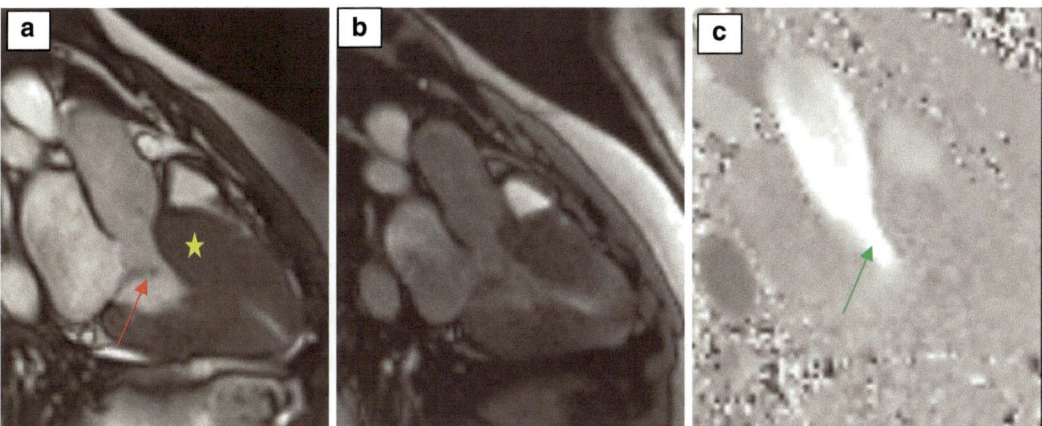

Fig. 2.7 (**a**) Hypertrophic cardiomyopathy with systolic anterior motion of the mitral valve (red arrow) and thickened septum (yellow star), and (**b**) corresponding magnitude image and (**c**) phase velocity encoded map used to assess flow in the left ventricular outflow tract (green arrow represents area of increased flow)

Hypertrophic Cardiomyopathy

CMR is a vital tool for assessment of hypertrophic cardiomyopathy. CMR allows clear identification of wall thickness, unlimited by imaging planes/windows, and further assessment of diffuse fibrosis as well as possible oedema using appropriate sequences. Aside from the unparalleled muscle assessment, it has also more recently been used to look at surgical planning for myectomy in the context of left ventricular outflow tract obstruction [18]. Echocardiography remains the modality of choice for haemodynamic assessment, including use of both exercise and Valsalva to look at obstruction, as well as concomitant mitral valve dysfunction, but haemodynamic assessment is possible, to a more limited extent, using CMR (Fig. 2.7).

Disease of the Aorta

CMR is a valuable modality for imaging the aorta, with no blind spot segments as in transthoracic echo and TOE. 3D rendered images of the whole length of the aorta, possible both with contrast (Fig. 2.8) and without contrast, allow for accurate assessment of diameter and correct alignment of the measurement plane perpendicular to the long axis of the aorta and axial to the vessel itself. Measurements at the LVOT, aortic sinus, sinotubular junction, level of the main pulmonary artery, arch, and descending aorta give a full profile for surgical planning. Unlike computed tomography angiography, CMR does not involve exposure to ionising radiation and as such is preferred, particularly for surveillance scans that can lead to high cumulative lifetime radiation doses. CMR has high diagnostic accuracy for assessment of aortic disease, readily identifying atherosclerosis, intramural haematoma, and aortic dissection [19]. Due to length of time required for scan and limited monitoring in a confined space, CMR is not the preferred option in case of acute aortic syndromes, particularly in cases of instability.

CMR also has an important role in the assessment of congenital heart diseases, scanning of these patients is complex and requires special considerations and expertise. This topic is beyond the scope of the current chapter; however, the interested reader may refer to dedicated publications on this subject.

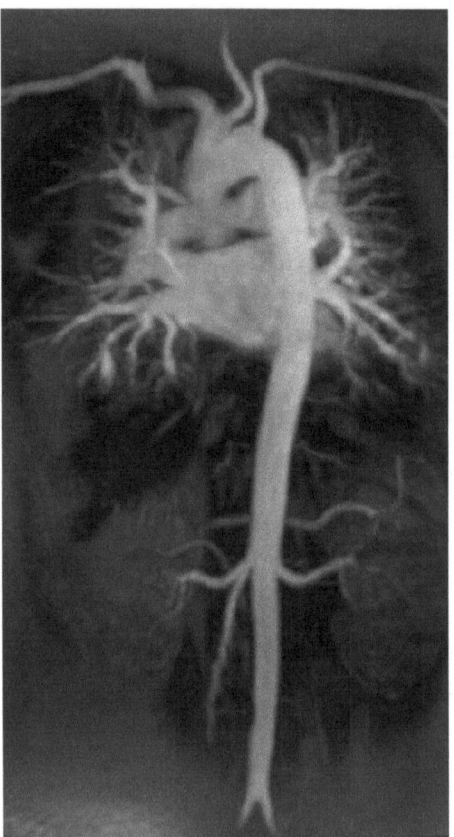

Fig. 2.8 Aortic angiogram performed using CMR. This can be rotated to obtain exact planes for measurement

Safety and Technical Considerations

Prior to referring patients for CMR imaging, several safety and technical points must be considered (Table 2.2). CMR scanning involves exposure to a strong magnetic field. Patients with ferromagnetic implants in their body cannot undergo CMR imaging. Particular caution is required regarding cerebral aneurysms clips, which are often ferromagnetic and an absolute contra-indication to CMR. Patients with intra-cardiac devices (pacemakers, intracardiac defibrillators, loop recorders) may be scanned at discretion of the CMR unit and with support of the cardiac physiology team [20].

A CMR scan typically lasts 30 min to 1 hour. During this time the patient lies flat inside the scanner. To control for respiratory and cardiac motion, the patient is required to maintain a series of breath holds and the images are ECG (electrocardiogram) gated. Images may be incomplete or of sub-optimal quality in patients who are unable to lie flat in this manner, maintain adequate breath-holds, or have significant arrhythmia. If this is a concern, consider alternative imaging modality or strive to control symptoms/arrhythmia prior to the scan. In patients with breath holding difficulties, free-breathing images may be acquired, however, such images are often degraded and are suitable, for the most part, for qualitative rather than quantitative assessment.

Administration of gadolinium in patients undergoing peritoneal dialysis would be contra-indicated, but most with even severe renal impairment would be candidates depending on local policies and following discussion with an imaging cardiologist/radiologist. If requesting a stress perfusion CMR, please be aware that patients with significant conduction disease (high grade heart block) are at risk of asystole, and those with severe and active pulmonary disease may develop bronchoconstriction with administration of adenosine and alternatives should be considered. Any form of caffeine should be avoided 24 hours prior to an adenosine stress CMR. We recommend clinical assessment of patients with known respiratory disease and consultation with the CMR unit in cases of uncertainty.

Table 2.2 Safety and technical consideration and recommended action

Safety/technical factor	Recommended action
Confirmed ferromagnetic object	Arrange alternative to CMR
Intra-cardiac device (permanent pacemaker, defibrillator)	Discuss with cardiac physiology team and CMR unit prior to arranging to allow checking of device and planning of pre/post programming plus additional monitoring of patient, if needed.
Implanted cardiac loop recorder	Discuss with cardiac physiology team- almost all are MR conditional, however magnetic field exposure may delete device memory, therefore it is advisable to download device memory before scanning.
Significant claustrophobia	Approximately 5% of patients cannot complete a CMR scan due to claustrophobia. Modifications to scanning technique or light sedative use may help- discuss with CMR unit.
Unable to lie flat	Consider alternative test
Unable to breath-hold	A CMR scan involves a series of breath-holds—Usually approximately 10s at a time over several minutes. Poor breath-holding can reduce quality of images and diagnostic accuracy. Try to control symptoms to improve breath-hold. Free-breathing sequences can be performed but at the expense of resolution.
Uncontrolled arrythmia	Fast and irregular heart rhythms can reduce image quality as they cause problems with ECG triggering of images and introduce cardiac motion artefact due to averaging and detracts from image quality. If possible, efforts should be taken to control arrhythmias prior to scanning.
Impaired renal function	Administration of gadolinium-based contrast agents requires caution in dialysis dependent patients– Discuss with cardiologist/radiologist.
Severe and/or active pulmonary disease	Adenosine agents can induce severe bronchospasm. Clinically assess for active wheeze and discuss with cardiologist.
Heart block	Adenosine should not be given to patients with second- or third-degree heart block as there is risk of asystole.

CMR cardiac magnetic resonance, *ECG* electrocardiogram, *eGFR* estimated glomerular filtration rate

Key Pearls and Pitfalls

- CMR is the reference standard for quantification of left and right ventricular structure and function.
- CMR allows visualisation and accurate diameter measurement of the entire length of the aorta without the use of ionising radiation.
- CMR has unique value in assessment of aortic regurgitation, by allowing true quantification of regurgitant volume.
- Stress perfusion CMR is an established technique for assessment of functional significance of coronary artery disease.
- Late gadolinium imaging allows reliable detection of myocardial infarction and inference of likelihood of myocardial viability.

End of Chapter Comprehension Questions

Question 1. A 35-year-old lady who was born in the republic of Congo attends following diagnosis of severe rheumatic mitral stenosis. She is reporting exertional breathlessness. Her electrocardiogram shows rate controlled atrial fibrillation. She has been unable to tolerate a transoesophageal echo. What information can a CMR provide in this scenario:

Exclude left atrial appendage thrombus
Mitral valve area by planimetry [x]
Quantification of sub-valvular apparatus calcification
Validated calculation of Wilkin's score to guide suitability for balloon Valvuloplasty

Explanation: CMR allows measurement of mitral valve area by direct planimetry. The sub-valvular apparatus is not well visualised on CMR. The Wilkin's score is not validated with CMR. Early gadolinium enhancement images may demonstrate a left atrial appendage thrombus, but cannot exclude thrombus.

Question 2. A 70-year-old gentleman is being considered for coronary artery bypass grafting. He reports symptoms of typical angina. Cine images show hypokinesia of the anterior and antero-septum from base to apex. Stress perfusion CMR shows adenosine induced perfusion defects in four segments of the left anterior descending (LAD) artery territory. There is sub-endocardial late gadolinium enhancement of these segments with 30% transmurality. What is the most accurate interpretation of this report:

Myocardial infarction with viability and isch-aemia in the LAD territory [x]
Multi-vessel coronary artery disease
Myocardial infarction with non-viability in four segments of the LAD territory
Myocardial infarction with underlying viable myocardium in the circumflex territory

Explanation: This patient has resting hypokinesia, stress induced perfusion defects, and myocardial infarction with <50% transmurality in the LAD territory. This suggests flow limiting coronary disease in the LAD with limited myocardial infarction (viable myocardium).

Question 3. A 40-year-old gentleman with a bicuspid aortic valve and moderate-severe aortic regurgitation has a dilated ascending aorta on transthoracic echo and is being considered for surgery. You would like to measure the entire length of the aorta and re-assess the severity of aortic regurgitation. What is the most suitable test to achieve this:

Cardiac magnetic resonance [x]
Computed tomography (CT) with ECG gating
Stress echocardiography
Trans-oesophageal echo

Explanation: All the echo modalities have blind spots for parts of the aorta. CT and CMR both allow imaging of the entire length of the aorta. However, only CMR also allows quantification of aortic regurgitation severity.

Question 4. You review a 47-year-old lady with asymptomatic severe mitral regurgitation. Assessment of left ventricular (LV) function is suboptimal due to poor transthoracic echo windows. You would like to accurately assess LV with CMR to guide timing of intervention. You note the patient has an implantable loop recorder (Medtronic Reveal LINQ). The manufacturer's guidelines state that the device is 'MR conditional'. What is the most appropriate course of action:

CMR is unlikely to improve visualisation of LV echo, arrange alternative test
Post-pone CMR after explantation of loop recorder
Proceed with CMR, after loop recorder download following discussion with cardiac electrophysiology team [x]
The loop recorder is not 'MR safe', arrange alternative test

Explanation: CMR is not reliant on acoustic windows, therefore it is likely to improve visualisation of the LV where echo has been suboptimal. 'MR conditional' means the patient may safely undergo MR under specified criteria, under which the manufacturer has tested the device. Exposure to the magnetic field deletes the memory of loop recorders, therefore it is best practice to arrange interrogation and download of the device memory prior to scanning.

References

1. Von Knobelsdorff-Brenkenhoff F, Schulz-Menger J. Role of cardiovascular magnetic resonance in the guidelines of the European Society of Cardiology. J Cardiovasc Magn Reson. 2016;18(1):1–18.
2. Von Knobelsdorff-Brenkenhoff F, Pilz G, Schulz-Menger J. Representation of cardiovascular magnetic resonance in the AHA/ACC guidelines. J Cardiovasc Magn Reson. 2017;19(1):1–21.
3. Greenwood JP, Maredia N, Younger JF, Brown JM, Nixon J, Everett CC, et al. Cardiovascular magnetic resonance and single-photon emission computed tomography for diagnosis of coronary heart disease (CE-MARC): a prospective trial. Lancet. 2012 Feb 4;379(9814):453–60.
4. Schwitter J, Wacker CM, Van Rossum AC, Lombardi M, Al-Saadi N, Ahlstrom H, et al. MR-IMPACT: comparison of perfusion-cardiac magnetic resonance

with single-photon emission computed tomography for the detection of coronary artery disease in a multicentre, multivendor, randomized trial. Eur Heart J. 2008;29(4):480–9.

5. Kim RJ, Wu E, Rafael A, Chen E-L, Parker MA, Simonetti O, et al. The use of contrast-enhanced magnetic resonance imaging to identify reversible myocardial dysfunction. N Engl J Med. 2000;343(20):1445–53.

6. Nishimura RA, Otto CM, Bonow RO, Carabello BA, Erwin JP, Fleisher LA, et al. 2017 AHA/ACC focused update of the 2014 AHA/ACC guideline for the Management of Patients with Valvular Heart Disease: a report of the American College of Cardiology/American Heart Association task force on clinical practice guidelines. J Am Coll Cardiol. 2017;70(2):252–89.

7. Baumgartner H, Falk V, Bax JJ, De Bonis M, Hamm C, Holm PJ, et al. 2017 ESC/EACTS guidelines for the management of valvular heart disease. Eur Heart J. 2017;38(36):2739–86.

8. Bing R, Cavalcante JL, Everett RJ, Clavel MA, Newby DE, Dweck MR. Imaging and impact of myocardial fibrosis in aortic stenosis. JACC Cardiovasc Imag. 2019;12(2):283–96.

9. Early Valve Replacement Guided by Biomarkers of LV Decompensation in Asymptomatic Patients With Severe AS–ClinicalTrials.gov. Available from https://clinicaltrials.gov/ct2/show/results/NCT03094143

10. Myerson SG, D'arcy J, Mohiaddin R, Greenwood JP, Karamitsos TD, Francis JM, et al. Aortic regurgitation quantification using cardiovascular magnetic resonance: association with clinical outcome. Circulation. 2012;126(12):1452–60.

11. Cawley PJ, Hamilton-Craig C, Owens DS, Krieger EV, Strugnell WE, Mitsumori L, et al. Prospective comparison of valve regurgitation quantitation by cardiac magnetic resonance imaging and transthoracic echocardiography. Circ Cardiovasc Imaging. 2013;6(1):48–57.

12. Kammerlander AA, Wiesinger M, Duca F, Aschauer S, Binder C, Zotter Tufaro C, et al. Diagnostic and prognostic utility of cardiac magnetic resonance imaging in aortic regurgitation. JACC Cardiovasc Imaging. 2019;12(8P1):1474–83.

13. Chan KJ, Wage R, Symmonds K, Rahman-Haley S, Mohiaddin RH, Firmin DN, et al. Towards comprehensive assessment of mitral regurgitation using cardiovascular magnetic resonance. J Cardiovasc Magn Reson. 2008;10(1):61.

14. Myerson SG, D'Arcy J, Christiansen JP, Dobson LE, Mohiaddin R, Francis JM, et al. Determination of clinical outcome in mitral regurgitation with cardiovascular magnetic resonance quantification. Circulation. 2016;133(23):2287–96.

15. Penicka M, Vecera J, Mirica DC, Kotrc M, Kockova R, Van Camp G. Prognostic implications of magnetic resonance-derived quantification in asymptomatic patients with organic mitral regurgitation: comparison with Doppler echocardiography-derived integrative approach. Circulation. 2018;137(13):1349–60.

16. Bui AH, Roujol S, Foppa M, Kissinger KV, Goddu B, Hauser TH, et al. Diffuse myocardial fibrosis in patients with mitral valve prolapse and ventricular arrhythmia. Heart. 2017;103(3):204–9.

17. Wilkins GT, Weyman AE, Abascal VM, Block PC, Palacios IF. Percutaneous balloon dilatation of the mitral valve: an analysis of echocardiographic variables related to outcome and the mechanism of dilatation. Heart. 1988;60(4):299–308.

18. Spirito P, Binaco I, Poggio D, Zyrianov A, Grillo M, Pezzoli L, et al. Role of preoperative cardiovascular magnetic resonance in planning ventricular septal Myectomy in patients with obstructive hypertrophic cardiomyopathy. Am J Cardiol. 2019;123(9):1517–26.

19. Erbel R, Aboyans V, Boileau C, Bossone E, Di Bartolomeo R, Eggebrecht H, et al. 2014 ESC guidelines on the diagnosis and treatment of aortic diseases. Eur Heart J. 2014;35:2873–926.

20. Ibrahim E-SH, Horwood L, Stojanovska J, Attili A, Frank L, Oral H, et al. Safety of CMR in patients with cardiac implanted electronic devices. J Cardiovasc Magn Reson. 2016 Dec;18(S1)

Systemic Inflammatory Response and Cardiopulmonary Bypass

3

Ahmet Rüçhan Akar, Bahadır İnan,
Karan P. Punjabi, and Sadettin Dernek

Abbreviations

ACT:	activated clotting time
CABG:	coronary artery bypass grafting
CPB:	cardiopulmonary bypass
CRRT:	continuous renal replacement therapy
DAMP:	damage associated molecular pattern
DIC:	disseminated intravascular coagulation
ET:	endothelin
FDPs:	fibrin degradation products
HBC:	heparin bonded circuits
HPA:	hypothalamic-pituitary-adrenal
IL:	interleukin
MECC:	minimized extracorporeal circulation
NO:	nitric oxide
PAMP:	pathogen associated molecular pattern
PGI_2:	prostacyclin
ROS:	reactive oxygen species
SDD:	selective decontamination of the digestive tract
SIRS:	systemic inflammatory response syndrome
TXA_2:	thromboxane

Learning Objectives

- Understand the etiopathogenesis of SIRS
- Understand the complexity of the CPB-associated SIRS
- Understand the results from a multitude of humoral, cellular, metabolic and endocrine mechanisms
- Understand the different treatment strategies to manage SIRS
- Understand the haemodynamic consequences of SIRS

Major surgery, trauma, sepsis, ischemia-reperfusion injury, or cardiac surgery with cardiopulmonary bypass (CPB) provoke a *"whole-body inflammatory response"* or *"systemic inflammatory response syndrome"* (SIRS) [1, 2]. SIRS is an exaggerated, nonspecific defense response of the body to a noxious stressor [3]. The etiopathogenesis of SIRS broadly divides into the damage-associated molecular pattern (DAMP) and pathogen-associated molecular pattern (PAMP) [3].

Currently, it is estimated that more than one million cardiac operations are performed each

A. R. Akar (✉) · B. İnan
Department of Cardiovascular Surgery, Ankara University School of Medicine, Ankara, Turkey

K. P. Punjabi
School of Medicine, St. George's University of London, London, UK

S. Dernek
Department of Cardiovascular Surgery, Osmangazi University, Ankara, Turkey

© Springer Nature Switzerland AG 2022
P. P. Punjabi, P. G. Kyriazis (eds.), *Essentials of Operative Cardiac Surgery*,
https://doi.org/10.1007/978-3-031-14557-5_3

year worldwide with CPB support using a heart-lung machine [4]. In CPB related SIRS early potential triggers are; (1) surgical trauma, (2) contact between heparinized blood components with the artificial surface of the CPB circuit, (3) nonendothelial cell surfaces in the mediastinum, (4) blood-air interface, (5) non-pulsatile blood-flow patterns, (6) ischemia and reperfusion injury, (7) endotoxemia [1, 5–10].

CPB associated SIRS is a complex process involving multiple humoral, cellular, and metabolic pathways involving autonomic, endocrine, hematological, and immunological alterations [3, 10]. Amplified inflammatory cascade and dys-regulated cytokine storm may exacerbate multiple organ dysfunction [3, 11, 12]. Clinical manifestations may involve pyrexia or hypothermia, increase in oxygen consumption, impaired hemodynamics, systolic and diastolic myocardial dysfunction, vasodilation, and increased capillary permeability, coagulopathy, neurocognitive defects, acute renal insufficiency, increased pulmonary reactivity, acute respiratory distress syndrome, increased gut permeability and increased susceptibility to infection both in adults and pediatric population [4, 5, 10, 11, 13–16].

SIRS is characterized by the activation of the endothelium, complement system, neutrophils, monocytes, platelets, kallikrein–bradykinin and fibrinolytic systems, cytokines, and coagulation pathways. SIRS may also cause disseminated intravascular coagulation (DIC) by aggravating the consumption of coagulation factors. Post-CPB SIRS is defined by the satisfaction of any two of the criteria below:

1. temperature > 38 °C or < 36 °C;
2. heart rate > 90 beats per minute,
3. respiratory rate > 20 act per minute; or, PaCO2 < 32 mmHg,
4. leukocyte count >12,000/mm^3; or, leukocyte count <4000/mm^3; or, over 10% immature forms or bands. However, some investigators suggest redefining the current definition of CPB-related SIRS by the leading societies of cardiothoracic surgery, anesthesia, and perfusion [17].

MacCallum NS et al. [18] showed that nearly all patients (96.2%) undergoing cardiac surgery fulfilled the standard two criterion definition within 24 hours of ICU admission. The investigators suggested that meeting at least three defining criteria for SIRS, or requiring that at least two criteria are met for six consecutive hours, would be more discriminatory in defining a cohort of patients with adverse clinical outcomes [18]. Recently, Squiccimarro E et al. [19] reported a 28.3% incidence of SIRS within 24 hours from cardiac surgery. Data from 28,763 patients from 20 centers in Australia and New Zealand who underwent coronary artery bypass grafting (CABG) and valve surgery demonstrated that increased patient age was strongly associated with reduced acute immune response and postoperative SIRS prevalence due to immunosenescence [20].

SIRS is also a frequent complication in the pediatric population after congenital heart surgery, which affects nearly one-third of children [13]. The investigators showed that the duration of CPB and the amount of fresh frozen plasma given were identified as significant risk factors for CPB-related SIRS [13]. Other investigators reported further independent risk factors for SIRS development in the pediatric population, including bodyweight below 10 kg and preoperative diagnosis of right to left shunt congenital heart disease [21].

SIRS is incited by some factors, including the interaction of blood with the foreign surfaces of the CPB circuit (i.e., contact activation), altered blood flow patterns (i.e., non-pulsatile flow), ischemia-reperfusion injury, and endotoxins (Fig. 3.1). Interaction between activated endothelial cells, leukocytes, and platelets, is mediated through the expression of three main groups of adhesion molecules: the selectins, the integrins, and the immunoglobulin superfamily [22].

Initiation results from a multitude of humoral, cellular, and metabolic processes:

1. **Humoral Response**
   - Kinin system and Hageman factor activation

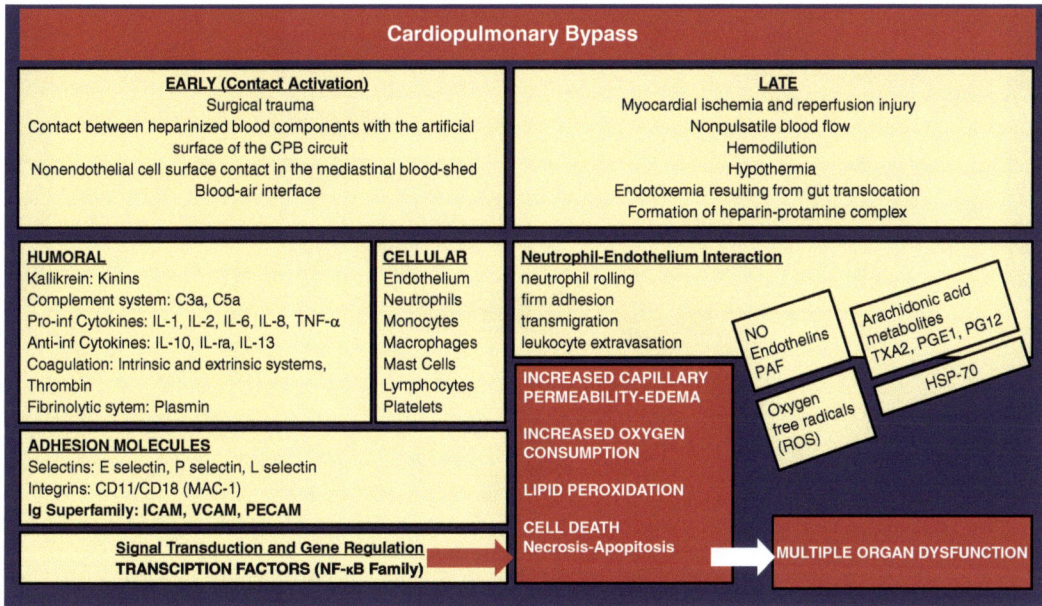

Fig. 3.1 Inflammatory response pathways in cardiopulmonary bypass-related SIRS

- Complement system activation
- Fibrinolytic system activation
- Synthesis of pro-inflammatory and anti-inflammatory cytokines

2. **Cellular Response**
   - Endothelium activation
   - Neutrophil activation
   - Platelet activation

3. **Metabolic and Endocrine Response**
   - Sympathetic nervous system and catecholamine response
   - Endocrine response

Humoral Response

Kinin System Activation and Hageman Factor

Exposure of blood to the extracorporeal circuit activates the contact system. Surface activation of the Hageman factor (Factor XII) may be the first critical event in the activation of other cascades. Activation of Hageman factor converts prekallikrein to kallikrein. Kallikrein has six main

actions; a) activation of plasma prekallikrein via a positive feedback loop, b) cleavage of HMWK to release bradykinin which is a potent vasodilator that increases vascular permeability, c) activation of complement system (C3 and C5), d) activation of the fibrinolytic pathway by stimulating tissue plasminogen activator, e) activation of the sympathetic nervous system and f) initiates the intrinsic coagulation cascade that leads to the formation of thrombin [2].

Thrombin plays a pivotal role in signaling inflammatory processes that directly activates complement factor 5 (C5) and neutrophils and also activates the endothelium [10]. Tissue factor and thrombin generation activation can also occur after ischemia-reperfusion injury [23].

The Complement System

The complement system consists of over 30 plasma proteins that are involved in chemoattraction, activation, opsonization, and cell lysis. Three major complement activation pathways have been described: the classical pathway, triggered by immune complexes; the mannose-binding lectin pathway, triggered when lectin

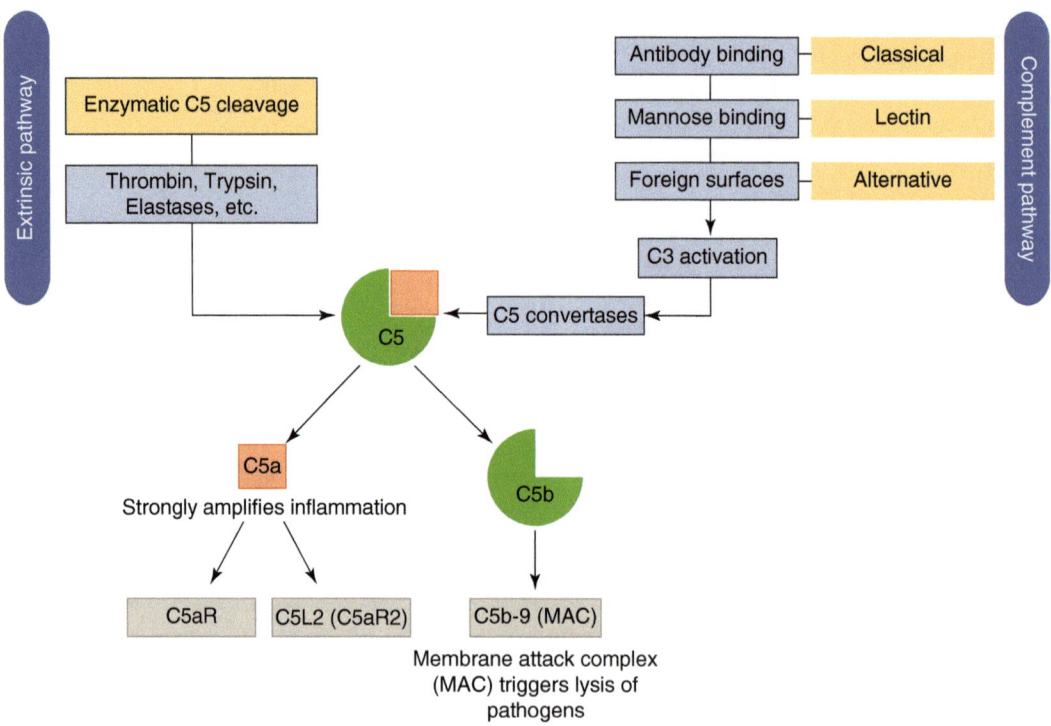

Fig. 3.2 Complement activation in response to cardiopulmonary bypass

binds mannose groups in bacteria; and the alternative or properdin pathway, triggered by contact with various viruses, bacteria, fungi, and tumor cells [24].

During CPB, the complement system is activated at three different times; a) blood contact with nonendothelial cell surfaces, b) after protamine administration, and formation of the protamine-heparin complex, c) during reperfusion of ischemic arrested heart [7, 25].

Contact with the CPB circuit provokes the formation of anaphylatoxins C3a and C5a soon after the institution of CPB (Fig. 3.2) [7, 25]. Activated complement products promote vasodilation, increased vascular permeability, leukocyte activation, leukocyte mobilization, chemotaxis and adhesion and phagocytosis of organisms by neutrophils and macrophages.

The classical pathway involves the activation of C1 by an antibody-antigen complex. The alternative pathway does not require an antibody for its activation: C3 fragments free-floating in serum attach directly to antigens, endotoxins, or foreign surfaces (otherwise known as contact activation). The standard step linking both pathways is the cleavage of C3. Cleavage of C3 to its activated form C3a stimulates the release of histamine and other inflammatory mediators from mast cells, eosinophils, and basophils, which results in smooth muscle constriction and an increase in vascular permeability. C5a is a potent chemotactic factor for neutrophils as it promotes its aggregation, adhesion, and activation. C3b and C5b interact on cell membranes with components C6–C9 to form a "membrane attack complex," which activates platelets and "punches" holes in cell membranes. This process is rapid: plasma levels of activated complement factors rise within 2 min of the onset of the bypass, and a second rise can be detected after the release of the aortic cross-clamp and rewarming. Levels decline postoperatively and generally return to average 18–48 hours postoperatively.

Fibrinolytic System Activation

Exposure of blood to the artificial surface of the CPB circuit, temperature changes, medications, mechanical trauma, or blood products trigger fibrin clot formation, resulting in activation of the fibrinolytic system. The fibrin clots are continuously proteolytically digested into fibrin degradation products (FDPs) by plasmin. Plasmin production is upregulated via two pathways:

(a) Bradykinin upregulates tissue plasminogen activator (tPA), which in turn converts plasminogen to plasmin. tPA levels peak with 30 minutes of CPB and return to baseline within 24 hours.

(b) Kallikrein and HMWK upregulate urokinase, which activates urokinase plasminogen activator (uPA), which in turn converts plasminogen to plasmin. Intravascular fibrin clots lead to impaired microcirculation and hypoxic cellular damage. FDPs compete with thrombin and slow down clotting by inhibiting the conversion of fibrinogen to fibrin. The net effect is endothelial and platelet dysfunction.

Synthesis of pro-Inflammatory and Anti-Inflammatory Cytokines

Cytokines are critical regulatory messengers released in response to local injury that generally acts in a paracrine fashion. They are secreted by immune cells, namely lymphocytes and macrophages, endothelial cells, neurons, glial cells, and other types of cells. Cytokines play a critical role in the pathophysiology of CPB-related SIRS.

Release of pro-inflammatory cytokines; interleukin-1 (IL1) and TNF-alpha results in dissociation of nuclear factor-kB (NF-kB) from its inhibitor [3]. NF-kB is thus able to induce the mass release of other pro-inflammatory cytokines, including IL-6, IL-8, and Interferon-gamma [3]. IL-6 induces the release of acute-phase reactants, including procalcitonin and C reactive protein. The compensatory anti-inflammatory response is also elevated and medi-ated by Interleukins IL-4 and IL-10, which tend to inhibit the production of TNF-alpha, IL-1, IL-6, and IL-8 [3]. These inflammatory mediators generally reach peak levels 2–4 h after termination of CPB [5, 26]. However, the balance among these cytokines is essential in determining the level of the inflammatory response following CPB [2]. Serum IL-19 and IL-22 were also induced during CPB concomitant with induction of IL-6 and TNF-alpha [27]. Excessive levels of cytokines lead to uncontrolled systemic inflammation causing tissue damage and acute kidney injury [3, 15]. Besides, they stimulate further expression of procoagulant and fibrinolytic enzymes.

Using coronary sinus blood sampling, Wan S. et al. [28] reported that myocardium is a significant source of pro-inflammatory cytokines in patients undergoing CPB. Another clinical study showed that CPB provokes a more significant pulmonary than systemic inflammatory response [29]. The investigators demonstrated that the production of all cytokines was 1.5–3 times higher in alveolar macrophages obtained at the end of surgery than in plasma monocytes obtained simultaneously in patients who underwent CPB [29].

Cellular Response

The Endothelium

The endothelium is an organ system [30], lines the interior surface of the vascular tree and lymphatic vessels. The endothelium is a genuinely pervasive cell layer, weighing 1 kg and covering a total surface area of 4000–7000 m^2 [31]. Physiologically, the endothelium is highly metabolically active organ sensing changes in the extracellular compartment and responding in ways that are beneficial or, at times, harmful to the host [30, 32]. In brief, endothelium not only functions as a barrier but also controls vascular tone and permeability, regulates coagulation, has the capacity for repair and regeneration.

Four key mediators mainly regulate vascular tone, namely nitric oxide (NO), prostacyclin PGI_2, thromboxane (TXA_2), and endothelin (ET).

Local vasodilation is mediated through nitric oxide and prostacyclin [33]. Nitric oxide (NO), corresponding to the endothelium-derived relaxing factor, is a significant regulator of vasomotor tone and blood flow. Extremely potent and long-lasting vasoconstriction is mediated by endothelin-1, which is a peptide with 21 amino acid residues, also released from the endothelium. A significant release of endothelin-1 after CPB has been shown in patients undergoing CABG.

Furthermore, the endothelium has the capacity for secreting anticoagulants such as tissue plasminogen activator (tPA), thrombomodulin, and heparin-like substances. The principal agonists for endothelial cell activation during CPB are thrombin, C5a, and the cytokines IL-1β and TNF-α, which bind to specific receptors on the endothelium.

Neutrophil Activation

Leucocytes play a fundamental role in the pathophysiology of CPB related inflammation [34]. Neutrophil-endothelium interaction via the expression of selectins is central to the development of the inflammatory process during CPB [4].

Activated endothelial cells, express on the cell (luminal) surface the adhesion molecule ligands corresponding to those being expressed in the activated neutrophil. The adhesion molecules family includes selectins (E selectin, L selectin, P selectin), integrins (CD11/CD18 (MAC-1)), and immunoglobulin superfamily (ICAM, VCAM, PECAM). The expression of integrin receptors results in tighter binding to the endothelial cells. The increased adhesive capability of activated circulating neutrophils flowing over activated vascular endothelial cells results in a step-wise interaction comprising three distinctive steps: neutrophil rolling, firm adhesion, and transmigration causing leukocyte extravasation [4]. Neutrophils and macrophages release reactive oxygen species (ROS) synthesized via the NADPH oxidase pathway with the stimuli of cytokines. Increased capillary permeability can lead to cell edema and cell necrosis or apoptosis.

Platelet Activation

Platelet dysfunction following CPB has been consistently demonstrated in several studies [35–38]. Platelet activation, degranulation, and adherence to vascular endothelium during CPB is evident by thrombin with the resultant clinical effects [38, 39]. Platelet aggregation stimulates serotonin (5-HT) release, which further enhances the interaction of platelets with circulating tissue factor-rich microvesicles [40]. Activated platelets also play an essential role in neutrophil adhesion and transmigration.

Metabolic and Endocrine Response

The extracellular fluid volume increases while body temperature decreases during CPB. Activation of the hypothalamic-pituitary-adrenal (HPA) axis and catecholamine release is evident with the unset of CPB [41]. Plasma epinephrine concentrations may increase up to ten-fold over the pre-bypass concentrations; norepinephrine levels typically increase to a lesser extent. Clinical studies showed that plasma cortisol, adrenocorticotropic hormones, and vasopressin or antidiuretic hormone (ADH) markedly increase during CPB [42, 43], which leads to peripheral vasoconstriction and shifts to visceral blood flow.

Genetic Predisposition

The interleukin 6–174 G/C polymorphism was demonstrated to have a role in the modulation of postoperative interleukin-6 levels and was associated with postoperative renal and pulmonary dysfunction [44]. Grunenfelder J. et al. [45] showed that the apolipoprotein E and the tumor necrosis factor-beta polymorphisms are associated with increased releases of interleukin-8 and tumor necrosis factor-alpha during CPB and risk factors for CPB-related SIRS.

Treatment Strategies for Sirs

Modulation of the inflammatory response in CPB can be broadly categorized into three groups, mainly pharmacological therapies, technical strategies, and endotoxemia-reducing strategies [2, 46].

Pharmacological Therapies

Corticosteroids

Preoperative use or the addition of methylprednisolone to the CPB circuit prime reduced the inflammatory response in experimental models [47]. Steroids suppress uncontrolled complement-mediated activation of neutrophils and lower pro-inflammatory cytokines TNFα, IL-6, IL-8, and E-selectin levels and increase IL-10 and IL-1ra. However, methylprednisolone has no measurable effect on recovery and increase anesthetic complications and impaired glucose tolerance in patients with SIRS. However, dexamethasone use during induction of anesthesia reduced gut permeability in pediatric patients undergoing cardiac surgery [48].

In a multicenter, randomized, double-blind, placebo-controlled trial (the DECS trial) of 4494 adult patients in the Netherlands enrolled between 2006 and 2011 patients were randomly assigned to receive a single intraoperative dose of 1 mg/kg dexamethasone (n = 2239) or placebo (n = 2255) [49]. The primary outcome measures of the study were the composite of death, myocardial infarction, stroke, renal failure, or respiratory failure within 30 days of randomization. However, the use of intraoperative dexamethasone did not reduce the 30-day incidence of major adverse events compared with placebo [49]. In another recent double-blind, randomized, controlled trial performed between 2007–2013 entitled The Steroids In caRdiac Surgery (SIRS) study [50], 7507 patients were randomly assigned to methylprednisolone (n = 3755) and placebo (n = 3752).

The investigators reported that methylprednisolone did not have a significant effect on mortality or significant morbidity after cardiac surgery [50].

In neonatal cardiac surgery, intravenous 30 mg/kg methylprednisolone administered before CPB resulted in a decreased systemic inflammatory response. However, the investigators could not demonstrate any cardioprotective effects of this strategy or effects on clinical outcomes [51].

Serine Protease Inhibitors (Aprotinin)

Aprotinin is a nonspecific serine protease inhibitor that was discovered in 1930 by a research group at the University of Munich. The research group isolated an inhibitor of kallikrein from bovine lung and pancreas tissues. The drug also binds directly to the fibrinolytic plasmin. Aprotinin inhibits platelet glycoprotein loss (GpIb and GpIIb/IIIa receptors) associated with CPB.

Royston et al. [52] randomized 22 patients undergoing repeat open-heart surgery to receive the serine proteinase inhibitor aprotinin (700 mg intravenously from the start of anesthesia to the end of the operation). Blood transfusion requirements were eightfold higher in the control group than in the aprotinin group [52]. Aprotinin also confers significant protection against platelet dysfunction and activation of the systemic inflammatory response [53].

Nitric Oxide

Nitric oxide (NO) is a soluble, non-flammable, free-radical gas reacts rapidly with oxygen to form nitrogen oxides. Primary functions of NO are vasodilation and antagonist properties for platelet activation and leukocyte recruitment [54–56]. In a prospective, randomized, blinded, placebo-controlled study, children were undergoing repair of tetralogy of Fallot enrolled to either 20 ppm of gaseous nitric oxide or placebo delivered to the membrane oxygenator during CPB [56]. Nitric oxide group resulted in better myocardial protection, improved fluid balance, and an improved postoperative intensive care unit course [56].

Antioxidants

During CPB, endogenous oxygen free radical scavengers like Vitamin E (alpha-tocopherol) and Vitamin C (ascorbic acid) diminish, which results in increased production of oxygen free radicals from neutrophils, leading severe endothelial damage. Although several randomized studies performed with the exogenous replacement of Vit C and D, none of these studies resulted in significant advantages affecting immune response after CPB [57–59].

In SIRS, due to other causes such as sepsis, use of Selenium, Glutamine, and Eicos-pentanoic acid as antioxidants are shown to be effective in reducing bowel permeability and reducing endotoxemia [60, 61].

Complement Inhibitors

Attempts to efficiently to control complement system in systemic inflammation include the application of endogenous soluble complement inhibitors (C1-inhibitor, recombinant soluble complement receptor 1- rsCR1), the administration of antibodies, either blocking critical proteins of the cascade reaction (e.g., C3, C5), neutralizing the action of the complement-derived anaphylatoxin C5a, or interfering with complement receptor 3 (CR3, CD18/11b)-mediated adhesion of inflammatory cells to the vascular endothelium [62].

The complement inhibitor that has achieved the most widespread attention as a therapeutic agent is a monoclonal antibody to C5. The advantage of this strategy is that it prevents the generation of C5a, the most potent of the anaphylatoxins.

Pexelizumab, a C5 complement inhibitor, was evaluated in a randomized, double-blind, placebo-controlled trial, including 3099 adult patients undergoing CABG with or without valve surgery at 205 hospitals in North America and Western Europe from 2002 to 2003 [63]. However, compared with placebo, pexelizumab was not sufficient for improving clinical outcomes [63]. A recent study in the pediatric cardiac surgical population, C1 esterase inhibitor given intravenously 60 min after CPB, was effective in reducing the inflammatory activation [64].

Phosphodiesterase Inhibitors

Phosphodiesterases are a class of enzymes that catalyze the hydrolysis of cAMP and cGMP into AMP and GMP. Phosphodiesterase inhibitors like milrinone, vesnarinone, and amrinone, inhibit the action of cyclic adenosine monophosphate (cAMP) phosphodiesterase. Specific inhibition results in an increased level of cAMP and also calcium levels causing positive myocardial inotropy [65].

cAMP and cGMP have an essential role in endothelial cells to maintain capillary endothelial barrier properties in acute inflammation. In a severe lipopolysaccharide (LPS)-induced systemic inflammation model in rats, Phosphodiesterase-4-inhibitors (PD-4-Is) rolipram or roflumilast increased endothelial cAMP, which reduces capillary permeability and breakdown of microcirculatory flow [66].

The phosphodiesterase inhibitors also directly affect interleukin production and release; vesnarinone and amrinone reduce endotoxin-induced IL-1b, TNF-a, and iNO releases [67], milrinone, reduces IL-6 and IL-1b production [68].

Cyclooxygenase Inhibitors

Leukotrienes, prostaglandins, and thromboxane are the products of cyclooxygenase (COX) and lipooxygenase pathways of arachidonic acid. They play an essential role in systemic inflammatory response; they decrease systemic vascular resistance, augment platelet aggregation, start membrane lysis, and increase capillary permeability. Most of the main events taking place during SIRS. Drugs that restrain or inhibit these pathways have been studied to treat SIRS.

Ibuprofen has been tested in a randomized trial in 455 patients with sepsis, reducing prostaglandin I2 and thromboxane levels, but there was no decrease in mortality [69]. However, in another study, ibuprofen administration decreased mortality in patients with sepsis and hypothermia [70].

Pentoxyphyline, as a COX inhibitor, increases thromboxane, and tissue plasminogen activator prevents endothelial cell dysfunction and suppresses of TNF-α, IL-1, and IL-10. A study by Otani et al. shows that preoperative daily administration of 900 mg/day Pentoxyphyline attenuates SIRS due to cardiopulmonary bypass and has a beneficial effect on the postoperative course after cardiovascular surgery [71]. Pentoxyphyline improves scores of organ dysfunction in a randomized, double-blind, placebo-controlled study [72], and reduces all-cause mortality in neonatal studies [73, 74].

Technical Strategies

Evolving technical strategies include reducing surgical tissue trauma by minimally invasive approaches, avoiding CPB altogether such as off-pump CABG or minimally invasive cardiac operations, inhibition of neutrophil and platelet activation, inhibition of complement activation, and leucocyte depletion [4, 46].

Minimized Extracorporeal Circulation System

Minimized extracorporeal circulation (MECC) system has been introduced to reduce surface area and the priming volume, coatings to improve the biocompatibility of extracorporeal surfaces, and optimization of suction blood management [75]. Koster A. et al., showed that avoidance of aspiration of blood via the cardiotomy suction line significantly reduces hemostatic activation during on-pump CABG [76]. Fromes Y. et al.

randomly randomized sixty consecutive patients undergoing CABG assigned to either standard normothermic CPB (n = 30) or the MECC system (n = 30). The investigators demonstrated a milder inflammatory reaction when compared to standard CPB. In another small randomized trial, Bical O. et al. also demonstrated the lesser inflammatory response of a miniaturized CPB compared to a standard CPB in patients undergoing aortic valve replacement.

Heparin Bonded Circuits (HBC) and Biocompatibility

In vitro and in vivo experimental studies in the 1960s showed that a colloidal graphite surface was capable of bonding heparin [77]. Subsequently, improved heparin coatings have been developed for bonding to various biomedical devices, including bileaflet valves, circuits, and oxygenators [78]. In addition to the antithrombotic property of heparin, potential biocompatibility properties include inhibition of contact and complement activation and adsorb lipoproteins, which may create a surface that can potentially stimulate cell membranes, and reduce the pro-inflammatory aspects of CPB. A meta-analysis of 41-randomized trials demonstrated a reduction in the incidence of blood transfusion required, decreased re-sternotomy rates, ICU length of stay, and hospital stays [79]. However, investigators showed only marginal differences for other outcomes [79].

Heparin Management

Heparin management may have an impact on hemostatic activation and inflammatory response during CPB. Koster A. et al., [80] compared heparin concentration-based anticoagulation management with activated clotting time (ACT)-based heparin management and showed that heparin concentration-based anticoagulation management during CPB leads to a significant reduction of thrombin generation, fibrinolysis, and neutrophil activation [80].

Leucofiltration and Leukocyte Depletion

The clinical benefit of white cell filters designed to remove polymorphonuclear cells (PMNs) and soluble mediators in patients who developed SIRS after CPB is still debatable [34, 81]. Several investigators support the cardioplegic leucocyte depletion strategy as the optimal method for attenuating neutrophil activation and myocardial ischemia-reperfusion injury [34].

Hemofiltration, Ultrafiltration and Hemoadsorption

Non-physiologic conditions during CPB, such as hypothermia, hemodilution, non-pulsatile flow, anticoagulation, and circulation of blood out of the body in non-endothelialized surfaces, are the leading causes of systemic inflammatory response. Hemodilution increases SIRS, and SIRS increases total body water, which results in hemodilution. Thus, the use of hemofiltration, hemodialysis, or ultrafiltration for the removal of cytokines has essential roles in preventing or treating SIRS [82].

The use of ultrafiltration during pediatric open-heart surgery has beneficial effects in reducing complement activation and pro-inflammatory cytokine release, together with hemodynamic, pulmonary, and hemostatic improvements [83–85]. In adults, ultrafiltration also reduces cytokines and adhesion molecules during and after CPB; however, this has not been associated with any clinical advantage [86].

In a retrospective case series study (n = 16), treatment of patients with a cytokine adsorber device (CytoSorb; CytoSorbents) combined with continuous renal replacement therapy (CRRT) who present with severe post-CPB SIRS resulted in a reduction of elevated cytokine levels and improved organ function [87].

Centrifugal Pumps

A comparison of the two pumps used in cardiopulmonary bypass systems is still controversial [88]. Some studies mention that Centrifugal pumps are superior to roller pumps because of less blood trauma, reduced activation of the coagulation cascade, and improved biocompatibility [89, 90]. However, in other studies, both show similarities in terms of platelet damage [91], and immune response [92]. Additionally, recent studies showed increased inflammatory response during CPB with a centrifugal pump [93, 94].

Not only pump type, but pulsatility is also a significant concern during cardiopulmonary bypass, some studies show reduced amounts of endotoxins and other mediators [95, 96] with pulsatility whereas others [97] do not have such results.

Cardiopulmonary Bypass Temperature

Bigelow described hypothermia as the most critical part of myocardial protection [98]. Although hypothermia significantly decreases cardiac metabolism, significant disadvantages were also reported [99–101].

There are several studies in the literature comparing hypothermia with normothermia, the main issue here is some authors mention 33–34 C as normothermic, while for others 36–37 C is normothermic. Most of these studies do not report any differences between normothermia and hypothermia. Menasche et al. have concluded that hypothermia delays but do not entirely prevent the expression of inflammatory mediators. They have found an increase in adhesion molecules and leukocyte proteolytic enzymes in normothermia [102–104] In another study, it has shown that during normothermia Nitric Oxide (NO) production is increased resulting in diminished systemic vascular resistance which limits the inflammatory response [105].

Endotoxemia Reducing Strategies

Selective Decontamination of the Digestive Tract

Selective decontamination of the digestive tract (SDD) is a strategy to prevent the colonization of the gut. Numerous randomized controlled trials have shown that SDD reduces the incidence of pneumonia and mortality in ICU patients [106, 107]. Martinez-Pellus et al., randomized one hundred consecutive patients undergoing CPB, allocated to two groups; gut decontamination (n = 50) who received oral non-absorbable antibiotics (polymyxin E, tobramycin and amphotericin B) and controls (n = 50). The investigators showed that SDD reduced the gut content of enterobacteria associated with the lower endotoxin and cytokine levels detected in SDD patients. A meta-analysis by Nathens AB. et al., demonstrated that SDD reduced mortality in critically ill surgical patients in whom rates of nosocomial infection are high and in whom infection contributes notably to adverse outcomes [108].

Disclosures The authors have no financial disclosures that would be a potential conflict of interest with the current manuscript.

Key Pearls and Pitfalls

SIRS is likely to have several causes. CPB produces multiple noxious stimuli which aggravate systemic inflammatory response in a unique fashion. The pathogenesis of CPB-associated SIRS is linked to surgical trauma, contact between heparinized blood components with the artificial surface of the CPB circuit, nonendothelial cell surfaces in the mediastinum, blood-air interface, non-pulsatile blood-flow patterns, ischemia and reperfusion injury, and endotoxemia. CPB associated uncontrolled inflammatory response is often a complex process involving humoral, cellular, and metabolic pathways.

Furthermore, the inflammatory response is modified by patient-specific factors. Novel pharmacological agents and technical strategies are under intense investigation for anti-inflammatory protection to improve patient outcomes. Several critical issues should be considered together to produce efficient prophylactic strategies to minimize SIRS.

Comprehension Questions

1. Which of the listed is <u>not</u> one of the primary triggers of CPB-related SIRS?
   - (a) myocardium
   - (b) ischemia-reperfusion injury
   - (c) immunomodulation
   - (d) endotoxemia
   - (e) contact between heparinized blood components with the artificial surface of the CPB circuit

2. Which one is the time where the complement system is mostly activated during CPB?
   - (a) cross-clamping
   - (b) after protamine administration, and formation of the protamine-heparin complex
   - (c) weaning of CPB
   - (d) anesthesia induction
   - (e) hypothermic cardioplegic cardiac arrest

3. Which description is <u>incorrect</u>?
   - (a) Post-CPB SIRS is defined by the satisfaction of all of the four criteria.
   - (b) Aprotinin, as a serine protease inhibitor, may cause SIRS.
   - (c) Phosphodiesterase inhibitors deplete cAMP and cause SIRS.
   - (d) The depletion of platelets is the primary mechanism responsible for SIRS during CPB.
   - (e) Methylprednisolone lowers cytokines TNFα, IL-6, IL-8, and increases IL-10 and IL-1ra levels and helps to limit the inflammatory response.

4. Which one is <u>not</u> one of the technical strategies that are involved in the modulation of the inflammatory response during CPB?

(a) Hemodilution
(b) Minimized extracorporeal circulation system (MECC)
(c) Leukocyte filtration
(d) Heparin bonded circuits (HBC)
(e) Hemofiltration
Answers.

1 (c), 2 (b), 3 (b), 4 (a).

References

1. Taylor KM. SIRS–the systemic inflammatory response syndrome after cardiac operations. Ann Thorac Surg. 1996;61(6):1607–8.
2. Paparella D, Yau TM, Young E. Cardiopulmonary bypass induced inflammation: pathophysiology and treatment. An update Eur J Cardiothorac Surg. 2002;21(2):232–44.
3. Chakraborty RK, Burns B. Systemic inflammatory response syndrome. Treasure Island (FL): StatPearls; 2019.
4. Punjabi PP, Taylor KM. The science and practice of cardiopulmonary bypass: from cross circulation to ECMO and SIRS. Glob Cardiol Sci Pract. 2013;2013(3):249–60.
5. Cremer J, Martin M, Redl H, Bahrami S, Abraham C, Graeter T, et al. Systemic inflammatory response syndrome after cardiac operations. Ann Thorac Surg. 1996;61(6):1714–20.
6. Lee WH Jr, Krumhaar D, Fonkalsrud EW, Schjeide OA, Maloney JV Jr. Denaturation of plasma proteins as a cause of morbidity and death after intracardiac operations. Surgery. 1961;50:29–39.
7. Chenoweth DE, Cooper SW, Hugli TE, Stewart RW, Blackstone EH, Kirklin JW. Complement activation during cardiopulmonary bypass: evidence for generation of C3a and C5a anaphylatoxins. N Engl J Med. 1981;304(9):497–503.
8. Wachtfogel YT, Kucich U, Greenplate J, Gluszko P, Abrams W, Weinbaum G, et al. Human neutrophil degranulation during extracorporeal circulation. Blood. 1987;69(1):324–30.
9. Edmunds LH Jr. Inflammatory response to cardiopulmonary bypass. Ann Thorac Surg. 1998;66(5 Suppl):S12–6. discussion S25-8
10. Levy JH, Tanaka KA. Inflammatory response to cardiopulmonary bypass. Ann Thorac Surg. 2003;75(2):S715–20.
11. Laffey JG, Boylan JF, Cheng DC. The systemic inflammatory response to cardiac surgery: implications for the anesthesiologist. Anesthesiology. 2002;97(1):215–52.
12. Day JR, Taylor KM. The systemic inflammatory response syndrome and cardiopulmonary bypass. Int J Surg. 2005;3(2):129–40.
13. Boehne M, Sasse M, Karch A, Dziuba F, Horke A, Kaussen T, et al. Systemic inflammatory response syndrome after pediatric congenital heart surgery: incidence, risk factors, and clinical outcome. J Card Surg. 2017;32(2):116–25.
14. Fransen E, Maessen J, Dentener M, Senden N, Geskes G, Buurman W. Systemic inflammation present in patients undergoing CABG without extracorporeal circulation. Chest. 1998;113(5):1290–5.
15. Zhang WR, Garg AX, Coca SG, Devereaux PJ, Eikelboom J, Kavsak P, et al. Plasma IL-6 and IL-10 concentrations predict AKI and long-term mortality in adults after cardiac surgery. J Am Soc Nephrol. 2015;26(12):3123–32.
16. Taylor KM. Brain damage during cardiopulmonary bypass. Ann Thorac Surg. 1998;65(4 Suppl):S20–6. discussion S7-8
17. Landis RC. 20 years on: is it time to redefine the systemic inflammatory response to cardiothoracic surgery? J Extra Corpor Technol. 2015;47(1):5–9.
18. MacCallum NS, Finney SJ, Gordon SE, Quinlan GJ, Evans TW. Modified criteria for the systemic inflammatory response syndrome improves their utility following cardiac surgery. Chest. 2014;145(6):1197–203.
19. Squiccimarro E, Labriola C, Malvindi PG, Margari V, Guida P, Visicchio G, et al. Prevalence and clinical impact of systemic inflammatory reaction after cardiac surgery. J Cardiothorac Vasc Anesth. 2019;33(6):1682–90.
20. Dieleman JM, Peelen LM, Coulson TG, Tran L, Reid CM, Smith JA, et al. Age and other perioperative risk factors for postoperative systemic inflammatory response syndrome after cardiac surgery. Br J Anaesth. 2017;119(4):637–44.
21. Guvener M, Korun O, Demirturk OS. Risk factors for systemic inflammatory response after congenital cardiac surgery. J Card Surg. 2015;30(1):92–6.
22. Asimakopoulos G, Taylor KM. Effects of cardiopulmonary bypass on leukocyte and endothelial adhesion molecules. Ann Thorac Surg. 1998;66(6):2135–44.
23. Hammon JW Jr, Vinten-Johansen J. Myocardial protection from surgical ischemic-reperfusion injury. Introduction Ann Thorac Surg. 1999;68(5):1897.
24. Michalski M, Pagowska-Klimek I, Thiel S, Swierzko AS, Hansen AG, Jensenius JC, et al. Factors involved in initiation and regulation of complement lectin pathway influence postoperative outcome after pediatric cardiac surgery involving cardiopulmonary bypass. Sci Rep. 2019;9(1):2930.
25. Kirklin JK, Westaby S, Blackstone EH, Kirklin JW, Chenoweth DE, Pacifico AD. Complement and the damaging effects of cardiopulmonary bypass. J Thorac Cardiovasc Surg. 1983;86(6):845–57.

26. Struber M, Cremer JT, Gohrbandt B, Hagl C, Jankowski M, Volker B, et al. Human cytokine responses to coronary artery bypass grafting with and without cardiopulmonary bypass. Ann Thorac Surg. 1999;68(4):1330–5.

27. Hsing CH, Hsieh MY, Chen WY, Cheung So E, Cheng BC, Chang MS. Induction of interleukin-19 and interleukin-22 after cardiac surgery with cardiopulmonary bypass. Ann Thorac Surg. 2006;81(6):2196–201.

28. Wan S, DeSmet JM, Barvais L, Goldstein M, Vincent JL, LeClerc JL. Myocardium is a major source of proinflammatory cytokines in patients undergoing cardiopulmonary bypass. J Thorac Cardiovasc Surg. 1996;112(3):806–11.

29. Kotani N, Hashimoto H, Sessler DI, Muraoka M, Wang JS, O'Connor MF, et al. Cardiopulmonary bypass produces greater pulmonary than systemic proinflammatory cytokines. Anesth Analg. 2000;90(5):1039–45.

30. Aird WC. Endothelium as an organ system. Crit Care Med. 2004;32(5 Suppl):S271–9.

31. Wolinsky H. A proposal linking clearance of circulating lipoproteins to tissue metabolic activity as a basis for understanding atherogenesis. Circ Res. 1980;47(3):301–11.

32. Aird WC. Endothelium and haemostasis. Hamostaseologie. 2015;35(1):11–6.

33. Lee WL, Slutsky AS. Sepsis and endothelial permeability. N Engl J Med. 2010;363(7):689–91.

34. Samankatiwat P, Samartzis I, Lertsithichai P, Stefanou D, Punjabi PP, Taylor KM, et al. Leucocyte depletion in cardiopulmonary bypass: a comparison of four strategies. Perfusion. 2003;18(2):95–105.

35. Friedenberg WR, Myers WO, Plotka ED, Beathard JN, Kummer DJ, Gatlin PF, et al. Platelet dysfunction associated with cardiopulmonary bypass. Ann Thorac Surg. 1978;25(4):298–305.

36. Ho LTS, Lenihan M, McVey MJ, Karkouti K. Transfusion avoidance in cardiac surgery study i. the association between platelet dysfunction and adverse outcomes in cardiac surgical patients. Anaesthesia. 2019;74(9):1130–7.

37. Czer LS, Bateman TM, Gray RJ, Raymond M, Stewart ME, Lee S, et al. Treatment of severe platelet dysfunction and hemorrhage after cardiopulmonary bypass: reduction in blood product usage with desmopressin. J Am Coll Cardiol. 1987;9(5):1139–47.

38. Weerasinghe A, Taylor KM. The platelet in cardiopulmonary bypass. Ann Thorac Surg. 1998;66(6):2145–52.

39. Zilla P, Fasol R, Groscurth P, Klepetko W, Reichenspurner H, Wolner E. Blood platelets in cardiopulmonary bypass operations. Recovery occurs after initial stimulation, rather than continual activation. J Thorac Cardiovasc Surg. 1989;97(3):379–88.

40. Lopez-Vilchez I, Diaz-Ricart M, White JG, Escolar G, Galan AM. Serotonin enhances platelet procoagulant properties and their activation induced during platelet tissue factor uptake. Cardiovasc Res. 2009;84(2):309–16.

41. Wallach R, Karp RB, Reves JG, Oparil S, Smith LR, James TN. Pathogenesis of paroxysmal hypertension developing during and after coronary bypass surgery: a study of hemodynamic and humoral factors. Am J Cardiol. 1980;46(4):559–65.

42. Taylor KM, Wright GS, Reid JM, Bain WH, Caves PK, Walker MS, et al. Comparative studies of pulsatile and nonpulsatile flow during cardiopulmonary bypass. II. The effects on adrenal secretion of cortisol. J Thorac Cardiovasc Surg. 1978;75(4):574–8.

43. Uozumi T, Manabe H, Kawashima Y, Hamanaka Y, Monden Y. Plasma cortisol, corticosterone and nonprotein-bound cortisol in extra-corporeal circulation. Acta Endocrinol. 1972;69(3):517–25.

44. Gaudino M, Di Castelnuovo A, Zamparelli R, Andreotti F, Burzotta F, Iacoviello L, et al. Genetic control of postoperative systemic inflammatory reaction and pulmonary and renal complications after coronary artery surgery. J Thorac Cardiovasc Surg. 2003;126(4):1107–12.

45. Grunenfelder J, Umbehr M, Plass A, Bestmann L, Maly FE, Zund G, et al. Genetic polymorphisms of apolipoprotein E4 and tumor necrosis factor beta as predisposing factors for increased inflammatory cytokines after cardiopulmonary bypass. J Thorac Cardiovasc Surg. 2004;128(1):92–7.

46. Raja SG, Dreyfus GD. Modulation of systemic inflammatory response after cardiac surgery. Asian Cardiovasc Thorac Ann. 2005;13(4):382–95.

47. Lodge AJ, Chai PJ, Daggett CW, Ungerleider RM, Jaggers J. Methylprednisolone reduces the inflammatory response to cardiopulmonary bypass in neonatal piglets: timing of dose is important. J Thorac Cardiovasc Surg. 1999;117(3):515–22.

48. Malagon I, Onkenhout W, Klok M, Linthorst L, van der Poel PF, Bovill JG, et al. Dexamethasone reduces gut permeability in pediatric cardiac surgery. J Thorac Cardiovasc Surg. 2005;130(2):265–71.

49. Dieleman JM, Nierich AP, Rosseel PM, van der Maaten JM, Hofland J, Diephuis JC, et al. Intraoperative high-dose dexamethasone for cardiac surgery: a randomized controlled trial. JAMA. 2012;308(17):1761–7.

50. Whitlock RP, Devereaux PJ, Teoh KH, Lamy A, Vincent J, Pogue J, et al. Methylprednisolone in patients undergoing cardiopulmonary bypass (SIRS): a randomised, double-blind, placebo-controlled trial. Lancet. 2015;386(10000):1243–53.

51. Keski-Nisula J, Pesonen E, Olkkola KT, Peltola K, Neuvonen PJ, Tuominen N, et al. Methylprednisolone in neonatal cardiac surgery: reduced inflammation without improved clinical outcome. Ann Thorac Surg. 2013;95(6):2126–32.

52. Royston D, Bidstrup BP, Taylor KM, Sapsford RN. Effect of aprotinin on need for blood transfusion after repeat open-heart surgery. Lancet. 1987;2(8571):1289–91.

53. Day JR, Landis RC, Taylor KM. Aprotinin and the protease-activated receptor 1 thrombin receptor: antithrombosis, inflammation, and stroke reduction. Semin Cardiothorac Vasc Anesth. 2006;10(2):132–42.

54. Lowson SM, Hassan HM, Rich GF. The effect of nitric oxide on platelets when delivered to the cardiopulmonary bypass circuit. Anesth Analg. 1999;89(6):1360–5.

55. Mellgren K, Mellgren G, Lundin S, Wennmalm A, Wadenvik H. Effect of nitric oxide gas on platelets during open heart operations. Ann Thorac Surg. 1998;65(5):1335–41.

56. Checchia PA, Bronicki RA, Muenzer JT, Dixon D, Raithel S, Gandhi SK, et al. Nitric oxide delivery during cardiopulmonary bypass reduces postoperative morbidity in children–a randomized trial. J Thorac Cardiovasc Surg. 2013;146(3):530–6.

57. Westhuyzen J, Cochrane AD, Tesar PJ, Mau T, Cross DB, Frenneaux MP, et al. Effect of preoperative supplementation with alpha-tocopherol and ascorbic acid on myocardial injury in patients undergoing cardiac operations. J Thorac Cardiovasc Surg. 1997;113(5):942–8.

58. Yau TM, Weisel RD, Mickle DA, Burton GW, Ingold KU, Ivanov J, et al. Vitamin E for coronary bypass operations. A prospective, double-blind, randomized trial. J Thorac Cardiovasc Surg. 1994;108(2):302–10.

59. Butterworth J, Legault C, Stump DA, Coker L, Hammon JW Jr, Troost BT, et al. A randomized, blinded trial of the antioxidant pegorgotein: no reduction in neuropsychological deficits, inotropic drug support, or myocardial ischemia after coronary artery bypass surgery. J Cardiothorac Vasc Anesth. 1999;13(6):690–4.

60. Angstwurm MW, Schottdorf J, Schopohl J, Gaertner R. Selenium replacement in patients with severe systemic inflammatory response syndrome improves clinical outcome. Crit Care Med. 1999;27(9):1807–13.

61. Quan ZF, Yang C, Li N, Li JS. Effect of glutamine on change in early postoperative intestinal permeability and its relation to systemic inflammatory response. World J Gastroenterol. 2004;10(13):1992–4.

62. Kirschfink M. Controlling the complement system in inflammation. Immunopharmacology. 1997;38(1–2):51–62.

63. Verrier ED, Shernan SK, Taylor KM, Van de Werf F, Newman MF, Chen JC, et al. Terminal complement blockade with pexelizumab during coronary artery bypass graft surgery requiring cardiopulmonary bypass: a randomized trial. JAMA. 2004;291(19):2319–27.

64. Miyamoto T, Ozaki S, Inui A, Tanaka Y, Yamada Y, Matsumoto N. C1 esterase inhibitor in pediatric cardiac surgery with cardiopulmonary bypass plays a vital role in activation of the complement system. Heart Vessel. 2019;

65. Rathmell JP, Prielipp RC, Butterworth JF, Williams E, Villamaria F, Testa L, et al. A multicenter, randomized, blind comparison of amrinone with milrinone after elective cardiac surgery. Anesth Analg. 1998;86(4):683–90.

66. Schick MA, Wunder C, Wollborn J, Roewer N, Waschke J, Germer CT, et al. Phosphodiesterase-4 inhibition as a therapeutic approach to treat capillary leakage in systemic inflammation. J Physiol. 2012;590(11):2693–708.

67. Takeuchi K, del Nido PJ, Ibrahim AE, Cao-Danh H, Friehs I, Glynn P, et al. Vesnarinone and amrinone reduce the systemic inflammatory response syndrome. J Thorac Cardiovasc Surg. 1999;117(2):375–82.

68. Hayashida N, Tomoeda H, Oda T, Tayama E, Chihara S, Kawara T, et al. Inhibitory effect of milrinone on cytokine production after cardiopulmonary bypass. Ann Thorac Surg. 1999;68(5):1661–7.

69. Bernard GR, Wheeler AP, Russell JA, Schein R, Summer WR, Steinberg KP, et al. The effects of ibuprofen on the physiology and survival of patients with sepsis. The ibuprofen in sepsis study group. N Engl J Med. 1997;336(13):912–8.

70. Arons MM, Wheeler AP, Bernard GR, Christman BW, Russell JA, Schein R, et al. Effects of ibuprofen on the physiology and survival of hypothermic sepsis. Ibuprofen in sepsis study group. Crit Care Med. 1999;27(4):699–707.

71. Otani S, Kuinose M, Murakami T, Saito S, Iwagaki H, Tanaka N, et al. Preoperative oral administration of pentoxifylline ameliorates respiratory index after cardiopulmonary bypass through decreased production of IL-6. Acta Med Okayama. 2008;62(2):69–74.

72. Staubach KH, Schroder J, Stuber F, Gehrke K, Traumann E, Zabel P. Effect of pentoxifylline in severe sepsis: results of a randomized, double-blind, placebo-controlled study. Arch Surg. 1998;133(1):94–100.

73. Lauterbach R, Pawlik D, Kowalczyk D, Ksycinski W, Helwich E, Zembala M. Effect of the immuno-modulating agent, pentoxifylline, in the treatment of sepsis in prematurely delivered infants: a placebo-controlled, double-blind trial. Crit Care Med. 1999;27(4):807–14.

74. Lauterbach R, Zembala M. Pentoxifylline reduces plasma tumour necrosis factor-alpha concentration in premature infants with sepsis. Eur J Pediatr. 1996;155(5):404–9.

75. Starck CT, Bettex D, Felix C, Reser D, Dreizler T, Hasenclever P, et al. Initial results of an optimized perfusion system. Perfusion. 2013;28(4):292–7.

76. Koster A, Bottcher W, Merkel F, Hetzer R, Kuppe H. The more closed the bypass system the better: a pilot study on the effects of reduction of cardiotomy suction and passive venting on hemostatic activation during on-pump coronary artery bypass grafting. Perfusion. 2005;20(5):285–8.

77. Gott VL, Whiffen JD, Dutton RC. Heparin bonding on colloidal graphite surfaces. Science. 1963;142(3597):1297–8.
78. Gott VL, Daggett RL. Serendipity and the development of heparin and carbon surfaces. Ann Thorac Surg. 1999;68(3 Suppl):S19–22.
79. Mangoush O, Purkayastha S, Haj-Yahia S, Kinross J, Hayward M, Bartolozzi F, et al. Heparin-bonded circuits versus nonheparin-bonded circuits: an evaluation of their effect on clinical outcomes. Eur J Cardiothorac Surg. 2007;31(6):1058–69.
80. Koster A, Fischer T, Praus M, Haberzettl H, Kuebler WM, Hetzer R, et al. Hemostatic activation and inflammatory response during cardiopulmonary bypass: impact of heparin management. Anesthesiology. 2002;97(4):837–41.
81. Treacher DF, Sabbato M, Brown KA, Gant V. The effects of leucodepletion in patients who develop the systemic inflammatory response syndrome following cardiopulmonary bypass. Perfusion. 2001;16(Suppl):67–73.
82. Jaffer U, Wade RG, Gourlay T. Cytokines in the systemic inflammatory response syndrome: a review. HSR Proc Intensive Care Cardiovasc Anesth. 2010;2(3):161–75.
83. Naik SK, Knight A, Elliott M. A prospective randomized study of a modified technique of ultrafiltration during pediatric open-heart surgery. Circulation. 1991;84(5 Suppl):III422–31.
84. Journois D, Pouard P, Greeley WJ, Mauriat P, Vouhe P, Safran D. Hemofiltration during cardiopulmonary bypass in pediatric cardiac surgery. Effects on hemostasis, cytokines, and complement components. Anesthesiology. 1994;81(5):1181–9. discussion 26A-27A
85. Wang S, Palanzo D, Undar A. Current ultrafiltration techniques before, during and after pediatric cardiopulmonary bypass procedures. Perfusion. 2012;27(5):438–46.
86. Grunenfelder J, Zund G, Schoeberlein A, Maly FE, Schurr U, Guntli S, et al. Modified ultrafiltration lowers adhesion molecule and cytokine levels after cardiopulmonary bypass without clinical relevance in adults. Eur J Cardiothorac Surg. 2000;17(1):77–83.
87. Trager K, Fritzler D, Fischer G, Schroder J, Skrabal C, Liebold A, et al. Treatment of post-cardiopulmonary bypass SIRS by hemoadsorption: a case series. Int J Artif Organs. 2016;39(3):141–6.
88. Parolari A, Alamanni F, Naliato M, Spirito R, Franze V, Pompilio G, et al. Adult cardiac surgery outcomes: role of the pump type. Eur J Cardiothorac Surg. 2000;18(5):575–82.
89. Steinbrueckner BE, Steigerwald U, Keller F, Neukam K, Elert O, Babin-Ebell J. Centrifugal and roller pumps–are there differences in coagulation and fibrinolysis during and after cardiopulmonary bypass? Heart Vessel. 1995;10(1):46–53.
90. Moen O, Fosse E, Dregelid E, Brockmeier V, Andersson C, Hogasen K, et al. Centrifugal pump and heparin coating improves cardiopulmonary bypass biocompatibility. Ann Thorac Surg. 1996;62(4):1134–40.
91. Misoph M, Babin-Ebell J, Schwender S. A comparative evaluation of the effect of pump type and heparin-coated surfaces on platelets during cardiopulmonary bypass. Thorac Cardiovasc Surg. 1997;45(6):302–6.
92. Perttila J, Salo M, Peltola O. Comparison of the effects of centrifugal versus roller pump on the immune response in open-heart surgery. Perfusion. 1995;10(4):249–56.
93. Ashraf S, Butler J, Tian Y, Cowan D, Lintin S, Saunders NR, et al. Inflammatory mediators in adults undergoing cardiopulmonary bypass: comparison of centrifugal and roller pumps. Ann Thorac Surg. 1998;65(2):480–4.
94. Baufreton C, Intrator L, Jansen PG, te Velthuis H, Le Besnerais P, Vonk A, et al. Inflammatory response to cardiopulmonary bypass using roller or centrifugal pumps. Ann Thorac Surg. 1999;67(4):972–7.
95. Orime Y, Shiono M, Hata H, Yagi S, Tsukamoto S, Okumura H, et al. Cytokine and endothelial damage in pulsatile and nonpulsatile cardiopulmonary bypass. Artif Organs. 1999;23(6):508–12.
96. Watarida S, Mori A, Onoe M, Tabata R, Shiraishi S, Sugita T, et al. A clinical study on the effects of pulsatile cardiopulmonary bypass on the blood endotoxin levels. J Thorac Cardiovasc Surg. 1994;108(4):620–5.
97. Taggart DP, Sundaram S, McCartney C, Bowman A, McIntyre H, Courtney JM, et al. Endotoxemia, complement, and white blood cell activation in cardiac surgery: a randomized trial of laxatives and pulsatile perfusion. Ann Thorac Surg. 1994;57(2):376–82.
98. Bigelow WG, Lindsay WK, Greenwood WF. Hypothermia; its possible role in cardiac surgery: an investigation of factors governing survival in dogs at low body temperatures. Ann Surg. 1950;132(5):849–66.
99. Martin DR, Scott DF, Downes GL, Belzer FO. Primary cause of unsuccessful liver and heart preservation: cold sensitivity of the ATPase system. Ann Surg. 1972;175(1):111–7.
100. McMurchie EJ, Raison JK, Cairncross KD. Temperature-induced phase changes in membranes of heart: a contrast between the thermal response of poikilotherms and homeotherms. Comp Biochem Physiol B. 1973;44(4):1017–26.
101. Russ C, Lee JC. Effect of hypothermia on myocardial metabolism. Am J Phys. 1965;208:1253–8.
102. Menasche P, Peynet J, Lariviere J, Tronc F, Piwnica A, Bloch G, et al. Does normothermia during cardiopulmonary bypass increase neutrophil-endothelium interactions? Circulation. 1994;90(5 Pt 2):II275–9.
103. Menasche P, Peynet J, Haeffner-Cavaillon N, Carreno MP, de Chaumaray T, Dillisse V, et al. Influence of temperature on neutrophil trafficking during clinical cardiopulmonary bypass. Circulation. 1995;92(9 Suppl):II334–40.

104. Le Deist F, Menasche P, Kucharski C, Bel A, Piwnica A, Bloch G. Hypothermia during cardiopulmonary bypass delays but does not prevent neutrophil-endothelial cell adhesion. A clinical study. Circulation. 1995;92(9 Suppl):II354–8.

105. Ohata T, Sawa Y, Kadoba K, Kagisaki K, Suzuki K, Matsuda H. Role of nitric oxide in a temperature dependent regulation of systemic vascular resistance in cardiopulmonary bypass. Eur J Cardiothorac Surg. 2000;18(3):342–7.

106. Ulrich C, Harinck-de Weerd JE, Bakker NC, Jacz K, Doornbos L, de Ridder VA. Selective decontamination of the digestive tract with norfloxacin in the prevention of ICU-acquired infections: a prospective randomized study. Intensive Care Med. 1989;15(7):424–31.

107. Rocha LA, Martin MJ, Pita S, Paz J, Seco C, Margusino L, et al. Prevention of nosocomial infection in critically ill patients by selective decontamination of the digestive tract. A randomized, double blind, placebo-controlled study. Intensive Care Med. 1992;18(7):398–404.

108. Nathens AB, Marshall JC. Selective decontamination of the digestive tract in surgical patients: a systematic review of the evidence. Arch Surg. 1999;134(2):170–6.

Basic Setup in Adult Cardiac Surgery

4

Panagiotis G. Kyriazis, Guiqing Liu, Nikhil Sahdev, and Prakash P. Punjabi

Abbreviations

CPB: Cardiopulmonary Bypass
SVC: Superior Venous Cava
IVC: Inferior Venous Cava
RA: Right Atrium
CABG: Coronary Artery Bypass Grafting
MV: Mitral Valve

Learning Objectives

- Understand the principles of set up in adult cardiac surgery
- Understand the set up for different cardiac surgical procedures
- Understand the differences between the arterial and the venous cannulation
- Understand the steps of decannulation
- Understand the steps of chest closure technique

P. G. Kyriazis · N. Sahdev
Department of Cardiothoracic Surgery, Hammersmith Hospital, Imperial College Healthcare NHS Trust, London, UK
e-mail: panagiotis.kyriazis@nhs.net; nikhil.sahdev@nhs.net

G. Liu · P. P. Punjabi (✉)
Department of Cardiothoracic Surgery, Hammersmith Hospital, Imperial College Healthcare NHS Trust, London, UK

National Heart and Lung Institute, Faculty of Medicine, Imperial College London, London, UK
e-mail: guiqing.liu@nhs.net; p.punjabi@imperial.ac.uk

Introduction

Standardized routine access for cardiac operation is essential, makes every operation more efficient and, in the case of emergency, allows surgeons to proceed with speed and accuracy. Most cardiac surgery is carried out through a median sternotomy, which is usually a straightforward procedure, but certain principles are important to ensure safe entry to the heart. Nowadays, more and more patients require second, third or fourth re-sternotomy. Most cardiac operations are performed on Cardiopulmonary bypass, during which, safe and effective methods of cannulation of the various vessels and venting the heart are important. An effective, secure technique of closing the chest is necessary to avoid the risk of subsequent sternal wound dehiscence or infection.

Incisions

Median Sternotomy

A midsternal incision (Median Sternotomy) is made for almost all cardiac operations. The midline incision begins below the sternal notch over the sternal manubrium and extends to the xiphoid process. It is essential to open the sternum via strict midline. Locating the intercostal spaces on either side of the sternum and the edges of the muscle fibres along the sternum helps to identify the midline of the sternum. The midline of the sternum can be marked on the periosteum of the sternum using diathermy prior to sternotomy. A superficial mark on the fibrous layer is sufficient, and it is not necessary to make deep mark on the sternum as this may cause sternum de-vascularisation [1].

The xiphisternum is cut with scissors, and the pericardium is freed from under the sternum with the right index finger. This manoeuvre is important to ensure the pericardium is below the plane of the sternotomy. The sternum saw is tested for proper operation before placing it again the bottom end of the sternum. The saw should be held firmly and slightly pushed forwards while dividing the sternum. The tip of the saw is kept elevated so that the toe of the saw hugs the back of the sternum. It is usually advisable to move the saw backwards and forwards once or twice during opening the sternum to release mediasternal tissue that may be caught up on the saw to cause resistance.

Alternatively, the sternum can be divided from the top to bottom.

The medium size swap was packed between the two sternal edges, and the haemostasis of periosteum is achieved using diathermy and a thin layer of bone wax is applied on the sternal marrow.

Redo Sternotomy

Prior to Redo Sternotomy surgery, the surgeon must estimate the chances that catastrophic haemorrhage will develop from repeat sternotomy. This affects the decision regarding whether to cannulate peripheral vessels and establish Cardiopulmonary Bypass (CPB) before sternotomy. It is essential to study the chest images (Chest X-Ray, CT or MRI) to identify the positions of sternal wires, the retro-sternal structures (Great Vessels, right ventricle, coronary artery bypass grafts…) and the relationship between those structures and sternum [2].

Six unit packed red cells should be available for immediate use. De-Fibrillation pads should be placed in the Anaesthetic room, bilateral femoral arteries should be marked for potential emergency femoral cannulation in case of uncontrolled bleeding.

In redo Sternotomy, the sternal skin incision and dissection of the sternum are carried out in the standard surgical manner. The previous sternal wires are untwisted and removed. We do not routinely recommend leaving wires in place to protect the retro-sternal structures during sternotomy as this not only limits the ability to control an injury upon sternal re-entry but also can result in multiple wire fragments that can injury underlying mediastinal structures.

Three thick strong sutures are placed through the costal cartilage on either side of the sternum about 2–3 cm from the midline. The assistant lifts these up during the redo sternotomy to separate the sternum from the underlying tissues. The dissection is started at the bottom under direct vision by lifting up the xiphisternum. Almost the lower third of the sternum can be freed of adhesions. The anaesthetist is then asked to hyperinflate the lungs to a maximum pressure of 30 cm H_2O. The Manoeuvre widens the potential retrosternal space between the sternum and the heart to minimise the injury. Furthermore, hyperinflation, by generating positive pressure inspiration, decreases caval flow and right ventricular dimensions. The sternum is divided with the oscillating saw. As the sternum is split, the sternal edges are separated and kept apart with the help of a flat instrument (e.g. flat end of sternal saw key) and underlying tissue is cut with curved Mayo scissors. The lungs are kept hyperinflated without deflation during sternotomy, although this may be repeated with intermittent normal ventilation to prevent hypoxia until complete sternal division. Once fully divided, standard ventilation is recommenced. A backhand or cat's paw retractor is then used to lift the posterior table of the sternum for further dissection on both sides. This is continued until the sternum is completely separate and can be safely retracted.

Dividing the Pericardium

Following sternotomy, the fat over the lower part of the pericardium can simply be pushed apart with a swab along its natural plane. This minimises cutting through fat with diathermy and bleeding. The pericardium is opened in the midline up to the pericardial reflection, superiorly. The pericardium over the aorta at the pericardial reflection should be left so as not to weaken the aorta.

In case of redo operation, careful mediastinal dissection is fundamental to success during cardiac reoperations. The primary goal of mediastinal dissection is to discuss available cardiopulmonary bypass and appropriate aortic cross-clamp sites. The 'golden rule' of reoperative cardiac dissection is that only areas necessary for the planned procedure should be dissected. For patients undergoing reoperations for isolated valve repair or replacements, it is not necessary to dissect out the left side of the heast, and it is acceptable to leave adherent pericardium to the right atrium to avoid injury if extensive adhesions are encountered. For difficult, high-risk reoperations, initiation of early CPB can also aid mediastinal dissection by decompression the heart.

If the sternum is osteoporotic or fractured as a result of an off-centre sternotomy, it can be supported by cutting either a 32 Fr chest drain or a venous drainage line in half longitudinally and placing this on the sternum on top of which the retractor blade is placed. This may limit further damage to the sternum.

Towels are placed on the sternal edge. The pericardium is lifted up using Roberts and the sternal retractor is placed on the pericardium to support it. The anaesthetist should be cautioned during this manoeuvre as the blood pressure may drop transiently due to kinking of the SVC and IVC. Should the patient be unstable, then pericardial stay sutures can be taken without lifting the heart. In general, patients with poor left ventricular function usually do not drop their blood pressure significantly on lifting the pericardium as the heart is usually well filled in these patients. Patients with good left ventricular function usually drop their blood pressure during this manoeuvre but it usually recovers quickly.

It may sometimes be desirable to place a Nylon Tape around the aorta. The aorta has to be mobilised for this and this ensures that when the cross-clamp is applied, it is placed across the full diameter of the aorta. The pulmonary artery is separated from the aorta, usually at the site where the curvature of the aorta is most anterior, by a combination of sharp and blunt dissection. Dissection should be parallel to the aorta and pulmonary artery to avoid damage to either of the great vessels. The pulmonary artery can sometimes be very thin-walled and care must be taken to avoid damage to it. The dissection in such cases should be more towards the aorta. Once a sufficient plane has been developed, the thumb and index finger is placed around the aorta in the transverse sinus to ensure that the back wall of the aorta is also free of tissue. A Semb clamp is then advanced around the back of the aorta while in contact with the index finger. It is withdrawn back after grabbing an nylon tape.

If the pulmonary artery is injured, it may be preferable to go on cardiopulmonary bypass to repair it. This allows blood conservation and visualisation as the right atrium and pulmonary artery will empty of blood.

Cannulation

Aortic Cannulation

The site for Aortic cannulation should be within the pericardial reflection whenever possible, as the aorta where the pericardium is fused onto the anterior surface is tougher and better for cannulation than the part outside the reflection. The cannulation site is proximal to the origin of the innominate artery. The cannulation site should be

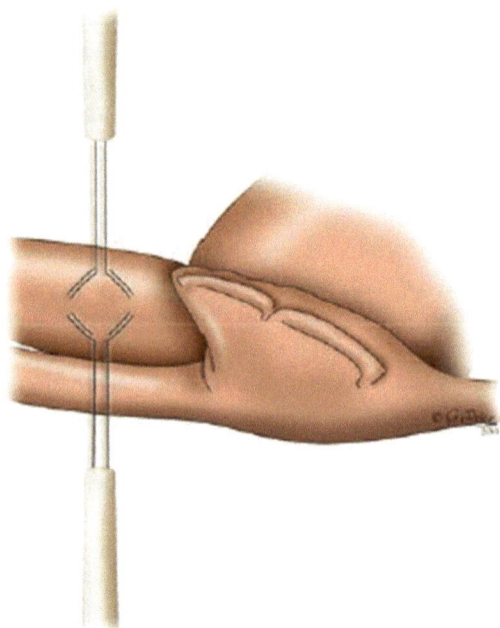

Fig. 4.1 Two purse string (diamond-shaped) used at opposite ends

The aortic incision should be just slightly smaller than the diameter of the aortic cannula to allow it to pass easily into the aortic lumen and without any leaks after cannulation. It is important to ensure that the systolic blood pressure is less than 100 mmHg when cannulating the aorta to avoid aortic dissection.

The snares on the pruse-string suture is secured, and the cannula is tied to it. The aortic cannula is then connected to the arterial tubing from the CPB circuit and carefully de-aired.

Aortic atherosclerosis is a risk factor for perioperative aortic dissection and post-operative stroke and renal dysfunction, therefore careful assessment of ascending aorta is essential. Potential Aortic cannulation complications include Intramural placement of cannula, persistent bleeding around the cannula, malposition of the tip to retrograde position or even across aortic valve, malposition against vessel wall or into aortic arch vessels, aortic dissection or haematoma and high CPB line pressure.

a little to the left side of the anterior aortic surface as an added precaution against the cannula tip entering the innominate artery. Initially palpitate the aorta to identify any areas that many contain atheromatous plaques which should be avoided. A diamond-shaped purse string is placed on the aorta just below the pericardial reflection (Fig. 4.1). Two purse strings are used, starting at opposite ends to each other. The inner purse string is usually placed starting at the assistant's side. The purse string should run through the aortic media. Should the stitch go right through into the aortic lumen, it should be removed and a new bite taken. A haematoma will inevitably form if this happens. The adventitia should be cut to relieve it.

After Heparin is given, the adventitia within the purse string is incised. A digitally controlled stab wound of sufficient length and width is made within the purse string using size 11 blade, then the stab wound is covered by operator' left index finger. The aortic cannula can then be slipped into the aorta easily and usually bloodlessly. If an angled cannula is used, it is positioned so that the opening faces distally into the aortic arch.

Venous Cannulation

Purse-string sutures for venous cannulation can be placed before or after heparinisation and aortic cannulation. Number and sites of these purse strings depend on the perfusion technique to be used. When a single venous cannula is used, only a right atrial appendage purse-string suture is needed (Fig. 4.2a). When two venous cannulae are used, the SVC, and IVC may be cannulated directly (Fig. 4.2b).

When single cannula is required, the two-stage cannula is normally used. "D"-shaped purse string is placed in the right atrium following the curve of the needle. Small bites should be taken around the right atrium. The right atrium is held medially with a Duval by an assistant and laterally by the surgeon with a pair of forceps. A 2-cm vertical incision is made in the right atrium with an 11 blade. This incision is then dilated with scissor or a Roberts until it is about the size of the venous cannula. The right atrium is then cannulated [3].

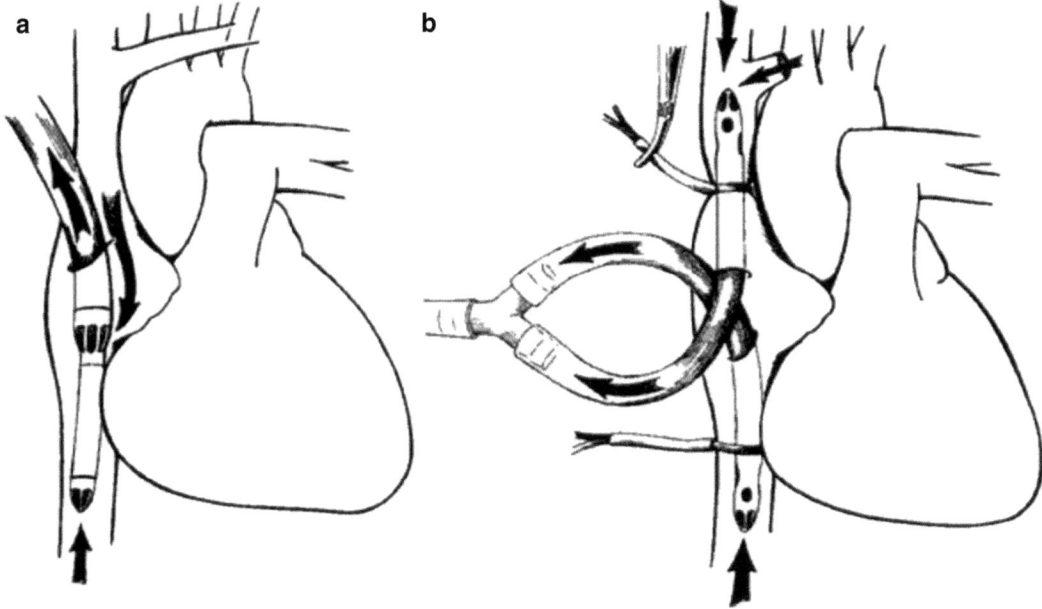

Fig. 4.2 (a) Single venous cannulation (b) Double venouscanullation

If double venous cannulation is required, the SVC and IVC should be cannulated separately. The SVC can be cannulated through an incision in the right atrium, with the cannula directed superiorly towards the SVC. It can also be cannulated directly through an incision on it. The IVC is cannulated through an incision placed about 2 cm above the junction of the IVC with the right atrium. After the venous cannulae are inserted, each tip must lie directly parallel to the walls of the vena cava, with tip of the SVC cannula pointing upward and that of the IVC downward. Otherwise, venous drainage will be compromised.

If right sided heart needs to be opened, both the SVC and IVC should be isolated and have nylon tapes placed around them. To isolate the SVC, the assistant applies gentle traction on the Nylon tape around the aorta, retracting it towards the left and exposing the pericardium covering the SVC on its left. The pericardium, at this point, is just above the right pulmonary artery. It is lifted up and cut to create a plane around the SVC. The pericardium on the right side of the SVC is also lifted up and cut. A right-angled clamp is then placed round the back of the SVC from right to left. A nylon tape is placed on it by an assistant and the clamp withdrawn. To isolate the IVC, the heart is mobilised gently by blunt dissection, near its junction with the IVC. The middle finger and thumb of the right hand can easily then go around the IVC, meeting each other, followed by passing a Semb clamp through this plane and grabbing a nylon tape with it on withdrawal. It is often easier to perform this on cardiopulmonary bypass.

When exposure of the IVC is particularly difficult, partial CPB maybe established first, and the IVC then can be exposed easily for placing the tape and purse string suture and cannulating the IVC.

Femoral Artery and Femoral Venous Cannulation

There are situations where arterial and venous access for initiating cardiopulmonary bypass is achieved by the cannulating peripheral vessels. Femoral cannulation for CPB is applicable in

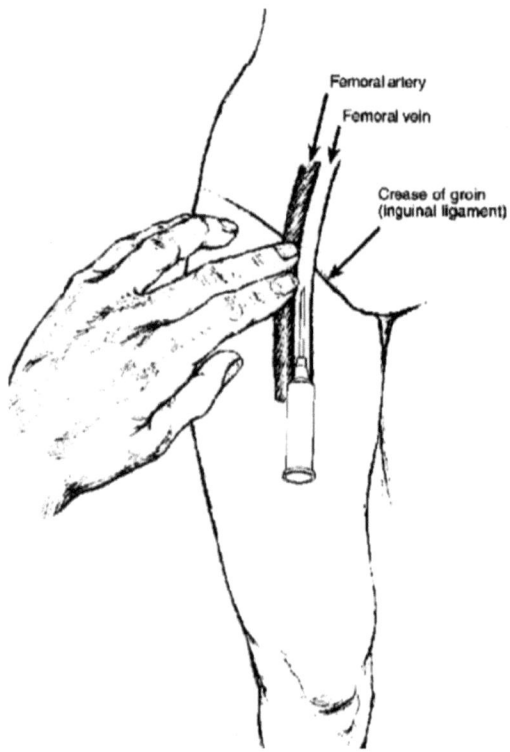

Femoral artery

Femoral vein

Crease of groin
(inguinal ligament)

Fig. 4.3 Femoral venous cannulation

cases of redo sternotomy when there are risks of cardiac or great vessel injury (Fig. 4.3); for operations when direct cannulation of ascending aorta is undesirable; and in some emergency situations.

It is easier to have these landmarks marked with a pen before draping the patient. An incision is made above the femoral artery in the groin crease in the femoral or mid-inguinal point (midway between the pubic symphysis and the anterior superior iliac spine). After the femoral artery is exposed, tapes are placed above and below the intended site of incision for cannulation. This site of cannulation should be above the origin of the profunda femoris. Vascular clamps may be applied above and below the intended cannulation site. An 8–10 mm arteriotomy is performed. The femoral cannula is then inserted. The tapes are then snugged down onto the cannula. The femoral vein can be cannulated in a similar way.

The general hazard associated with cannulation of the femoral artery is dissection of the arterial wall, which could extend to the entire aorta after blood is perfused through the cannula. Absolute care during the insertion of the cannular is essential to reduce the risk of arterial wall dissection. The intima of the artery must be accurately viewed, especially in cases of degenerative arterial disease. The cannula is introduced with the bevel directed toward the intact back wall of the artery up to the point of vascular clamp occlusion.

Decompressing the Heart

When the heart is no longer pumping or is fibrillating there may be blood returning to the ventricles causing distended and rewarming. This can have determinantal effects to the future contractility of the heart and can cause myocardial ischaemia. This is not an issue for the right ventricle as it is already vented by venous cannulation. The left ventricle can be vented through the right superior pulmonary vein, the pulmonary artery or the left ventricle (it is not recommend decompressing the heart using the left ventricle vent as the risk of bleeding with this vent is much higher compared with the others).

Aortic Root Vent

A 4–0 polypropylene purse string suture is placed in the ascending aorta, proximal to where the cross clamp will be applied. In CABG procedures, this cannula is positioned the site where it is used for one of the proximal anastomoses. 'Y' shape antegrade cardioplegia cannula is then inserted into the ascending aorta. One end of the cannula is connected to cardioplegia giving tube, the other end of the cannula is connected to the CPB pump suction as the aortic root.

Right Superior Pulmonary Vein Vent

A purse string is placed around the right superior pulmonary vein. It is important to place full thickness bites through the right superior pulmonary vein and not just through the pericardium.

An incision is then made with an 11 blade. This incision is then dilated with a Roberts. In most cases, a long, soft, angled catheter is used to be inserted into left atrium, directing towards the left ventricle. This must be done precisely if the heart is beating, in view of the possibility that air can be introduced into it and embolise to the brain unless the aorta is cross clamped. When inserting the vent, venous pressure is increased by reducing venous drainage to increase the volume of blood in the heart.

Pulmonary Artery Vent

A horizontal incision is made on the pulmonary artery just distal to the pulmonary valve. A bullet pump suction is inserted into it. Drainage and decompression of the left heart may be suboptimal with this technique.

Left Ventricle Apex Vent

The heart is lifted up and a stab incision is made at the apex of the left ventricle with an 11 blade. A bullet pump suction is placed into this. This incision is closed at the end of the operation using two felt pledgeted mattress suture of 2–0 or 3–0 polypropylene on either side of the incision.

De-Airing the Heart

With the aortic cross-clamped, patient is placed in a 30-degree head-down position, the IVC and SVC isolation nylon tapes are released, and the perfusionist fill the right heart, the anaesthetist inflate the lungs. The heart is gently massaged while the vent in the LV continues to drain. The aortic root vent is put on suction and some air will be removed via the antegrade cardioplegic cannula. Once de-airing is satisfactory, CPB flow is reduced, the aortic cross clamp is removed while the root suction is maintained on the antegrade cardioplegia cannula. Transoesophageal Echocardiography is useful to determine if there is residual air within the heart and where is the air.

Rocking table from side to side, gently massaging heart, shaking the sternal retractor and making heart ejecting blood normally will help de-airing effectively. When Echocardiography confirms the left heart is free of air, the operating table can be restored to normal position. The vent cannula and aortic cardioplegia cannula can be removed.

Discontinuing Cardiopulmonary Bypass and Decannulation

During re-warming and de-airing process, two temporary ventricular pacing wires are placed to the right ventricular myocardium on the anterior or inferior surface. Coronary artery and vein branches should be avoided while placing the ventricular pacing wires. Two atrial pacing wires sometimes are required and are secured to the right atrium surface using 5–0 sutures with adequate separation.

When patient body temperature reaches to 37C, perfusion flow rate is gradually decrease until the right and left atrial and aortic pressure are adequate, and CPB is then discontinued. The venous cannulae are removed, and protamine is administered slowly. Then the purse string sutures are tied if there isn't reaction to protamine. The venous cannulation sites are oversewn using 4–0 polypropylene. If patients have severely impaired heart function, or had prolonged or complex surgery, weaning down CPB should be carried on gradually, with constant communication between surgeon, perfusionist and anaesthetist. If the heart dose not function effectively after termination of CPB, CPB is restarted to prevent overdistention of LV or hypoxia. When inotropic support is administrated, cardiac function is recovered and haemodynamic stability is achieved, CPB can be weaned down gradually.

The aorta can either be decannulated while still fully heparinised or after the administration of protamine. We prefer decannulating the aorta after the administration of protamine as fluid volume can be given during protamine-related vasodilation if there is hypotension. Some surgeons prefer decannulation of aorta prior to giving protamine as it prevents potential clot formation on the aortic cannula prior to decannulation. It is important to ensure that the systolic blood pressure is less than 120 mmHg when decannulating the aorta to avoid aortic dissection.

To decannulate the aorta, the aortic cannula is clamped and held securely to prevent it from dislodging from aorta. The retaining sutures are cut, and aortic cannula is removed while gently snugging on the purse string to achieve haemostasis. Following decannulation, the inner purse string is tied first (assistant's side) followed by the outer purse string (surgeon's side). It is then oversewn with another stitch using 4–0 or 3–0 polypropylene.

Positioning Chest Drains and Chest Closure

In general, chest drains are inserted just before chest closure. The number and type of chest drains depends on the type of operation and choices of surgeons. We normally electively insert bilateral pleural chest drains if patients had poor heart function and or had Mitral Valve and or Tricuspid Valve surgery, as this group patient tend to develop pleural effusion post operatively. If left side pleural cavity is open, we routinely perform pericardial window to left chest cavity to reduce post-operative cardiac tamponade, and position drains to left pleural cavity and mediastinum.

Secure sternal closure is critically important. Stainless steel wires are normally used. Various techniques for closing the chest have been described for example, Single Trans-sternal (Fig. 4.4a), Single Peristernal (Fig. 4.4b), figure of 8 (Fig. 4.4c), etc. or single interrupted wire technique) or Ethibond.

The technique shown below (Fig. 4.5a, b, c, d) has been used extensively at our centre in more than 2000 cases, with excellent results.

First place a swab under the sternum to prevent any damage to the mediastinum from wire insertion. A minimum of at least 6 wires should be passed. The wires should run around the sternum in the intercostal spaces except in the manubrium where it has to be passed through the bone (Fig. 4.5a).

When going around the sternum it is important to stay close to the sternal bone to prevent damage to any unharvested internal mammary vessels. Adjacent wires on the surgeon's side are wrapped around each other (Fig. 4.5b).

Adjacent wires on the assistant's side are then also wrapped around each other. Clip any wires to prevent any needlestick injury. The wires on the surgeon's side are then pulled towards the assistant's side by the assistant so that the sternum is re-approximated. The wrapped wires on both sides are then wrapped around each other (Fig. 4.5c).

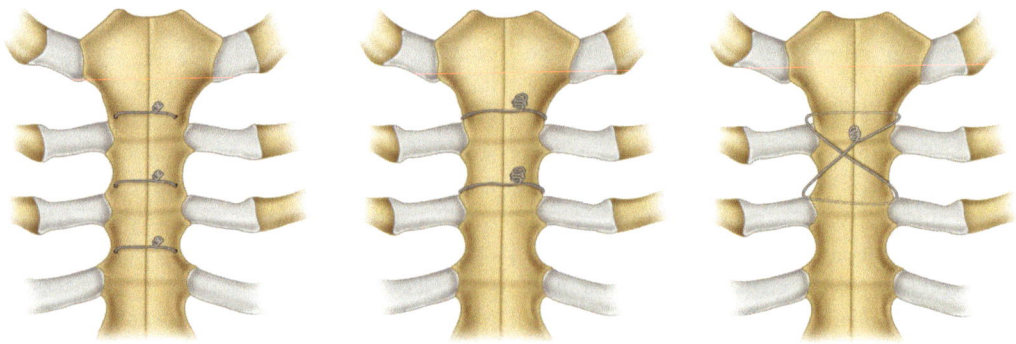

Fig. 4.4 Various techniques for closing the chest. (Printed with permission—Gemma Price)

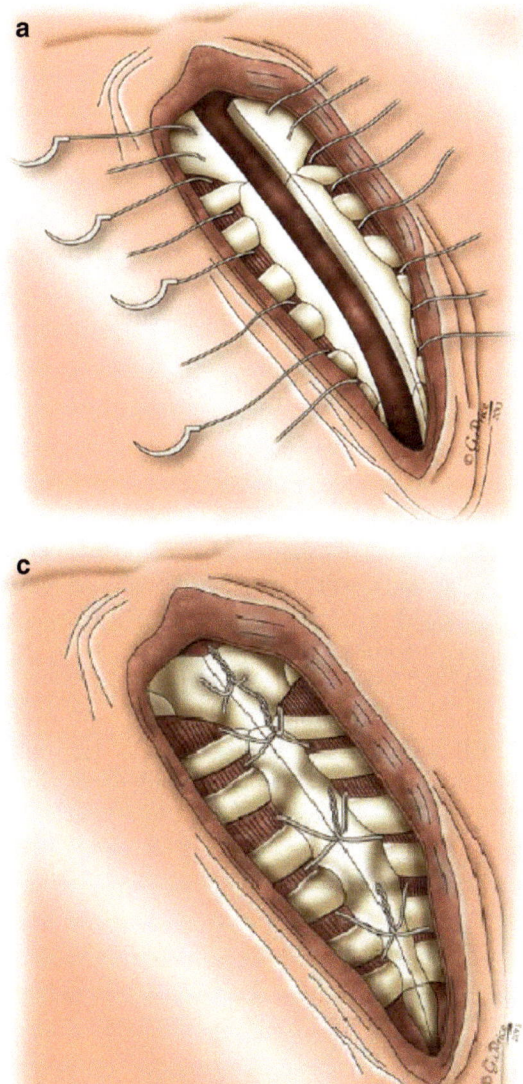

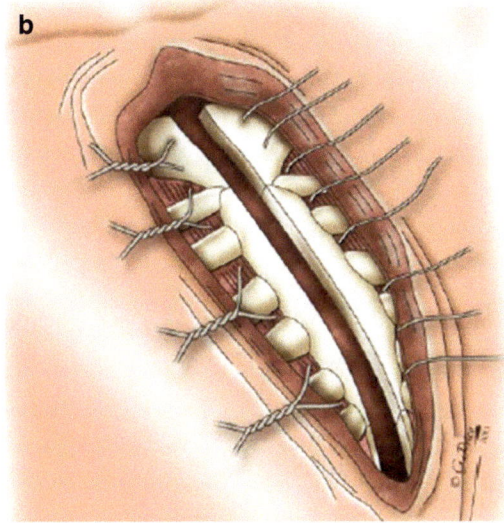

Fig. 4.5 (**a**) Sternal wires are passed around the sternum. (**b**) The sternal wires on the surgeon's side are twisted first. (Printed with permission—Gemma Price). (**c**) The wrapped wires on both sides are then wrapped around each other. (Printed with permission—Gemma Price)

Using a wire twister pull upwards to remove any slack below the sternum and twist loose ends 2–3 times. Bend the wire stumps so the tips are embedded into the periosteum. Close the soft tissue using a 2-layered closure technique, vertical sutures for the deep layer and horizontal sutures for the superficial layer to ensure strong wound healing.

If the sternal edges are thin or fragmented, Robiscek Sternal Closure technique can be used. Wires are passed through vertically in the parasternal position in front of and behind to costal cartilages on one or both sides. These vertical wires can provide extra strength to the sternal and can be incorporated into the closure by the transverse wires (Fig. 4.6).

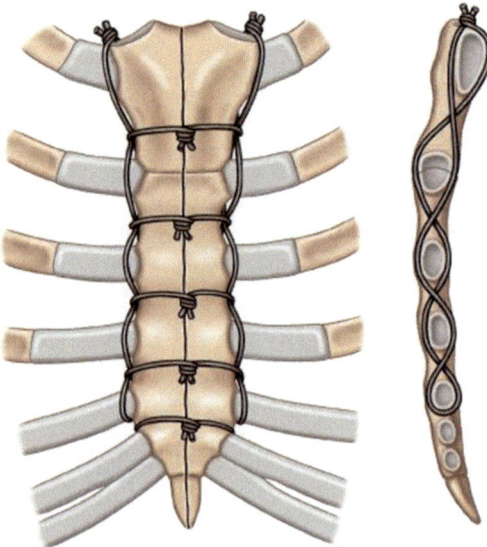

Fig. 4.6 Robiscek Sternal Closure technique

Key Pearls & Pitfalls

- Standardized routine access for cardiac operation is essential, ensuring every operation is safe and, in case of an emergency, done with speed and accuracy
- Locating the intercostal spaces on either side of the sternum and the edges of the muscle fibres along the sternum helps to identify the midline of the sternum
- The xiphisternum is cut with scissors, and the pericardium is freed from under the sternum with the right index finger
- In case of redo operation, careful mediastinal dissection is fundamental to reduce risk
- The pulmonary artery can sometimes be very thin-walled and care must be taken to avoid damage to it

Review QS

1) Where does the midline incision begin?
   a. **Below the sternal notch**
   b. Below the sternal manubrium

c. At the xiphoid process

2) The pericardium is freed from the sternum at the xiphoid by
   a. A pair of scissors
   b. **The right index finger**
   c. A haemostatic forceps
3) Which is the 'golden rule' of reoperative cardiac dissection?
   a. **Careful mediastinal dissection**
   b. Careful mediastinal incision
   c. Careful mediastinal excision
4) Once a sufficient plane has been developed, the thumb and index finger is placed around the aorta in the transverse sinus to ensure that the back wall of the aorta is also free of tissue. What kind of clamp is used around the back of the aorta while in contact with the index finger?
   a. A Satinsky clamp
   b. A Lees clamp
   c. **A Semb clamp**
5) Based on the technique used in our centre which is the minimum number of wires passed for chest closure?
   a. 5
   b. **6**
   c. 7

References

1. Vo TX, Juanda N, Ngu J, Gawad N, LaBelle K, Rubens FD. Development of a median sternotomy simulation model for cardiac surgery training. JTCVS techniques. 2020;2:109–16. https://doi.org/10.1016/j.xjtc.2020.03.007.
2. Rupprecht L, Schopka S, Keyser A, Lunz D, Sossalla S, Hilker M, Schmid C. 25 Years' experience with redo operations in cardiac surgery-third-time sternotomy procedures. Thorac Cardiovasc Surg. 2020 Dec 24; https://doi.org/10.1055/s-0040-1719157.
3. Yildiz Y, Ulukan MO, Erkanli K, Unal O, Oztas DM, Beyaz MO, Ugurlucan M. Preoperative arterial and venous cannulation in redo cardiac surgery: from the safety and cost-effectiveness points of view. Braz J Cardiovasc Surg. 2020 Dec 1;35(6):927–33. https://doi.org/10.21470/1678-9741-2019-0472.

Coronary Artery Bypass Graft with Cardiopulmonary Bypass

5

Panagiotis G. Kyriazis, Habib Khan, Guiqing Liu, and Prakash P. Punjabi

Learning Objectives

Several considerations when performing Coronary Artery Bypass Grafting (CABG):

1. Is CABG the best treatment option for this patient?
2. Which coronary arteries need to be grafted
3. Where the anastomosis should be on the coronary arteries
4. The site of proximal anastomosis (Aorta, T or Y grafts onto another conduit)
5. Any other procedures need to be done at the same time, whether the additional procedure or device would compromise the grafts
6. The choices of conduit (Left internal mammary artery, bilateral internal mammary artery, saphenous vein, radial artery or/and other conduits)

7. On Cardiopulmonary Bypass or Off Cardiopulmonary Bypass

Introduction

CABG surgery is a surgical intervention that improves blood flow to the heart muscle by bypassing the severely narrowed or blocked vessels that affect the normal function of the heart. The decision to perform a CABG surgery lies on multiple factors and decisions to be considered by the surgical team including the suitability of the patient and if CABG is the best option for the patient among others. Nowadays this is usually confirmed by a multidisciplinary meeting discussion. A bypass graft can be performed using one or more vessels including internal mammary arteries, radial arteries, saphenous veins and other conduits.

Pre-operative preparation is a vital part of all operations; initial assessment of the patient is similar to conventional CABG: a full history of the patient is taken, and a comprehensive clinical examination is performed. Then, investigations such as blood tests, CXR, coronary angiography and echocardiograms are carried out or reviewed, in order to better understand the patient's baseline, and indications for surgery. As well as these investigations, patients who are thought to be at a high risk of having carotid artery disease should have a carotid duplex ultrasound scan. After

P. G. Kyriazis · P. P. Punjabi (✉)
Department of Cardiothoracic Surgery, Hammersmith Hospital, Imperial College Healthcare NHS Trust, London, England, UK

National Heart and Lung Institute, Faculty of Medicine, Imperial College London, London, England, UK
e-mail: panagiotis.kyriazis@nhs.net;
p.punjabi@imperial.ac.uk

H. Khan · G. Liu
Department of Cardiothoracic Surgery, Hammersmith Hospital, Imperial College Healthcare NHS Trust, London, England, UK
e-mail: guiqing.liu@nhs.net; hkhan1@nhs.net

P. P. Punjabi, P. G. Kyriazis (eds.), *Essentials of Operative Cardiac Surgery*,
https://doi.org/10.1007/978-3-031-14557-5_5

reviewing this information, and confirming the need for intervention, the next step is to obtain informed consent.

When performing coronary artery bypass grafting (CABG), several decisions need to be made:

1. The coronary vessel to be grafted.
2. The choice of conduit (left internal mammary artery, bilateral internal mammary artery, saphenous vein, radial artery).
3. The site of proximal of anastomosis (aorta, T or Y grafts onto another conduit).
4. The approach (on cardiopulmonary bypass, off pump) Currently, most surgeons perform CABG on cardiopulmonary bypass although off-pump CABG is also an established approach.

Which Coronary Vessel Needs Graft

Coronary Angiogram is reviewed carefully, vessels are grafted if they have a stenosis of more than 70% (50% in left main stem stenosis) or if they are occluded, provided there is a distal vessel of reasonable size, generally 1 mm or greater in diameter. Grafting vessels with only minor or mild stenosis or very small vessels should be avoided as early graft failure will result.

Target coronary arteries have been determined through preoperative angiography, providing an anatomical assessment of the lesion as well as the haemodynamic significance of the stenosis; however, fractional flow reserve (FFR) can also be used to gain a functional assessment of the lesion, comparing the maximal blood flow in stenosed vessel to a normal vessel. Several studies have investigated the value of this functional assessment through the use of FFR guidance prior to CABG; although, this method is currently not widely used in the preoperative CABG assessment. Instantaneous wave-free ratio (iFR) is a similar measure to FFR that assesses coronary stenosis. Focus has increased on the role of iFR-guided CABG, and whether the differences between iFR and usual assessment play a role in the outcomes observed in studies.

Several studies have investigated the benefits of FFR and physiological guidance for PCI and CABG; however, there is limited literature exploring the role of iFR, particularly when comparing iFR and angiography-guided CABG [1]. iFR is a physiological index that measures the severity of coronary artery stenosis, calculated as the distal: proximal pressure ratio. Introduced with the aim of making stenosis assessment quicker and easier to conduct, iFR has been tested in a range of studies, from confirming its fundamental properties and validity to exploring its potential role in clinical practice.

In a retrospective study of 109 patients, Moscona et al. compared procedural and clinical outcomes over an 18 month follow up period between iFR or FFR guided, and angiography-guided CABG [2]. In the functionally guided group (iFR/FFR), three-vessel anastomoses and venous grafting rates were significantly higher ($p < 0.05$), with reduced major adverse cardiac events (MACCE) or angina incidence. As a result, they concluded that physiological guidance can be effectively used for CABG for complete revascularisation, and may also influence the revascularisation method used. However, as a retrospective study this may have been subjected to selection bias, whilst sample sizes were unbalanced between the intervention groups. Moreover, this study did not differentiate between results following iFR and FFR guidance, limiting the understanding of the specific role of iFR in improving CABG outcomes.

Recently, Wada et al. retrospectively analysed positive and negative iFR and FFR values and subsequent graft failure at 1 year post-CABG [3]. It was found that even when FFR was positive, if the vessel had a negative iFR, graft failure would be more likely to occur than if the vessel had a positive iFR. This suggests that iFR may be a useful prognostic marker for CABG. Although as a retrospective study, these findings may have been subjected to bias, the clear differences in measurement requirements between iFR and FFR also suggest that iFR may have a beneficial role in guiding CABG. As accurate assessment of CAD and stenosis severity determines CABG outcomes, we have explored the differences between iFR and FFR below to understand how iFR guidance may assist CABG.

Where the Anastomosis Should Be on the Coronary Arteries

Ideally, immediately distal to the diseased part, but depending on the coronary artery's quality, size and difficulties of exposure. The anastomosis site on the coronary arteries should be minimally diseased. Heavily calcified areas should be avoided. Endarterectomy can be performed in the extremely difficult situation, but long-term result is not optimal.

Choice of Conduit

Traditionally, the left internal mammary artery is used to graft the left anterior descending coronary artery and saphenous veins are used to graft the other coronary arteries. The use of the right internal mammary artery and the use of both internal mammary arteries in improving long-term survival, especially in the young, nondiabetic patient population have been extensively highlighted. The benefits of total arterial revascularization using radial artery as the third bypass conduit have been shown to have excellent 4-year patency. It has been reported by some centers that there is no significant difference in 1 year patency between the radial artery grafts and saphenous vein grafts.

In addition to the above named conduits, the gastroepiploic arteries, the lesser saphenous vein, the inferior epigastric artery and cephalic veins are the alternatives.

Harvesting the Left Internal Mammary Artery

Coronary artery bypass using the internal mammary artery for the bypass conduit has become established practice, and shown to have excellent long-term patency and improves survival. However, in emergency situation for unstable patients, the internal mammary artery is not

appropriate choice as it is necessary to minimize the time of the operation, and restoring myocardial reperfusion is the first priority. In very elderly patients, it's very important to reduce the operation time to reduce mortality and morbidity, harvesting the internal mammary artery may also not be advisable. Internal Mammary artery can be harvested as a pedicle with two internal mammary veins on either side of it or skeletonized.

Harvesting Pedicle Internal Mammary Artery

The dissection starts at the distal end of the internal mammary artery (IMA) using diathermy set at 30% of full power. The fascia is cut with diathermy about half a centimetre medial to the distal end of the IMA and its vein and parallel to it. The incision is continued for about an inch parallel to the IMA and its vein. Once a plane has been developed, the facia is then pulled downwards and the IMA and its two veins separated from the chest wall by blunt dissection using the diathermy blade. Any IMA branches are clipped on the artery side and diathermied on the chest-wall side. The distal end of the IMA is then tied off with silk ties and divided, leaving a reasonable length of silk tie attached to the IMA. Gentle traction is applied to the silk tie, pulling the IMA superiorly towards the head. A point diathermy is used, set power at 30, cutting the fascia on either side of the IMA and its veins. This frees up the IMA and its veins. The IMA branches are diathermied close to the chest wall. The IMA and its veins are harvested past the first IMA branch until very near to its junction with the subclavian artery. It should lie freely in the chest. The IMA is then placed on a wet swab and papaverine applied to it. Any branches are then clipped. Harvesting of the IMA can usually be completed in about 5–10 min using this technique. It is safe and there is minimal contact with the IMA during harvesting. The important principle using this technique is to get into the right plane where the IMA and its veins are relatively free of the fascia.

A more conventional method to harvest the IMA is not to divide it until the end. The initial dissection on the fascia parallel to the IMA and its vein is continued all along its length. The vein and then the IMA are then dissected off the chest wall using blunt dissection with the diathermy blade. Any IMA branches are clipped on the artery side and diathermied on the chest-wall side. A disadvantage with this technique is there is more contact between the diathermy blade and the IMA during the blunt dissection to separate it from the chest wall, thus, increasing the risk of trauma to the IMA. It is also a much slower technique.

Harvesting Skeletonized Internal Mammary Artery

The IMA can be harvested as a skeleton, i.e. without its two surrounding veins and fascia. An incision is first made with diathermy parallel to the IMA and its vein about an inch along its length and about half a centimetre medial to it. The fascia is then pulled downwards, and the media vein is pushed upwards to leave the vein attached to the chest wall, but pulling the IMA off the chest wall. Branches on the IMA are clipped on both the IMA side and the chest-wall side and cut with scissors. The dissection is continued all along the length of the IMA. This method of harvesting the IMA is more challenging and there is increased risk of trauma to the IMA. The advantages of it are an increased length of the IMA and also possibly preservation of the blood supply to the sternum, which may reduce the risk of wound infections in obese diabetics, particularly if the right internal mammary artery is also harvested. Curve tipped forceps are useful during harvesting skeletonized internal mammary artery.

Radial Artery Harvesting

Before harvesting the radial artery, it is important that an Allen's test has been performed before surgery to ensure that there is reasonable flow through the ulnar artery. The radial artery is always harvested as a pedicle with its two surrounding veins. The radial artery is very prone to vasospasm and, so, there should be minimal handling of it. The radial artery is held via its two surrounding veins and not directly. Previous

attempts at harvesting the radial artery as a skeleton has resulted in early occlusion due to vasospasm.

The radial artery pulse is located proximally and distally. The skin incision is made, starting from the distal radial pulse just proximal to the skin crease at the wrist and then extending proximally, medial to the brachioradialis, ending just before the elbow crease. The fat and then the fascia attaching the brachioradials to the pronator teres and flexor carpi radialis are divided. Once this fascia is divided, the radial artery is easily seen and lies free in areolar tissue. It is then grasped via its vein on either side. Any branches are clipped on the radial artery side and diathermied on the arm side. Depending on the length of the conduit required, the radial artery can be harvested until its junction with the brachial artery, i.e. just before the origin of the ulnar artery with the brachial artery. Once the radial artery is completely mobilized, a bulldog clamp is placed on the mid to distal artery, and final confirmation of a retrograde radial pulse is confirmed distal to the bulldog clamp before dividing the radial artery (Fig. 5.1a, b).

Endoscopic Technique for Radial Artery Harvesting has been rising in popularity in recent years. There are currently two categrories of systems for endoscopic radial artery harvest: the open system and the sealed system. The open system uses a specialized retractor for endoscopic exposure. The closed system delivers CO_2 insufflation at a controlled pressure to aid visualization, the wound is sealed at the scope entry site with a special balloon (Fig. 5.2).

Harvesting the Saphenous Vein

The saphenous vein is usually harvested from the ankle and continued upwards. The vein is identified just above the medial malleolus. The skin above it is cut and the vein freed from the enclosing facia. Any branches are tied and then divided. Depending on the length of conduit needed, the entire vein can be harvested up to the groin.

Interrupted small skin incision bridging technique is used widely in our unit. This allow better closure of the wound, minimize ischemic changes

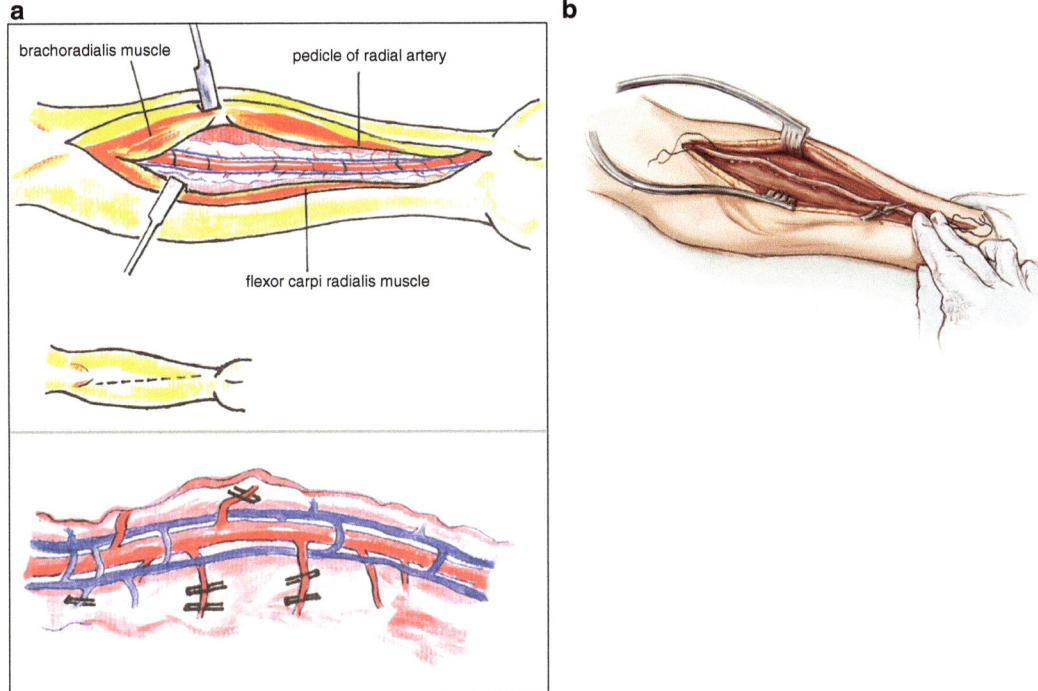

Fig. 5.1 (**a**) Important landmarks in harvesting of radial artery as pedicle conduit. (**b**) Radial artery harvested in skeletonized fasion

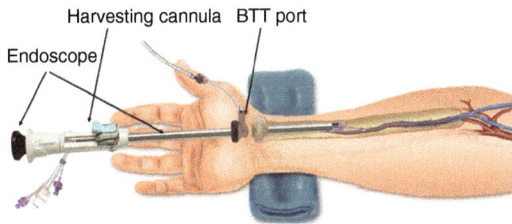

Fig. 5.2 Endoscopic technique of harvesting radial artery

along skin edges and reduce infection rate, especially for patients who are diabetic or peripheral vascular disease which are prone to poor wound healing (Fig. 5.3).

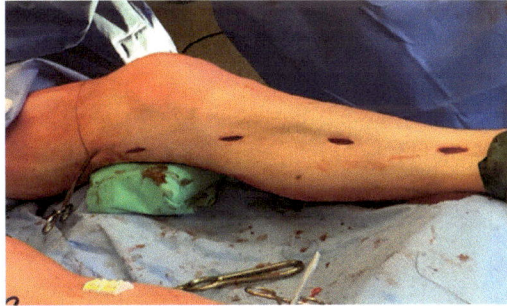

Fig. 5.3 Harvesting of Long Saphanous vein via skin bridge technique

The stripper can be also used to minimize the length of the skin incision on the leg and, hence, reduce wound infections and the time for recovery. The incision is usually begun in the groin and the proximal end of the saphenous vein is ligated at the sapheno-femoral junction, keeping a reasonable length of silk tie attached to the saphenous vein. The tissue surrounding the vein is freed by blunt dissection such that the saphenous vein lies free. The vein is then passed into the

stripper which is advanced distally until some resistance is met. This corresponds to the position of saphenous vein branches. A 1-cm incision is then made in the skin above where the end of the stripper is. The vein is brought out through this incision, the branches are ligated and divided and the stripper placed again into the vein through this incision and advanced further distally. Use of the stripper requires considerable experience. If too much force is used, especially when resis-

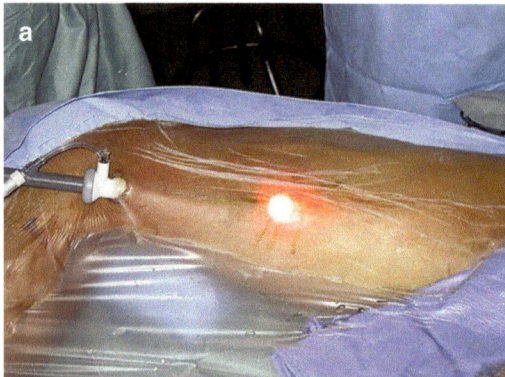

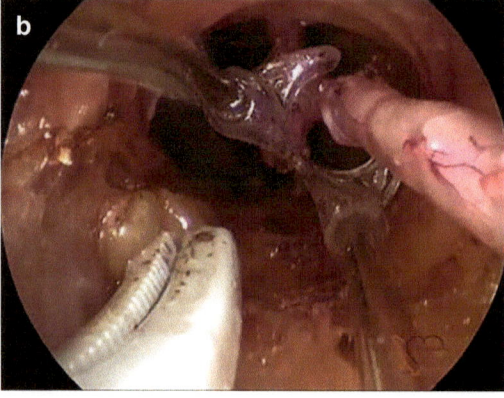

Fig. 5.4 (**a**) Ednoscopic harvesting of long saphanous vein-external view. (**b**) Ednoscopic harvesting of long saphanous vein-internal view

tance is encountered, the branches can be avulsed off the vein, resulting in an unusable vein. Considerable trauma can also result if too much force is used.

Endoscopic harvesting of the saphenous vein is very similar to the use of a stripper. It is usually harvested from the knee or, sometimes, the groin. The use of the endoscope allows direct visualisation of the vein and its branches and so trauma to the vein is minimised. Only two incisions are needed: one at the proximal end and the other at the distal end (Fig. 5.4a, b).

Setup for on-Pump Coronary Artery Bypass

After performing the midline sternotomy and left internal mammary artery is been harvested. The Pericardium is lifted up on both side to provide good exposure to heart. To institute cardiopulmonary bypass (CPB) aortic and right atrial cannulation is performed. Before going on CPB the conduit harvest should be prepared and checked. Once on bypass the targeted vessels should be identified or if needed can be marked by using size 11or 15 blade. Cross clamped to the ascending aorta is applied and antegrade cold cardioplegia given via aortic root and repeated every 15–20 min. Retrograde cardioplegia can be used if required specially in patient who had very severe proximal left main coronary artery stenosis. The other option to perform the operation is using cross clamp fibrillation technique without using cardioplegia. In this technique each anastomosis is performed within 10 min time and once the distal anastomosis is performed the cross clamp is removed and top end anastomosis is performed.

Prior to instituting CPB Left internal mammary artery and long saphenous vein graft conduits are prepared. The left internal mammary artery is cut at the distal end and a soft bull dog is applied proximally to stop the flow of the blood. The LIMA is attached to the left upper edge of the sternal incision by a hemostat clip. Using the potts scissors the distal end of the LIMA is cut, creating a "V" shaped opening. The long saphenous vein is occluded by placing a fine forcep at the distal end by a assistant. A pair of scissors than cut the end at a slight angle and inferiorly creating a "V"shapped opening.

A general principal of anastomosing perform the right coronary anastomosis first and work your way up towards the left side and perform LIMA to LAD last. In case if the right coronary artery is blocked at the ostia it is worth considering giving cardioplegia through the vein graft once the anastomosis is performed. To bring the heart out and perform the anastomosis either few small wet or a large swabs are placed behind the heart. Stay sutures can be used proximally and distally to the intended arteriotomy to ensure blood less field. The same stay sutures can be moved around to position the heart to provide best exposure. Once satisfied with the position of the heart a clip can be placed at the end of the suture and line clamp is hung through one of the holes of the clip's handle and allowed to hang by the patient side, thereby securing the heat in the required position.

Positioning the Heart for Anastomosis of the Right Posterior Descending Coronary Artery (PDA)

To visualize PDA the heart is lifted up and either four small swabs or one large swabs is placed behind the heart. The heart is than retracted towards the right shoulder to visualize PDA, one end of which lie towards 2 0'clock position and the other end at the 8 o'clock position. 2/0 Ethibond stitches can be placed proximally and distally to the intended arteriotomy. One end of the clip is placed towards the right shoulder and the other end towards the left shoulder. Line clamp can be passed through one of the hole of the clips on each side and let them hang on each side of the patient to stabilize the heart and keep a bloodless field.

Positioning the Heart for Anastomosis of the Circumflex Obtuse Marginal Coronary Artery (OM)

Positioning the heart for OM is slightly more challenging than PDA. There are few option to position the heart while performing OM anastomosis. Heart is lifted up and four small swabs are placed behind and the anastomosis is performed on an upside down heart. In this position table can be rotated towards the surgeon to help for better exposure. The other option is to put either four small or two large swabs and rotate the heart towards the surgeon and place 2/0 Ethibond stiches proximally and distally of the intended arteriotomy and pull proximal end towards the assistant and distal end towards the surgeon securing the positon of the heart.

Positioning the Heart for Anastomosis of the Left Anterior Descending Coronary Artery (LAD) and the Diagonal Artery

To position the heart for left anterior descending artery either four small swabs or one large swab can be placed behind the heart. 2/0 Ethibond stich can be used if needed with same principle as described above. If diagonal has to be grafted than 2/0 Ethibond stiches can be placed proximally in the LAD before the bifurcation and another one in the diagonal distal to anastomosis site.

Performing the Coronary Arteriotomy

After identifying the coronary artery the fat and fascia is separated. The intended arteriotomy can be performed by either using size 11 or 15 blade. The care has to be given the arteriotomy has to be done in the middle. If there is excess tissue or fat, a fat retractor or 5/0 prolene can be used to provide good exposure. Before performing the arteriotomy the surgeon and assistant hold each side of the tissue up with fine forceps and perform the arteriotomy. This is further enlarged by using forward and backward cutting Potts scissors.

Performing the Distal Anastomosis

There are several ways of performing distal coronary anastomosis. The general principle stays the same which include taking the stitch from outside in into the conduit and inside out in the coronary artery. Generally an 8/0 or 7/0 polypropylene suture is used to anastomosis especially for LAD and 7/0 for other anastomosis. Once 3–5 suture are placed in this way than holding both end of the suture gently bring the conduit down on to the coronary artery and continue either a forehand or backhand as per surgeon convenient. General principle is that all the bites in to the conduit and coronary artery are taken separately ensuring good visibility of the coronary artery. The stiches taken either in the conduit or in the coronary should not be very deep and attention is given all the time that back wall of the coronary artery is not taken. Emphasis is given to match the conduit and coronary exactly and at the end of heal and toe all the bites are taken separately and carefully to avoid any narrowing of the anastomosis.

A safe technique, particularly in small coronary arteries, is to place a 1-mm probe into the coronary artery before placing sutures at the heel and toe, which would ensure that the back wall of the vessel is not inadvertently caught. Once the anastomosis is complete, a syringe of cardioplegia or saline can be flushed through the venous graft or if it is the LAD than the bull dog can be release to see the flow in the coronary artery and any leakage around it.

Short Left Internal Mammary Artery or Hyperinflated Lungs

Situation can arise where either the left internal mammary artery length is not adequate or the lungs are hyperinflated secondary to pulmonary disease. This will become apparent after cardiopulmonary bypass once the lungs are fully inflated. In this situation to avoid any tension on the LIMA to LAD graft the pericardium can be fixed to the left chest wall superiorly. (Fig. 5.5).

A vertical slit is made in the pericardium, creating a short superior limb and an inferior limb continuous with the rest of the pericardium. The inferior limb of the pericardial slit is lifted caudally and laterally and sutured to a costal cartilage as caudally as possible (approximately two intercostal spaces caudal to its original position and just medial to the lateral margin of the LIMA harvest site), using a 2/0 Ethibond® suture (Ethicon, Somerville, NJ, US) (Fig. 5.5). This manoeuvre bring the heart anteriorly toward the chest wall and caudally thereby reducing the tension on the LIMA to LAD anastomosis.

Performing the Proximal Anastomosis

There are different techniques to perform the proximal anastomosis. It can be performed once all the distal anastomosis are performed or it can be done as single cross clamp technique where after each distal anastomosis the top end is performed. When performing after the all the distal anastomosis are done, before taking out the aortic root cannula the vein grafts are measured. This done by infusing either a heparinized blood or saline into the vein. The heart is lifted and vein graft are measured ensuring that the graft are not twisted and not in tension. The left side graft are brought above the pulmonary artery. The right side graft can either be brought in front of right atrial cannula or behind it.

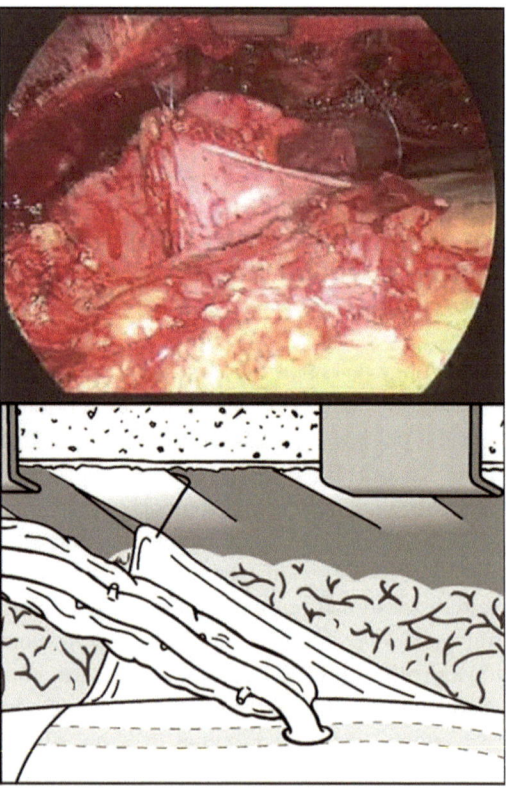

Fig. 5.5 Securing the left pericardium to the chest wall to reduce or avoid tension on the LIMA LAD anastomosis (Reproduced with permission. Chan et al. [4])

Once measured the cardioplegia cannula is removed and depending on the number of proximal anastomosis the size of side clamp is chosen. The author prefers large side clamp and perform all the anastomosis on one side clamp. The fat on the ascending aorta is excised and the whole is created using No 11 blade and this is enlarged using 3.5 to 4 mm hole puncher. The vein is then cut at an angle to enlarge it to the same size as the aortotomy and a bull dog is applied. The anastomosis is then performed in a similar fashion to the distal coronary anastomoses following the general principle of anastomosis. A method to ensure secure anastomoses is to ensure that the edge of the vein overlaps the surface of the aorta by 1–2 mm and reasonably deep bites are taken on the aorta, spaced evenly.

Size mismatch may occur between the conduit and the aortotomy, more commonly with a radial artery graft or free internal mammary artery grafts (Fig. 5.6a). In such situations, it is important to stop the bleeding without compromising the anastomosis or the blood flow from the aorta to the coronary arteries through the graft. If there is generalised bleeding or ooze around the anastomosis, a separate stitch (6/0 polypropylene) is placed as a separate purse string concentrically around the aortotomy, approximately 5 mm from the anastomotic edge. The perfusionist or anaesthetist is requested to reduce the blood pressure and the purse string is then tied, leading to a reduction of the aortotomy in a uniform style, thereby, causing the bleeding or ooze to stop (Fig. 5.6b).

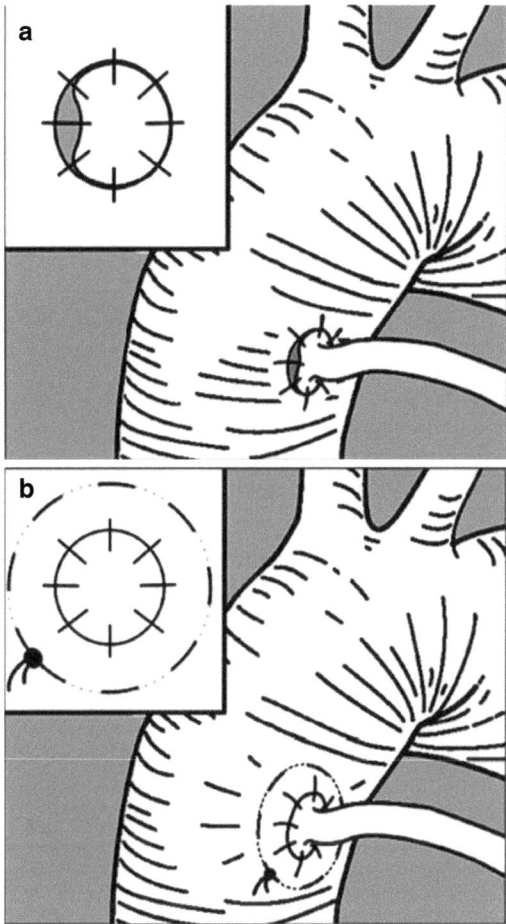

Fig. 5.6 (**a**) Size mismatch between a conduit and the aortotomy causing bleeding (Reproduced with permission. Jarral et al. [5]) (**b**) Purse string suture placed around the aortotomy to reduce its size (Reproduced with permission. Jarral et al. [5])

Key Pearls & Pitfalls

- Vessels are grafted if they have a stenosis of more than 70% (50% in left main stem stenosis) or if they are occluded
- Traditionally, the left internal mammary artery is used to graft the left anterior descending coronary artery and saphenous veins are commonly used to graft the other coronary arteries
- Cross clamp to the ascending aorta is applied and antegrade cold cardioplegia given via aortic root and repeated every 15-20 min
- Using the potts scissors the distal end of the LIMA is cut, creating a "V" shaped opening
- Positioning the heart for OM is slightly more challenging than PDA

Review QS

1. Which of the following tests should patients at high risk of having carotid artery disease should have?
   a. Cardiac ultrasound scan
   b. **Carotid duplex ultrasound scan**
   c. Carotid angiogram

2. Which graft is used for revascularisation of the left anterior descending coronary artery, traditionally?
   a. **Left internal mammary artery**
   b. Saphenous vein
   c. Radial artery
3. The IMA and its veins are harvested past the first IMA branch until its junction with the subclavian artery
   a. **Very near to**
   b. It reaches
   c. It's half way from
4. The intended arteriotomy can be performed by using
   a. Either 11 or 14 blade
   b. Either 9 or 15 blade
   c. **Either 11 or 15 blade**
5. What suture type is used for LAD anastomosis
   a. **7/0 or 8/0 polypropylene**
   b. 4/0 or 5/0 polypropylene
   c. 5/0 or 6/0 polypropelene

References

1. Wada T, Shiono Y, Higashioka D, Kashiwagi M, Shimamura K, Kuroi A, et al. P2700Impact of instantaneous wave-free ratio on graft failure after coronary artery bypass graft surgery. European Heart J. 2019;40(Supplement_1)   https://doi.org/10.1093/eurheartj/ehz748.1017.
2. Jarral OA, Jarral RA, Chan KMJ, Punjabi PP. Use of a purse string suture in proximal coronary anastomosis to reduce size mismatch between conduit and aortotomy. Ann R Coll Surg Engl. 2011;93:414–21.
3. Chan KMJ, Jarral OA, Jarral RA, Punjabi PP. Avoiding tension in the left internal mammary artery to left anterior descending coronary artery anastomosis during coronary artery bypass surgery. Ann R Coll Surg Engl. 2013;95:73–81.
4. Götberg M, Cook CM, Sen S, Nijjer S, Escaned J, Davies JE. The Evolving Future of Instantaneous Wave-Free Ratio and Fractional Flow Reserve. J Am College Cardiol. 2017;70(11):1379–402. https://doi.org/10.1016/j.jacc.2017.07.770.
5. Moscona JC, Stencel JD, Milligan G, Salmon C, Maini R, Katigbak P, et al. Physiologic assessment of moderate coronary lesions: a step towards complete revascularization in coronary artery bypass grafting. Ann of Transl Med. 2018;6(15):300. https://doi.org/10.21037/atm.2018.06.31.

Off Pump Coronary Artery Bypass Grafting

6

Nikhil Sahdev, Osama Hamid,
Panagiotis G. Kyriazis, and Prakash P. Punjabi

Introduction

Off-pump coronary artery bypass grafting (CABG) surgery is performed without the use of a cardiopulmonary bypass machine which was primarily developed in the early 1990s; however, this soon became not only a financial enticement but the choice of many surgeons worldwide as it was thought to reduce the risk of adverse clinical outcomes associated with bypass. As off-pump surgery avoids cardiopulmonary bypass, it prevents the systemic inflammatory response and impaired haemostasis that is associated with an extracorporeal circulation. However, as the heart remains beating throughout the procedure it can

be more technically challenging. Therefore, many surgeons still prefer on pump CABG as it provides a motionless field with more haemodynamic and respiratory control.

Despite continuous improvements in both technology and our understanding of inflammation and coagulation, there remains much debate surrounding the use of off-pump. There is strong evidence in the literature (including NICE guidelines) that the risk of mortality, stroke and myocardial infarction in off-pump surgery is now comparable to on-pump when performed by experienced surgeons [1]. In fact, some groups suggest there is a significant reduction in stroke in the off pump operations [2]; however, off-pump is still debated by some due to concerns regarding early revascularisation [3] and in addition some data suggests longer-term survival in patients undergoing on-pump CABG [1]. Current indications for off-pump include patients with a very atherosclerotic or heavily calcified aorta.

Off pump CABG is a widely performed invasive approach suggested to patients suffering from aortic disease, chronic lung disease and those at higher risk of complications from CPB such as renal insufficiency. The benefits of avoiding bypass, and hence cross-clamp time, include lower risk of myocardial infarction, aortic dissection, pulmonary embolism, atrial injury and arrhythmias. Since there's no activation of coagulation and inflammation caused by cannulation, off-pump has the advantage of less bleeding and

N. Sahdev
Department of Cardiothoracic Surgery, Harefield Hospital, Royal Brompton & Harefield NHS Foundation Trust, London, UK
e-mail: nikhil.sahdev@nhs.net

O. Hamid
Department of Cardiothoracic Surgery, Gloucestershire Royal Hospital, Gloucestershire Hospital NHS Foundation Trust, Gloucester, UK

P. G. Kyriazis · P. P. Punjabi (✉)
Department of Cardiothoracic Surgery, Hammersmith Hospital, Imperial College Healthcare NHS Trust, London, UK

National Heart and Lung Institute, Faculty of Medicine, Imperial College London, London, UK
e-mail: panagiotis.kyriazis@nhs.net;
p.punjabi@imperial.ac.uk

© Springer Nature Switzerland AG 2022
P. P. Punjabi, P. G. Kyriazis (eds.), *Essentials of Operative Cardiac Surgery*,
https://doi.org/10.1007/978-3-031-14557-5_6

as a consequence minimal transfusion is required during surgery. Hence, off pump CABG is overall a more cost-effective approach compared to on pump CABG; however, off pump CABG approach is followed by other challenges, obstacles and difficulties. This type of surgery requires very skilled surgeons with more technical knowledge as the risk of anastomotic bleeding, suboptimal revascularization and myocardial ischaemia is increased; not all coronary arteries are well reached by the technique due to the pumping heart which restricts the surgeons access to the heart muscle from different sites, it is more likely for the patient to have an MI due to cardioplegia absence and there is a higher tendency of graft failure when undergoing off pump CABG. To adopt the off-pump technique into the repertoire of a cardiothoracic unit it is vital for appropriate patient selection, individualized grafting strategy, peer-to-peer training of the entire team, and graded clinical experience [4]. The learning curve is thought to be around 50 to 75 cases and good proficiency with the technique is usually associated with a low 1% to 2% conversion rate to bypass [5].

Akhrass and Bakaeen support the idea of performing primarily CABG on-pump and reverting to off pump CABG when the aorta is more calcified or in the case of a high risk for CPB [6]. Published studies around the topic have failed to provide evidence in supporting an advantage for off pump CABG and have -in the contrary- raised concerns regarding suboptimal outcomes of increased numbers of incomplete revascularization compared to on pump CABG as well as higher late mortality rate when the surgery was performed by inexperienced surgeons. Although, as previously stated above, the off pump CABG is suitable for a group of patients with significant aortic calcification or those who are at higher risk for CPB.

Lastly, surgeons already experienced with off pump CABG surgery may implement multiarterial grafting and continue with their off-pump practice; however, it is probably prudent for the on-pump surgeons to become proficient with multiarterial grafting surgery prior to making another change in their daily practice.

Total Lesion Revascularisation (TLR)

Performance of total arterial off-pump coronary revascularization would offer the benefits of reduced morbidity and need for re-intervention with better long-term survival [7]. The published experience to date validates this hypothesis. An extension of the concept of total arterial off-pump CABG is total arterial anaortic off-pump CABG. This strategy by avoiding aortic manipulation significantly reduces the risk of neurological complications compared with both conventional CABG and off-pump CABG with aortic manipulation and brings the stroke rate on par with PCI. Total arterial anaortic off-pump CABG can be achieved by using either a combination of in-situ bilateral mammary arteries (BIMA) only, in-situ BIMA and right gastroepiploic artery or composite grafts using the BIMA and radial artery ('T-graft' and composite extension grafts).

Pre-Operative Considerations

The pre-operative considerations are the same as mentioned in the introduction of the previous chapter.

Steps should be taken to minimise complications such as hypothermia and haemodynamic compromise during surgery. Strategies to tackle hypothermia include: using a heating mattress or warming blanket, applying a fluid warmer, as well as ensuring the operating theatre temperature is well regulated. Cardiac positioning and manipulation occurs throughout the procedure which can result in haemodynamic compromise. The anaesthetic team should conduct regular monitoring of vitals such as blood pressure and heart rate. They should respond to any deterioration via medications such as vasopressors, fluids or temporary epicardial pacing. Without a doubt, excellent communication between the surgeon and the anaesthetist is essential in a successful operation.

Preparation for off-pump should involve a multidisciplinary approach. Patients should be discussed during briefings, to ensure suitable equipment such CO2 blower, stabiliser, appropriate intracoronary shunts and cell salvage machines are all available.

Operative Technique

Incision and Anticoagulation

In the majority of cases a traditional median sternotomy is performed. All conduits are harvested as per a traditional CABG procedure, but care must be taken to ensure that the left internal mammary (LIMA) is harvested as long as possible to avoid later excessive tension when the heart is elevated after the graft to the LAD is performed (Fig. 6.1).

Following conduit harvest and before coronary anastomosis, 100 U/kg of unfractionated heparin is administered to achieve an ACT of >300 seconds. The ACT should be monitored every 30 minutes with heparin supplemented as needed. Cardiopulmonary bypass is set-up but not primed and the perfusionist should be on

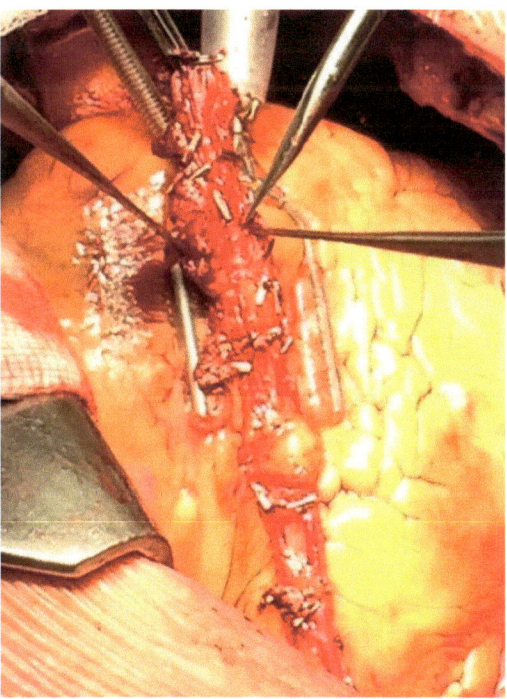

Fig. 6.1 LIMA harvest and length

stand-by and always present in the operating room.

Exposure & Stabilisation

Correct positioning and stabilisation are critical steps for enabling successful outcomes in off-pump surgery as it allows optimal anastomotic suturing. To position the heart so that there is a good exposure of the target coronary artery, as well as to prevent haemodynamic compromise, different techniques and adjuncts such as pericardial sutures, stabilising devices and intraluminal shunts are used.

Sutures
Deep pericardial sutures are placed to create a ridge of pericardium that supports the base of the lateral wall and allows the heart to assume an apex up position. This is accomplished by placing one or two silk (2/0) posterior to the left phrenic nerve and anterior to the pulmonary veins, another suture is placed in the oblique sinus behind the left atrium and a final one can be placed to the left and posterior to the IVC.

The placement of these deep sutures can be associated with the risk of injury to underlying structure therefore it is crucial to pull that segment of the pericardium with a Roberts to avoid injury to the structures behind the pericardium. When placing these sutures there may be severe haemodynamic compromise as retraction is required to expose the posterior pericardium. The blood pressure should recover quickly as long as the patient is head down.

Modified Swab Technique
Some surgeons prefer not to use traction sutures as they lift the pericardial cavity and can therefore reduce the freedom of movement of the heart which is later needed to manipulate the position so that the coronary arteries can be accessed. A half-folded swab (12 cm wide and 70 cm long) is snared to the posterior pericardium (using a single stitch 0-silk suture), halfway between the inferior vena cava and the left inferior pulmonary vein. Traction is applied on the two limbs of the

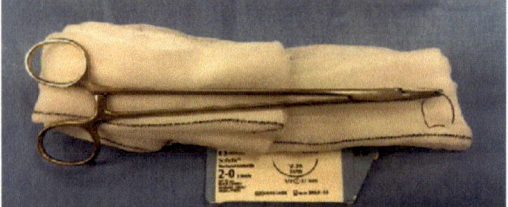

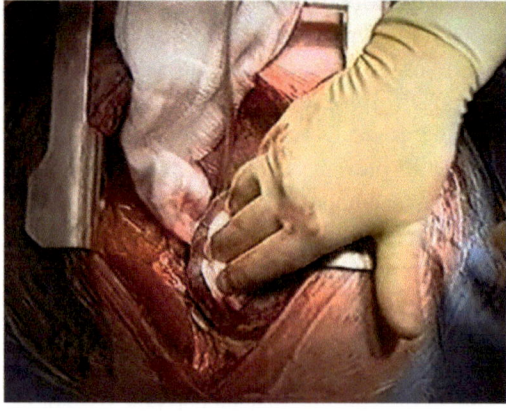

Fig. 6.2 Modified deep pericardial swab/suture

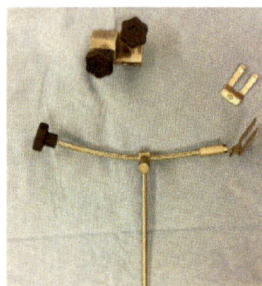

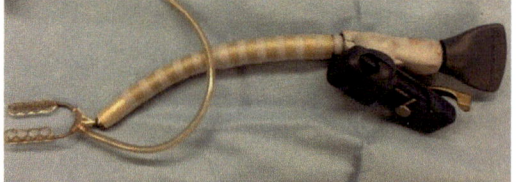

Fig. 6.3 Compression stabiliser (above). Suction stabiliser (below)

swab and the snare (Fig. 6.2). These are then fixed to the surgical drapes to facilitate exposure of the target coronary vessels.

Stabilisers

Stabilisation of the target coronary artery is achieved by either mechanical compression or suction devices. These devices hold the heart in position to expose the vessel and create an immobile field (Fig. 6.3).

Bloodless Site

To avoid myocardial ischaemia and instability of the target vessel during off-pump surgery intra-coronary shunts are used (Fig. 6.4). These intraluminal shunts are placed within the vessel after arteriotomy and allow distal perfusion as well as a bloodless field. These shunts have a role in training as the anastomosis can be fashioned with plenty more time.

Blower/Mister

The use of a CO_2 blower/mister by the assistant throughout the coronary anastomosis allows improved visualisation by gently clearing blood from the site and therefore providing a near

bloodless surgical field (Fig. 6.5). It is important the assistant must only blow during stitch placement at a flow rate not >5 L per minute. This is to prevent damage to the coronary endothelium as well as avoiding directing the gas jet directly into the vessel lumen to prevent gas embolus which can induce ventricular fibrillation.

Sequence of Anastomosis

When grafting the coronary arteries, more cardiac displacement is tolerated as the heart becomes more revascularized. Hence the coronary arteries should be grafted in order of increasing cardiac displacement so that it is better tolerated by the myocardium (anterior wall vessels followed by inferior wall vessels and finally lateral wall vessels).

Positioning the Heart

Anterior Wall Presentation

This allows exposure of the anterior wall coronary arteries (LAD, diagonal and ramus intermedius). The LIMA to LAD graft is usually done first, as the LAD can be exposed with minimal manipulation of the heart.

The operating table is kept flat, and a deep pericardial retraction suture is placed a couple of

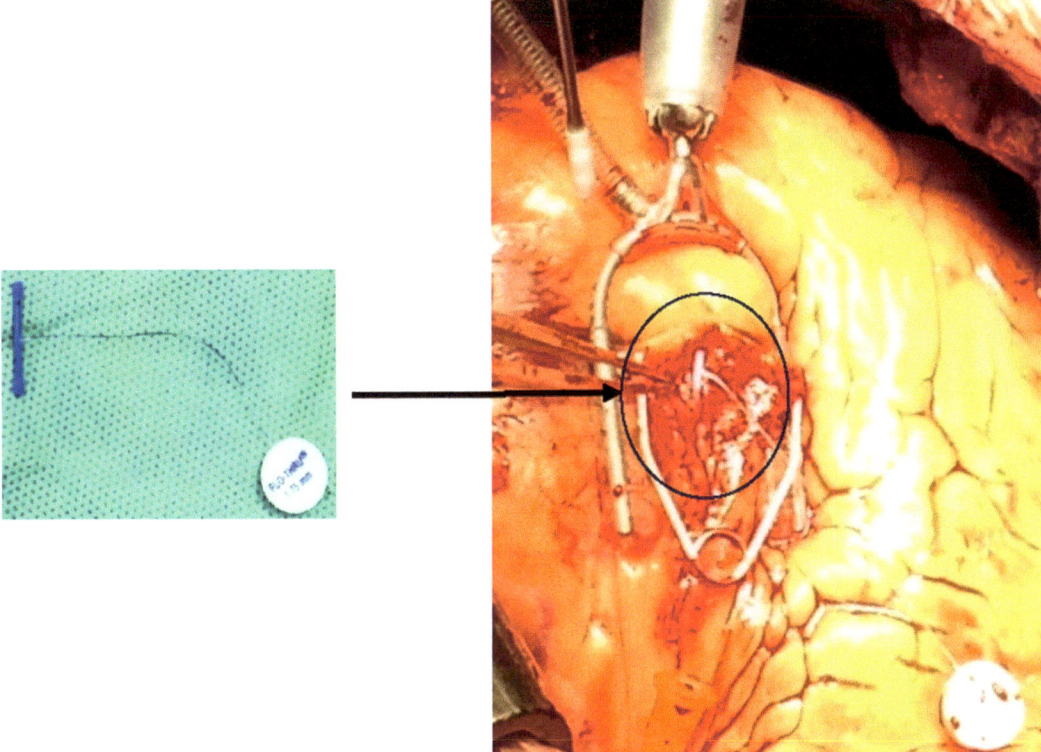

Fig. 6.4 Intraluminal shunt

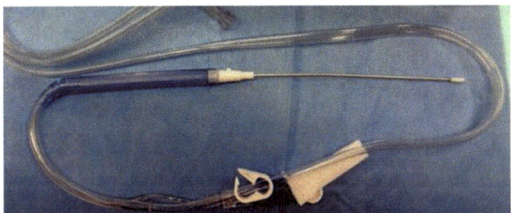

Fig. 6.5 Mister blower

centimetres above the left superior pulmonary vein, pulled firm and secured to the drape on the left side of the patient. This has the result of lifting the pericardium and therefore the apex of the heart, upwards. If a modified swab technique is used, both limbs of the swab are pulled to the left towards the assistant side to rotate the heart anti-clockwise. The snare is pulled caudally to lift the pericardium and consequently the heart apex upward. Once the heart is satisfactorily positioned, the segment of the LAD that is to be grafted is carefully selected, and the mechanical stabiliser is fastened (Fig. 6.6). A 4–0 prolene suture and a soft plastic snugger is used to perform temporary proximal occlusion of the LAD, and the arteriotomy incision is made. Then an appropriately sized intra-coronary shut is inserted with the aid of the CO_2 blower and distal anastomosis made. A similar technique is used to graft the diagonal coronaries. The ramus intermedius, however, may be intramyocardial and require grafting near the heart base, therefore moving the heart into a vertical position can allow better visualisation and easier access.

Inferior Wall Presentation

This allows exposure of the distal RCA and PDA. The PDA is the preferred side for grafting the right coronary distribution. Similar to the lateral wall approach, the operating table is positioned in the steep Trendelenburg position (20°) and rotated towards the surgeon (10–20°).

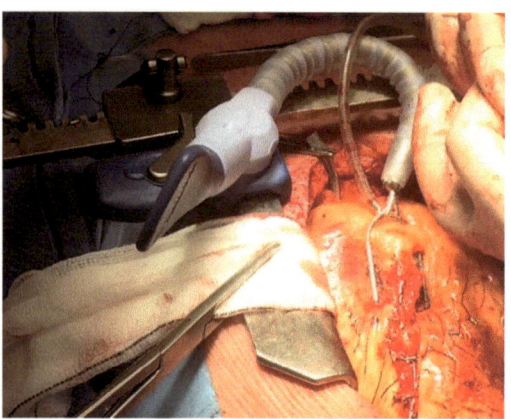

Fig. 6.6 A. Position of heart and stabiliser for LAD

The deep pericardial retraction sutures are repositioned so as to place the target vessel in the center of the operative field.

If swabs are used, both limbs of the snared swab are positioned to hold the heart with its apex upward, and are fixed to the surgical drapes at the top end of the sternotomy incision. The plastic snare is pulled caudally and fixed to the left of the midline. The stabiliser is placed at the cranial end of the right arm of the sternal retractor, whilst its foot is directed downwards in order to stabilize the exposed PDA. Temporary occlusion of the RCA proximal to the bifurcation is necessary in order to perform the arteriotomy. This can compromise blood supply to the AV node which can result in AV node block and bradycardia, leading to heart distension and haemodynamic instability. This is prevented via the placement of temporary epicardial pacing wires.

For grafting the right coronary artery, the operating table is put in the flat position, and the deep pericardial retraction sutures are relaxed, causing the heart to fall to the left side. The stabiliser is positioned according to surgeon preference, either to the left or the right of the retractor, and the tips directed downward along the course of the artery. Arteriotomy is then performed, and the anastomosis performed.

Lateral Wall Presentation

This allows exposure of obtuse marginals and posterolateral branches of right coronary artery. The operating table is positioned in Trendelenburg at about 20° and rotated towards the right (10–20°) this will allow gravity to displace heart to the right and apex anteriorly as well as increase venous return and facilitate the spontaneous anti-clockwise rotation of the beating heart to the right. At this stage remove any pericardial sutures on the right side. It may be desirable to open the right pleural space. This manoeuvre allows the heart to move more to the right without compressing the right ventricle and causing haemodynamic instability. If pericardial retraction sutures are used, they should be placed on the posterior pericardial surface. This should be half-way between an imaginary line drawn from the left inferior pulmonary vein to the inferior vena cava. The mechanical stabiliser is positioned at the cranial end of the right arm of the sternal retractor, whilst its foot is directed downward toward the base of the heart to stabilise the exposed PDA.

Key Pearls & Pitfalls

- Current indications for off-pump include patients with a very atherosclerotic or heavily calcified aorta
- To adopt the off-pump technique into the repertoire of a cardiothoracic unit it is vital for appropriate patient selection, individualized grafting strategy, peer-to-peer training of the entire team, and graded clinical experience
- Total arterial anaortic off-pump CABG can be achieved by using either a combination of in-situ bilateral mammary arteries (BIMA) only or in-situ BIMA and right gastroepiploic artery or composite grafts using the BIMA and radial artery ('T-graft' and composite extension grafts)
- The activation of coagulation and inflammation caused by cannulation is reduced, thus

off-pump may have the advantage of less bleeding

- Lateral wall coronary arteries – The operating table is positioned in Trendelenburg position at about 20° and rotated towards the right (10–20°) this will allow gravity to displace heart to the right and apex anteriorly as well as increase venous return and facilitate the spontaneous anti-clockwise rotation of the beating heart to the right

Review QS

1. Why many surgeons still prefer on pump CABG surgery compared to off pump?
   a. Requires more challenging technique
   b. **Provides more haemodynamic control**
   c. Avoids SIRs
2. What are the current indications for off pump?
   a. **Very atherosclerotic or heavily calcified aorta**
   b. Significant bleeding
   c. Significant increase in stroke
3. For which patients is off pump surgery more suitable?
   a. Those with higher BP
   b. **Those with significant aortic calcification**
   c. Those with multiple underlying diseases
4. Deep pericardial sutures are placed to create a ridge of pericardium that supports the base of the lateral wall and allows the heart to assume an apex up position. How many and what kind sutures are being used?

a. One or two nylon 2/0 sutures
b. Two polypropylene 2/0 sutures
c. **One or two silk 2/0 sutures**

5. What is the recommended CO_2 flow rate by the assistant throughout the coronary anastomosis?
   a. **Not >5L**
   b. Not <5L
   c. Not > 6L

References

1. Møller CH, Penninga L, Wetterslev J, Steinbrüchel DA, Gluud C. Off-pump versus on-pump coronary artery bypass grafting for ischaemic heart disease. Cochrane Database Syst Rev. 2012 Mar 14;3:CD007224.
2. Afilalo J, Rasti M, Ohayon SM, Shimony A, Eisenberg MJ. Off-pump vs. on-pump coronary artery bypass surgery: an updated meta-analysis and meta-regression of randomized trials. Eur Heart J. 2012 May;33(10):1257–67.
3. Lamy A, Devereaux PJ, Prabhakaran D, Taggart DP, Hu S, Paolasso E, et al. Off-pump or on-pump coronary-artery bypass grafting at 30 days. N Engl J Med. 2012 Apr 19;366(16):1489–97.
4. Halkos ME, Puskas JD. Teaching off-pump coronary artery bypass surgery. Semin Thorac Cardiovasc Surg. 2009;21(3):224–8.
5. Caputo M, Reeves BC, Rogers CA, Ascione R, Angelini GD. Monitoring the performance of residents during training in off-pump coronary surgery. J Thorac Cardiovasc Surg. 2004 Dec;128(6):907–15.
6. Akhrass R, Bakaeen G. The 10 Commandments for Multiarterial Grafting. Innovations: Technology and Techniques in Cardiothoracic and Vascular Surg. 2021 May/Jun;16(3):209.
7. Shahzad GR. Total arterial off-pump coronary revascularization the holy grail? Curr Opinion Cardiol.

Aortic Valve Repair/Replacement

Panagiotis G. Kyriazis, Nikita P. Punjabi,
and Prakash P. Punjabi

Learning Objectives

- Understand how to distinguish the need between AV repair and replacement
- Understand the setup for an aortic valve surgery
- Understand the steps to expose the aortic valve
- Understand different surgical techniques including Nick's, Manouguian and Konno/Rastan procedure to enlarge aortic root
- Understand the difference between the 2-layered and the pericardial patch closure

Introduction

The most common indication for aortic valve replacement in the Western world is degenerative calcified aortic stenosis. In developing countries, rheumatic heart disease remains and continues to be an important indication.

Setup

The approach can be a standard sternotomy or a mini sternotomy incision. The ascending aorta should be cannulated as distally as possible, at or above the pericardial aortic reflection, so as to maximise the space available for subsequent placement of the aortic cross-clamp as well as the aortotomy. A single two-stage venous cannula is placed into the right atrium. Cardiopulmonary bypass is commenced. To optimise visualisation during the operation, a vent may be placed through the right superior pulmonary vein via the left atrium and into the left ventricle. The aortic cross-clamp is applied as close to the aortic cannula as possible. In the absence of significant aortic regurgitation, antegrade cardioplegia may be delivered to arrest the heart prior to aortotomy. Retrograde cardioplegia can also be delivered if desired for continued myocardial protection. This may also be helpful in cases of aortic regurgitation.

Exposing the Aortic Valve

An oblique or transverse aortotomy approximately 15–20 mm above the origin of the right coronary artery is made. An oblique incision may be

P. G. Kyriazis · P. P. Punjabi (✉)
Department of Cardiothoracic Surgery, Hammersmith Hospital, Imperial College Healthcare NHS Trust, London, UK

National Heart and Lung Institute, Faculty of Medicine, Imperial College London, London, UK
e-mail: panagiotis.kyriazis@nhs.net;
p.punjabi@imperial.ac.uk

N. P. Punjabi
Academic Foundation Programme, Imperial College London, London, UK
e-mail: nikita.punjabi1@nhs.net

P. P. Punjabi, P. G. Kyriazis (eds.), *Essentials of Operative Cardiac Surgery*,
https://doi.org/10.1007/978-3-031-14557-5_7

extended into the middle of the non-coronary sinus of Valsalva to increase the exposure or to facilitate subsequent aortic root widening. The incision should stop at least 10 mm from the aortic annulus to facilitate easy placement of sutures and closure of the aortotomy. Pump suction is placed through the aortic valve leaflets to remove blood from the left ventricle. Cardioplegia is given at this stage, directly to the coronary ostia if it has not already been given. Typically, 600–800 ml of cold blood cardioplegia is delivered to the left coronary ostia and 250–400 ml to the right coronary ostia. Stay sutures can be placed on the aorta and an assistant can further retract the aortic wall with a leaflet retractor to maximise exposure.

Decalcification and Excision of Leaflet

The aortic valve leaflets are completely excised and can often be removed intact with the attached calcification. Residual calcification on the aortic annulus is then removed with the help of a Ronguers or similar instrument to crush the calcium, followed by the use of scissors and forceps to cut and remove the calcium. In some cases, the use of a scalpel with a No. 11 blade may be helpful. Removal of all calcium deposits is important to allow proper seating of the valve prosthesis and avoid or reduce the incidence of paraprosthetic leaks.

Care must be taken during leaflet excision and decalcification so that the deeper and surrounding structures of the aortic annulus are not damaged. In general, it is safest to leave a 1-mm rim of leaflet tissue during excision. Any remaining calcium deposits can be subsequently removed. Care must be taken not to perforate the aorta, particularly in the region between the commissure of the non-coronary and left coronary leaflet and the middle of the left coronary leaflet. Other structures at risk include the right and left coronary ostia, the anterior leaflet of the mitral valve which lies below the non-coronary sinus and conduction tissues in the region of the membranous septum around the commissure between the right and non-coronary sinus.

High-powered suction is used throughout the decalcification to remove calcium debris and ensure that these do not enter the coronary ostia or the left ventricle chamber. Placement of a small wet gauze into the left ventricle prior to decalcification can be helpful to catch any calcium deposits which may fall into the left ventricle. A washout with cold saline delivered with a 50 ml syringe is used at the end to flush out and remove any calcium deposits which may have fallen into the left ventricle.

Valve Replacement

The annulus is sized using valve obturators of the desired valve prosthesis. The valve should fit snugly onto the aortic annulus. Too loose a fit would suggest that the patient could benefit from a larger sized prosthesis while too tight a fit would make seating the prosthesis difficult and also risk disruption of the aortic annulus and closure of the aortotomy. In small aortic roots or where patient-prosthesis mismatch may occur, for example, in a large patient with a small aortic root, patch enlargement of the aortic root may be necessary, using either an anterior (Nick's, Manouguian procedure) or a posterior (Konno/Rastan) approach.

Suture Placement

The valve may be replaced by using semi-continuous Prolene sutures or interrupted Ethibond sutures, with or without pledgets. Simple interrupted non-pledgeted sutures and nonpledgeted horizontal mattress sutures have the advantage of allowing a larger sized valve prosthesis to be placed, but at a possible risk of increased paraprosthetic leaks. Semicontinuous suturing techniques are also used, which are quicker to perform, but may be less secure than interrupted techniques.

Our preference is to use interrupted pledgeted horizontal mattress non-absorbable 2/0 sutures (e.g. Ethibond) in all patients undergoing aortic valve replacement for degenerative calcification; semi-continuous sutures may be used in non-calcific aortic regurgitation.

The sutures are placed, starting at the commissure between the non-coronary and left coronary leaflets and moving in a clockwise direction along the left coronary leaflet, the right coronary leaflet and ending at the non-coronary leaflet. A double-ended pledgeted suture is used. The needle passes through the annulus with sufficient depth so as to be secure, but care must be taken to avoid injury to deeper structures with a deeper bite of the suture. The suture must pass through annular tissue and not just through leaflet remnants. The mattress sutures are placed appropriately by applying traction to the preceding suture to facilitate visualisation of the aortic annulus for placement of the next suture. Alternating sutures of two colours (e.g. blue and white) will help identification of each suture pair. The sutures of each sinus are grouped together to allow easy subsequent placement.

An alternative technique is to place everting horizontal mattress sutures where the pledgets are placed above the annulus rather than below it. This technique has the disadvantage of narrowing the aortic annulus, necessitating the use of a smaller sized valve. However, it may be advantageous if the aortic annulus is large or dilated and it may lower the risk of paraprosthetic leaks. It is also technically easier to perform and avoids the risk of a loose pledget in the left ventricle if the suture breaks, either during placement or knot tying.

Once the sutures have been placed around the aortic annulus, they are then passed through the sewing ring of the valve prosthesis, starting with the sutures from the commissure of the right and left coronary sinus and moving towards the commissure of the left and non-coronary sinus, then with the sutures from commissure of the left and right sinus and moving towards the commissure of the right and noncoronary sinus and ending with the sutures from the noncoronary sinus. Care is taken to ensure equal spacing of the sutures.

Securing the Valve

The sutures are held taut and the valve is lowered into the annulus. The sutures may be relaxed as the valve passes into the aorta and the valve is angled through the aortotomy. The sutures are then pulled taut again while supporting the valve prosthesis to ensure a correct placement on the aortic annulus.

The valve holder is then removed. Sutures are tied, starting at the commissure of the non-coronary and left coronary sinus and moving in a clockwise direction along the left coronary sinus and the right coronary sinus and ending at the non-coronary sinus, following the pattern of placement. Sutures should be tied in a direction parallel to the sewing ring to avoid injury to the leaflet tissue. A minimum of five knots are used. The coronary orifices are inspected to ensure that they are not obstructed by the valve or its struts and the valve leaflets are inspected for optimum opening and closure without obstruction.

Aortic Root Enlargement

Nick's Procedure

Nick's (Fig. 7.1) procedure is generally preferred. The aortotomy is extended downwards through the middle of the non-coronary sinus onto the subaortic fibrous curtain (Fig. 7.1a). It is preferable not to cross aortic annulus and into the mitral valve to avoid any disruption of the mitral valve function (Fig. 7.1b). A pericardial patch is then used to close this defect, using continuous 3/0 Prolene (Fig. 7.1c). The valve prosthesis is stitched onto the annulus and either one or two stiches are inserted on the pericardial patch using a pledgeted horizontal mattress suture with the knot tied onto the pledget outside the pericardial patch [1].

Manouguian's Procedure

Alternatively, the Manouguian's (Fig. 7.2) procedure can be used. The aortotomy incision is extended downwards through the commissure between the left and non-coronary sinuses into the inter-leaflet triangle and ending just above the anterior mitral leaflet edge (Fig. 7.2a). There is little fibrous support in this region and the edges of the aortotomy can separate widely. The left atrium is dissected away and may or may not be opened. Depending on the degree of aortic root

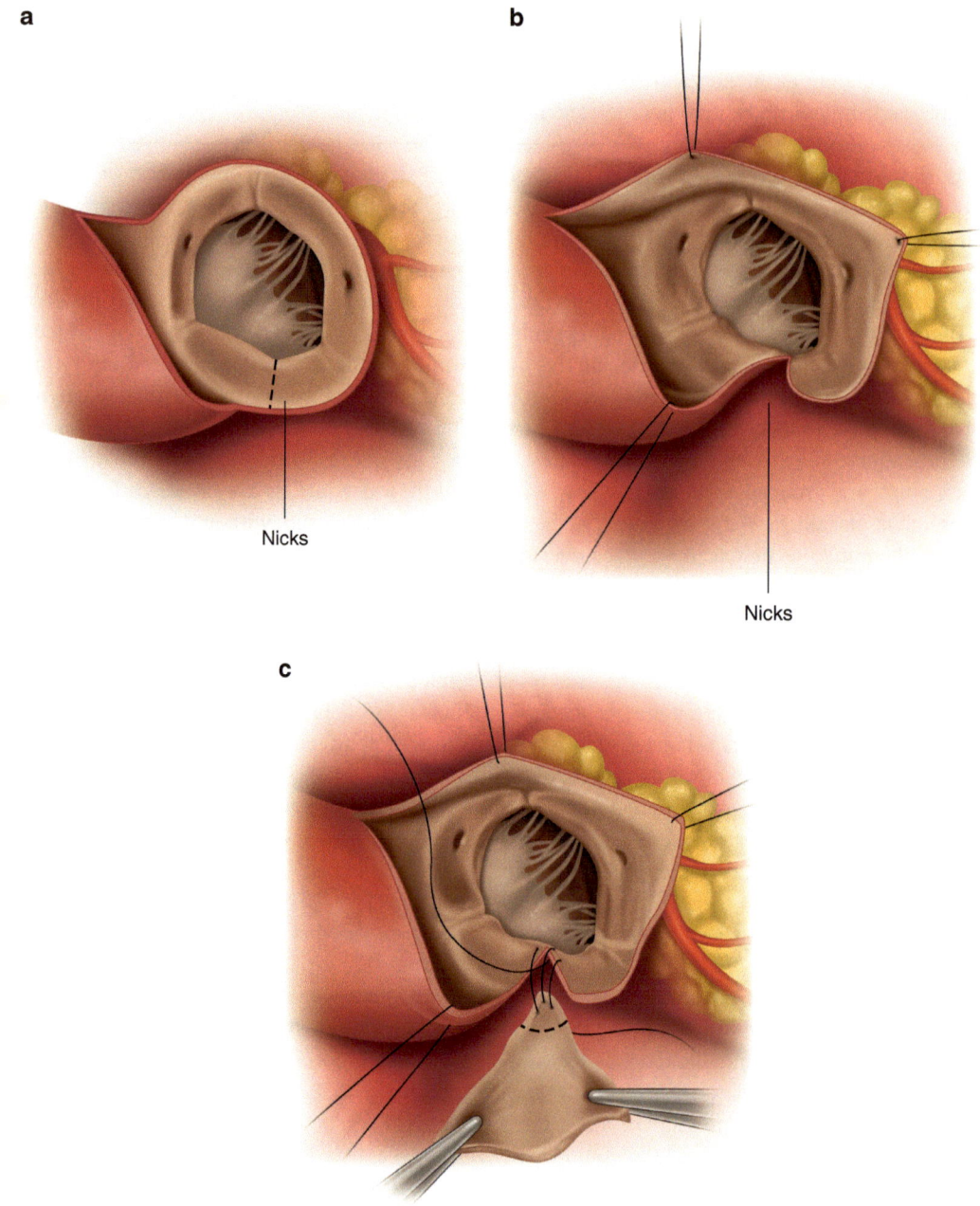

Fig. 7.1 (**a, b, c**) Nick's technique—aortic root enlargement

enlargement needed, some or all of the non-coronary sinus can be excised (Fig. 7.2b). An appropriate sized pericardial/prosthetic patch, usually about 4 cm in diameter, is used to fill the defect created (Fig. 7.2c). A pericardial/prosthetic strip is placed along the incision, outside the aortic wall. Continuous 3/0 Prolene sutures or multiple interrupted horizontal mattress 3/0 Ethibond sutures are then placed through the strip, the aorta and the patch. If the left atrium is opened, this will need to be closed by suturing to the pericardial/prosthetic patch [2].

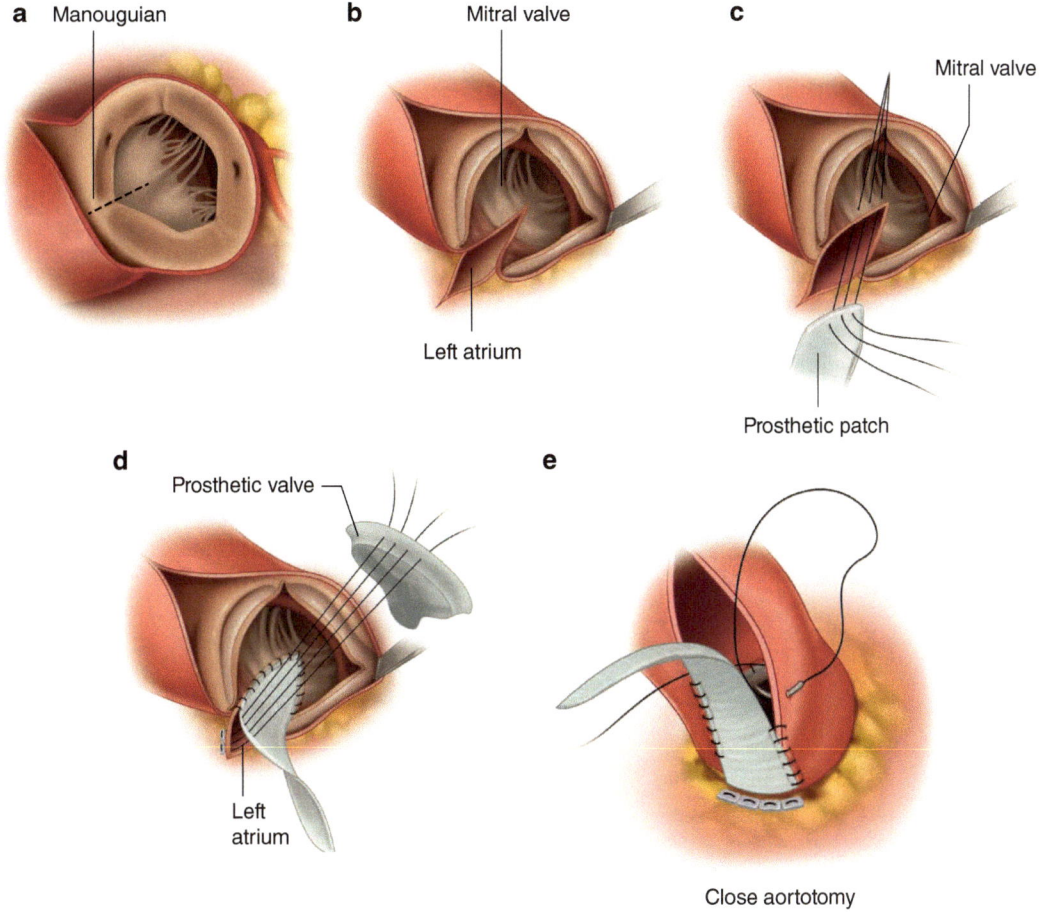

Fig. 7.2 (**a**, **b**, **c**, **d**, **e**) Manouguian technique—aortic root enlargement

The prosthetic valve is then sutured to the patch using interrupted horizontal matress 2/0 Ethibond sutures with the sutures passing through the patch and tied on the outside, supported by pledgets (Fig. 7.2d). The sutures can also pass through the anterior mitral annulus in this region for additional support. The aorta is then closed with the patch (Fig. 7.2e).

Konno/Rastan Procedure

The anterior approach described by Konno/Rastan (Figs. 7.3 and 7.4) is generally used in the paediatric population. A longitudinal aortotomy is made and is extended into the right coronary sinus of Valsalva, as far to the right of the right coronary ostia as possible, but not reaching the commissure between the right and non-coronary sinuses and onto the anterior wall of the right ventricle. The ventricular septum is incised. An appropriately sized oval pericardial patch is then sutured on the right ventricular side of the incised septum, continuing up to the level of the aortic annulus using interrupted pledgeted horizontal matress 3/0 Ethibond sutures. The valve sutures are then placed through the patch as a horizontal mattress suture supported by pledgets, with the knot tied on the outside of the patch. A separate continuous 3/0 Prolene suture is used to stich the patch to the aorta, closing the aortotomy. Another patch is then used to close the right ventricular outflow tract. This is sewn onto the edges of the right ventricular outflow tract and across the first patch at the level of the prosthetic valve, using continuous 3/0 Prolene [3].

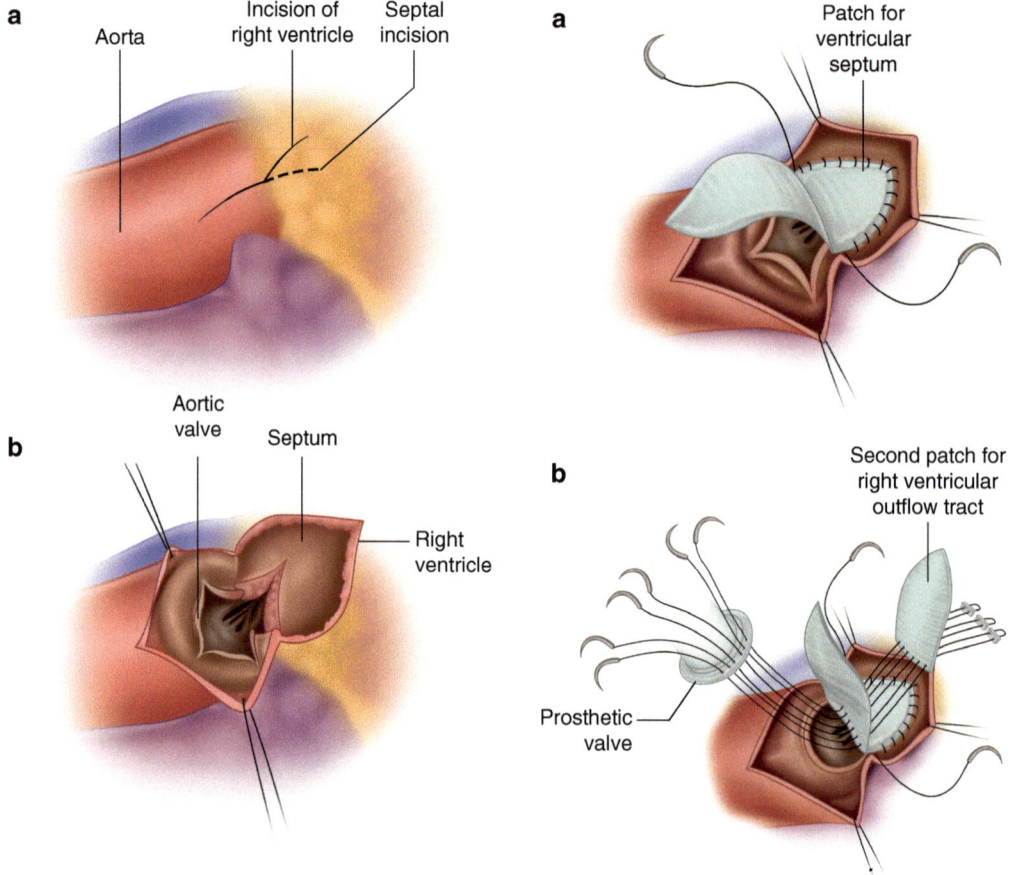

Fig. 7.3 (**a, b**) Konno-Rastan aortoventriculotomy

Fig. 7.4 (**a, b, c, d**) Konno-Rastan aortoventriculoplasty. Patch placement. The left ventricular outflow tract (LVOT) is reconstructed using a diamond-shaped patch, and a second triangular patch is used to widen the right ventricular outflow tract (RVOT). The suture line of the LVOT is continued to the level of the aortic annulus (**a**). Interrupted mattress stitches with Teflon felt pledgets are used to join the RVOT patch to the prosthetic LVOT patch, and the stitches are continued through the prosthetic aortic valve (**b**). The RVOT patch is sewn to the right ventriculotomy with a running 4–0 polypropylene suture. Aortic valve replacement in progress (**c**). Subsequent to Aortic valve replacement, closure of aorta and right ventricular outflow tract (**d**)

c

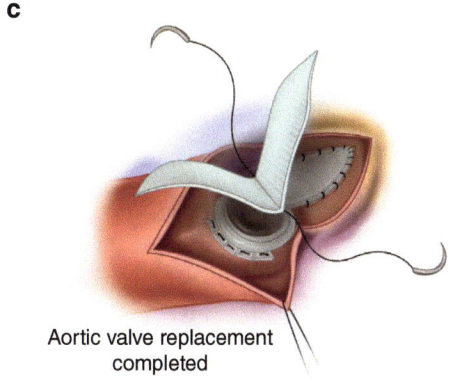

Aortic valve replacement
completed

d

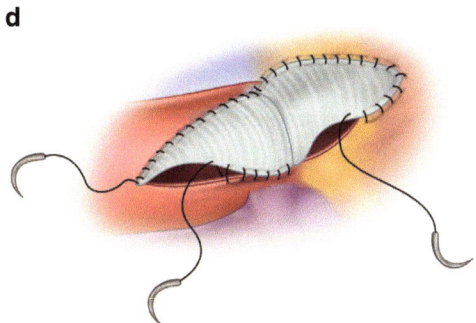

Aortic and right ventricular outflow tract enlarged

Fig. 7.4 (continued)

Aortotomy Closure (2 Layered)

In our technique of aortotomy closure a two-layered closure is used. A double-ended pledgeted 4/0 Prolene suture is used, starting at one end of the aortotomy. An everting horizontal mattress stich is first placed (Fig. 7.5a). Both needles are passed through both edges of the aortic wall about 5 mm apart and 5 mm in depth and another pledget is placed through these and the two ends of the sutures are tied down. A rubbershot clip is applied to one end of the sutures while the other end is used to close the aorta. A continuous horizontal mattress suture is used, approximating the two edges of the aortic wall and everting them. The sutures are placed about 5 mm in depth and moved about 5 mm at a time along the aortic wall. This is continued until about halfway along the aortotomy. The procedure is then repeated, using another double-ended suture, starting at the other end of the aortotomy and moving towards the first suture (Fig. 7.5b). The two ends are then tied in the middle, approximately half way along the aortotomy (Fig. 7.5c). Next, the other remaining sutures at either ends are also sutured towards the centre of the aortotomy over the everted edges such that the second layer is above the horizontal mattress layer; thus, providing more strength and ensuring a better seal (Fig. 7.5d). The two ends are then tied together again (Fig. 7.5e).

If the aortotomy has extended too close to the annulus, it may be necessary to **close the aortotomy using a pericardial patch** (Fig. 7.5). In such cases, it is better to suture the pericardial patch to the aortic wall before lowering the valve prosthesis onto the annulus. If a pericardial patch is not used, it is advisable to place the first stitch for aortotomy closure first before lowering the valve.

Once the second suture has reached the first suture, the aorta is de-aired. The patient is placed in a head-down position, the anaesthetist is asked to inflate the lungs and hold them in inflation, the perfusionist is asked to fill the heart and the aortic cross-clamp is removed. Forceps can be placed in the space between the two sutures to allow the escape of trapped air. The two sutures are then tied together once de-airing is complete. One end of the suture is then used as a continuous suture towards one end of the aortotomy. The depth of the suture should be above the previous horizontal matress suture. The suture is tied to the suture remaining at one end of the aortotomy and the procedure is repeated for the other side of the aortotomy.

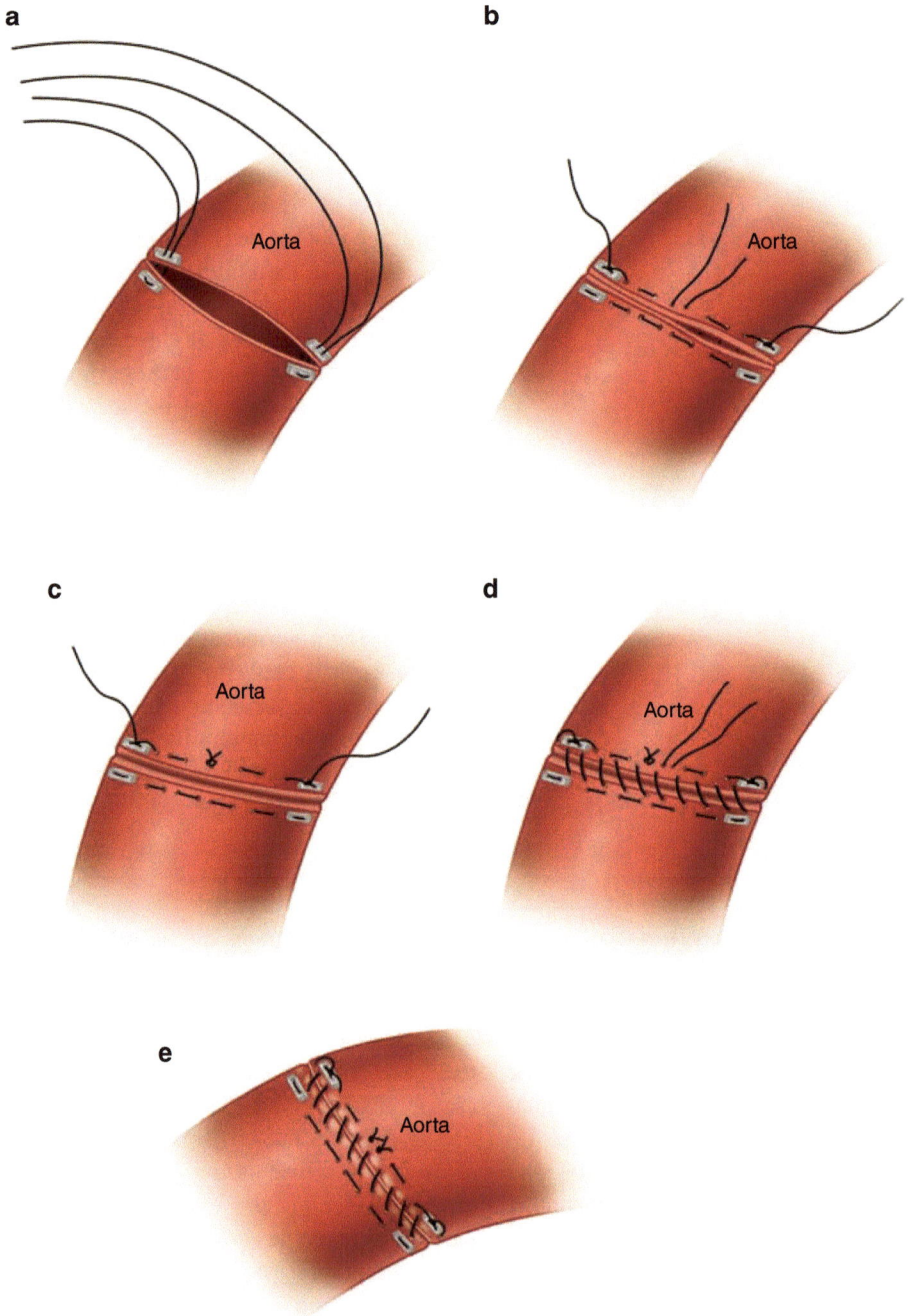

Fig. 7.5 (**a, b, c, d, e**) Aortotomy closure technique (2 layered)

Indications

Patients considering a bioprosthetic AVR have to make a choice between surgical aortic valve replacement (SAVR) and transcatheter aortic valve implantation (TAVI). Patients in higher or prohibited risk for SAVR lean towards TAVI instead of palliative care; however, in patients with lower risk, procedure-specific evaluations will be assessed. In the case where both procedures are available for a patient there is constrain due to lack of durability evidence about TAVI. SAVR is a well-established surgical procedure for over a period of more than 50 years with research data supporting durability for specific valve types among a range of ages compared to TAVI where research extends to only about 10 years. SAVR valve deterioration typically occurs after >10 years, so longer-term TAVI durability data are needed. Age is considered as one of the most important factors in the decision-making process when comparing with life expectancy to known valve. For a woman in the United States, the average additional expected years of life are 25 at age 60 years, 17 at age 70 years, and 10 at age 80 years. For a man, expected additional years of life are 22 at age 60 years, 14 at age 70 years, and 8 at age 80 years. Some younger patients with comorbid conditions have a limited life expectancy, whereas some older patients have a longer-than-average life expectancy. It is believed that decision-making should be individualised on the basis of patient-specific criteria such as quality of life, frailty, dementia and other factors. Also, the decision-making process should focus in accounting the patient's values and preferences offering all the available options for each approach and the potential need for and risks associated with valve reintervention [4].

Key Pearls & Pitfalls
- The ascending aorta should be cannulated as distally as possible, at or above the pericardial aortic reflection, so as to maximise the space available for subsequent placement of the aortic cross-clamp as well as the aortotomy

- An oblique or transverse aortotomy approximately 15-20 mm above the origin of the right coronary artery is made
- An oblique incision may be extended into the middle of the non-coronary sinus of Valsalva to increase the exposure or to facilitate subsequent aortic root widening
- Removal of all calcium deposits is important to allow proper seating of the valve prosthesis and avoid or reduce the incidence of paraprosthetic leaks
- If the aortotomy has extended too close to the annulus, it may be necessary to close the aortotomy using a pericardial patch

Review QS
1) Cardioplegia is given at this stage, directly to the coronary ostia if it has not already been given. Typically, what volume of cold blood cardioplegia is delivered to the left coronary ostia?
   a. **600-800 ml**
   b. 400-600 ml
   c. 250-400 ml
2) Cardioplegia is given at this stage, directly to the coronary ostia if it has not already been given. Typically, what volume of cold blood cardioplegia is delivered to the right coronary ostia?
   a. 600-800 ml
   b. 400-600 ml
   c. **250-400 ml**
3) In Nick's technique a pericardial patch in used to close the defect using what kind of suture?
   a. **3/0 prolene**
   b. 3/0 polypropylene
   c. 3/0 ethibond
4) In Manouguian's procedure, which cardiac chambers are entered into
   a. **Left ventricle and left atrium**
   b. Right ventricle
   c. Right atrium
5) In Konno/Rastan procedure, which cardiac chambers are entered into
   a. Left ventricle
   b. **Right ventricle**
   c. Left atrium
   d. Right atrium

References

1. Grubb KJ. Aortic root enlargement during aortic valve replacement: nicks and Manouguian techniques. Oper Tech Thorac Cardiovasc Surg. 2015;20(3):206–18.
2. Bhutani AK, Gupta CH, Abraham KA, Desai RN, Balakrishnan. Aortic root Enlargement by Manouguian's technique. J Thorac Cardiovasc Surg. 1994;108(4):788.
3. Urganci E, Aliabadi-Zuckermann A, Sandner S, Herbst C, Gokler J. Laufer Gunther and Zimpfer D. The Konno-Rastan procedure Multimedia manual of cardiothoracic surgery. 2019; https://doi.org/10.1510/mmcts.2019.017.
4. Otto CM, Nishimura RA, Bonow RO, Carabello BA, Erwin JP III, Gentile F, Jneid H, Krieger EV, Mack M, McLeod C, O'Gara PT, Rigolin VH, Sundt TM III, Thompson A, Toly C. 2020 ACC/AHA guideline for the Management of Patients with Valvular Heart Disease: a report of the American College of Cardiology/American Heart Association joint committee on clinical practice guidelines. Circulation. 2021;143:e72–e227.

Surgery for Mitral Valve Disease: Degenerative Repair

Philip Hartley, Panagiotis G. Kyriazis, and Prakash P. Punjabi

Learning Objectives

- Pathophysiology of mitral valve disease and its relation to surgical strategies for treatment of the mitral valve.
- Surgical approaches to the mitral valve and principles of setting up a mitral valve surgery case.
- Techniques for reconstruction of the posterior and anterior mitral valve leaflets.
- Adjuncts to leaflet resection including use of neochordae and annuloplasty in the treatment of mitral regurgitation.

P. Hartley
Department of Cardiothoracic Surgery, Hammersmith Hospital, Imperial College Healthcare NHS Trust, London, England, UK
e-mail: philip.hartley1@nhs.net

P. G. Kyriazis · P. P. Punjabi (✉)
Department of Cardiothoracic Surgery, Hammersmith Hospital, Imperial College Healthcare NHS Trust, London, England, UK

National Heart and Lung Institute, Faculty of Medicine, Imperial College London, London, England, UK
e-mail: panagiotis.kyriazis@nhs.net;
p.punjabi@imperial.ac.uk

Pathophysiology

Degenerative disease affecting the mitral valve is the commonest cause of mitral regurgitation requiring surgical intervention in Western countries. Myxomatous degeneration leads to elongation or rupture of the chords and consequently the development of severe mitral regurgitation. Mitral regurgitation may also be caused by other pathologies which directly affect the structure of the valve including endocarditis and rheumatic valve disease.

Mitral regurgitation may also occur where the valve is structurally normal but leaflet coaptation is inhibited by abnormalities in the surrounding structures. Dilation of the left atrium secondary to chronic atrial fibrillation or left ventricle due to ischaemic cardiomyopathy alters the balance between the closing force experienced by the valve during systole and tension in the subvalvular apparatus, preventing leaflet coaptation.

In primary mitral regurgitation valve failure is due to structural abnormalities of the valve or subvalvular apparatus itself. Surgical strategies for repair of the mitral valve correspondingly focus restoring coaptation of the valve leaflets by restoring the functional anatomy of the leaflets, annulus and chords. Symptomatic severe primary mitral regurgitation or asymptomatic severe primary mitral regurgitation in the context of left ventricular failure are Class I indications for surgery [1]. Mitral valve repair in this context remains the gold standard treatment and is preferred to valve replacement due to improved mortality, morbidity and post-operative left ventricular function. In secondary, or functional mitral regurgitation, where the valve is structurally normal, the indications for surgery are less well established. Mitral valve repair is usually reserved for patients undergoing concurrent coronary artery bypass surgery.

Rheumatic mitral valve disease is the commonest mitral valve lesion seen in developing countries. Chronic leaflet thickening and calcification leads ultimately to fusion of the commissures and stenosis of the mitral valve. Restriction in the movement of the valve leaflets may give a mixed picture of stenosis and regurgitation. Severe symptomatic mitral stenosis is an indication for percutaneous mitral commissurotomy with surgery the preferred option where unsuitable valve anatomy prohibits percutaneous intervention. Repairing mitral valves affected by rheumatic disease is challenging and for patients with severe symptomatic mitral stenosis mitral valve replacement is typically the best surgical option.

In addition to chronic disease processes which may affect the mitral valve, acute valve failure may also lead to severe mitral regurgitation. This may occur due to papillary muscle rupture following myocardial infarction or due to leaflet perforation in endocarditis. Sudden failure of the mitral valve causes acute volume overload of the left ventricle. Without the compensatory dilation of the left atrium and ventricle seen in chronic severe mitral regurgitation cardiogenic shock results. These patients are invariably symptomatic and require urgent mitral valve replacement.

Setup

Access to the mediastinum is gained through either a midline sternotomy or a minimally invasive approach using a right anterior thoracotomy.

In cases where a minimally invasive incision is preferred, cannulation of the femoral artery and vein is typically used for initiation of cardiopulmonary bypass. If a midline sternotomy incision is used, however, the aorta is cannulated directly followed by bicaval venous cannulation. Once cardiopulmonary bypass has been established the aorta is cross clamped and an antegrade cardioplegia line is inserted to allow for cold blood cardiolplegia to be delivered through the aortic root. Further cardioplegia is then delivered approximately every 20 minutes using a retrograde cardioplegia line, while venting the aortic root, or through the existing antegrade cardioplegia line.

Surgical Access to the Mitral Valve

Left Atriotomy

The pericardium is elevated on the right side and an incision of the pericardium perpendicular to the superior vena cava is made. This has the effect of rotating the heart upwards and towards the surgeon bringing the mitral valve into view once the left atrium is opened. An incision is made immediately posterior to the interatrial groove and extended inferiorly through the posterior wall of the left atrium (Fig. 8.1a and b). Retraction of the atrial wall using a Cosgrove retractor allows for optimisation of this view. Excessive retraction may distort the normal anatomy of the mitral valve and complicate its assessment prior to repair and risks damaging the left atrial wall especially if the tissue here is friable.

Transeptal Approach

A transeptal approach may be preferred for access to the mitral valve particularly if concomitant tricuspid valve surgery is indicated or a small left atrium would provide inadequate visualisation. The right atrium is opened using a vertical incision from the right atrial appendage to the

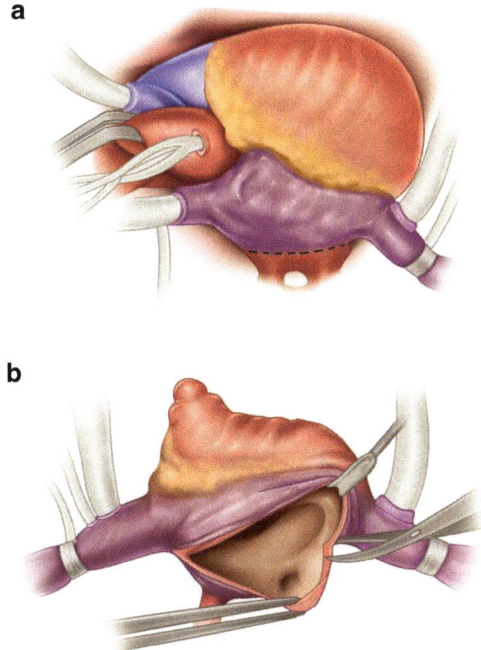

Fig. 8.1 (**a**) Position of left atriotomy. (**b**) Extension of atriotomy onto the posterior wall of the left atrium

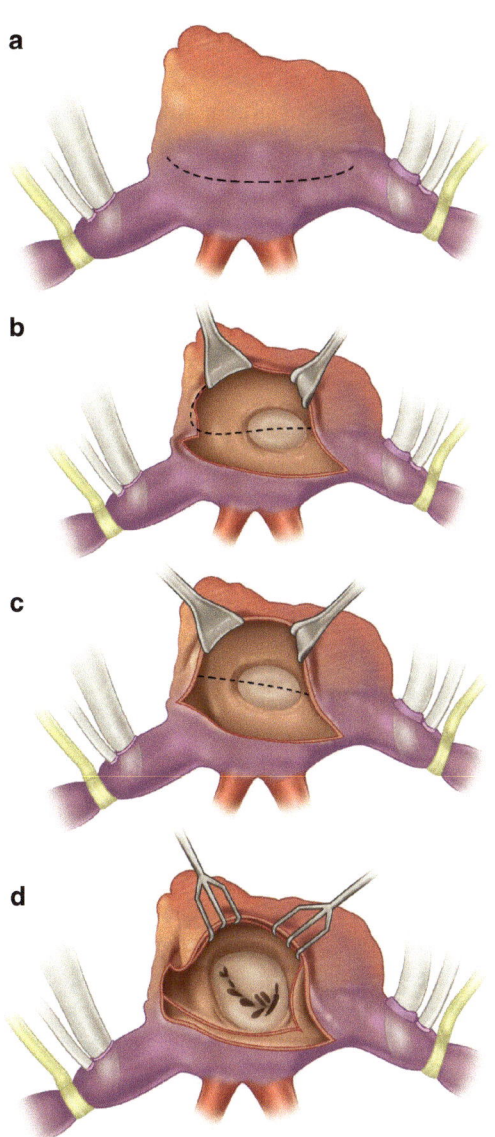

interatrial septum. Alternatively, an incision 2 cm superior and parallel to the interatrial groove is made and extended to the junction of the left atrium. The septum is then excised horizontally at the lower edge of the foramen ovale and extended superiorly to join the right atrial incision. The incision may be extended onto the roof of the left atrium as far as the base of the left atrial appendage to optimise exposure (Fig. 8.2). The mitral valve can then be visualised using a retractor placed on the septum or by using a stay suture.

Fig. 8.2 Transseptal approach (**a**) A position of right atriotomy (**b**) extension of incision onto the roof of the left atrium (**c**) Septal incision (**d**) Exposure of the mitral valve

Assessing the Mitral Valve

Once the mitral valve is adequately exposed a systematic assessment of the mitral valve is performed. A pair of nerve hooks are used to sequentially interrogate the range of motion of the leaflets determining if each anatomical division is normal (type I), prolapsed (type II), restricted opening (type IIIa) or restricted closure (type IIIb) [2]. The annulus and subvalvular apparatus should also be assessed at this stage to determine the integrity of the chords and their papillary muscle attachments. These findings are correlated with the expected anatomy of the valve as determined by preoperative echocardiography.

Planning the preferred surgical strategy based on the morphology and pathophysiology of mitral valve disease is crucial in performing a successful repair. Multi-segment prolapse, disease secondary to infective endocarditis or primary systolic anterior motion lesions are more likely to represent challenging surgical repair than isolated single segment prolapse.

Reconstruction of the Posterior Leaflet

The principle of mitral leaflet repair is to restore the surface of coaptation between the anterior and posterior leaflets. In posterior leaflet repair this can be achieved through several techniques which involve excision of the prolapsing portion of the leaflet.

The Mi-P Repair (Fig. 8.3)

T 'P' repair is inspect-respect-incise and repair or resect and repair. The 'P' repair is dominantly applicable to P2 prolapse, which is the most common lesion affecting degenerative mitral regurgitation. The principle being that the height and the width have to be appropriately reduced. Various other methods also exist, triangular excision, quadrangular excision etc. These are described later, but what we have found most appropriate and useful is simply to make an incision at the point of the maximum prolapse of the leaflet.

Subsequently, suture the two ends of the cut leaflet in such a way that we reduce the width by incorporating the leaflet edges below the left atrial surface on the ventricular side and over suture around the edge of the P2 incised leaflet and reduce the height.

The main principle, benefit and advantage of this technique is that you maintain a good amount of mobility of the posterior leaflet and the risk of fixing the posterior leaflet is almost minimised or negated. Most of the times, we have found that you can do more than one site of incise and repair,

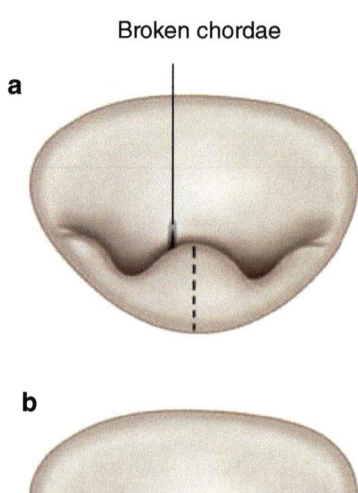

Broken chordae

a

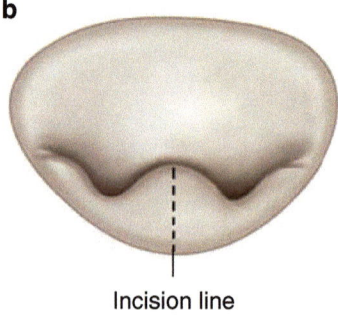

b

Incision line

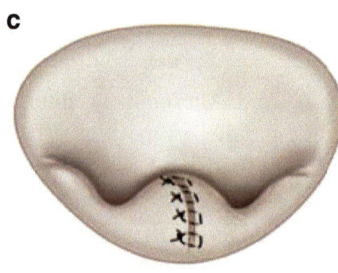

c

Fig. 8.3 Mi-P repair (**a**) Excision of broken chord (**b**) Incision (**c**) Repair

if need be. Should there be uneven prolapse leaflets or either end of the leaflet or in different parts of the valve in P1, P2, P3 and sometimes on the A2 segment, multiple incisions and repairs can be done.

Leaflet excision is almost never necessary. However, in a small minority of cases, there is a necessity to reduce the height and width by excision of repair. In that case, we follow the inspect-respect, resect. This has been our principle technique with good results over the last 10 years.

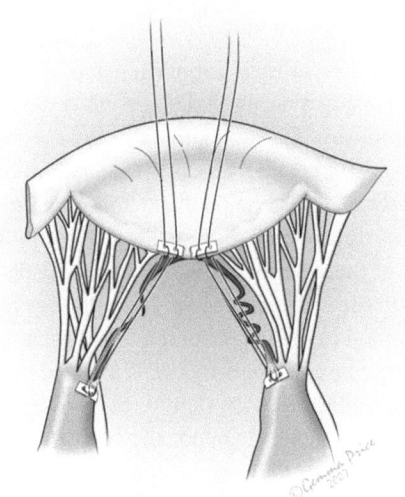

Fig. 8.4 Artificial Neocirdae

Quadrangular Repair

Alternatively, the prolapsed leaflet segment can be resected in a quadrangular fashion prior to re-approximation of the leaflets (Fig. 8.4). The posterior annulus at the base of the resection can be reduced in length using two or three interrupted sutures to decrease tension in the final repair. In cases where it is necessary to excise a large portion of leaflet tissue a sliding plasty to facilitate leaflet approximation may be required.

Triangular Repair

In cases where excision of the affected leaflet portion using a quadrangular or 'P' excision would leave insufficient leaflet tissue for a competent repair a triangular excision may be used. This simplifies the repair by avoiding annular re-approximation.

Reconstruction of the Anterior Leaflet

Anterior leaflet repair is typically more challenging than repair of the posterior leaflet. Our preferred method is incision and repair or a triangular resection of the prolapsing portion of the anterior leaflet combined with resuspension of the anterior leaflet using artificial neochordae. Although the technique described for artificial neochordae implantation is applied to the anterior leaflet it may be generalised for use in the repair of any prolapsed portion of the mitral valve. All repairs whether incision or resection repair are supported by insection of at least two neochordae with at least 1 on each papillary muscle.

Artificial Neochordae

In this technique the elongated or ruptured native chords to the anterior leaflet are functionally replaced using 5/0 Gor-Tex neochordae (Fig. 8.4). The prolapsed portion of the anterior leaflet is identified and the papillary muscle to which the neochordae should be attached is chosen. The pledgeted neochordae is placed through the fibrous tip of the papillary muscle, locked on itself and passed in the direction to which the leaflet is prolapsing. Equal distribution of length, and therefore tension, in the completed neochordae repair is ensured by leaving the neochordae untied at its attachment to the papillary muscle.

The neochordae is then passed through the prolapsing leaflet portion from below at the site of attachment of the pathological native chord and reinforced with a pledget. The stitch is then passed around the edge of the mitral valve leaflet, through it and the pledget again. The required length of the neochordae is estimated by approximating the free edge of the anterior leaflet onto the anterior annulus [3]. Alternatively, the anterior leaflet is retracted into apposition with the posterior leaflet using nerve hooks, bringing the remaining native chords into tension. The length of the neochordae is then adjusted to match that of the adjacent healthy native chords before locking the neochordae on itself and fixing the length of the neochoardae. If the Gor-Tex suture is not correctly locked it will be shortened as the neochordae are pulled up during tying leading to over correction of the prolapsing leaflet segment and restricted opening of the valve resulting in residual mitral regurgitation.

More recently strategies for the placement of neochordae using minimally invasive techniques have been developed. This has benefited patients with severe degenerative mitral regurgitation for whom conventional cardiac surgery and use of cardiopulmonary bypass is prohibitively high risk. The NeoChord system, for example, allows placement of neochordae through the apex of the left ventricle following a left anterior thoracotomy [4]. The prolapsed mitral valve portion is grasped by the artificial chords using live transoesphageal echocardiography images. The length of the neochordae are then optimised to minimise or eliminate mitral regurgitation before fixing their length.

Use of Native Chords

Other techniques have been described using the native chords to restore the normal tethering function on the mitral valve leaflets. Although good long-term results have been reported using native chord mitral valve repair the involvement of the chords in the pathophysiology of mitral regurgitation remains a concern, particularly in degenerative mitral valve disease.

Chordal Transposition

In chordal transposition elongated or ruptured chords of the affected prolapsed mitral valve segment are reinforced by transposition of adjacent healthy chords. In anterior leaflet repair chords from the opposing posterior leaflet are commonly detached in the 'flip-over' technique. A segment of the posterior leaflet is resected with associated primary chords. This is then attached to the anterior leaflet and secured using Prolene sutures. The resulting defect in the posterior leaflet must then be repaired using one of the techniques described above. Alternatively, chords may be transposed from an adjacent anterior leaflet segment.

Papillary Muscle Repositioning

The papillary muscle supporting the chords of the prolapsing anterior leaflet are cut vertically at the fibrous tip. The cut papillary muscle, to which the chords are attached, is then sutured more inferiorly on the same papillary muscle. The distance moved should be equal to the prolapsed height of the anterior leaflet to accurately correct the prolapse. The degree of correction is therefore limited to the length of the papillary muscle. Papillary muscle repositioning is avoided in ischaemic papillary muscle rupture as necrotic muscle will be unable to anchor the repositioned tip of papillary muscle.

Neochordae is our favoured technique and the advantage is by not utilising any native diseased or seemingly undiseased native cords.

Annuloplasty

Mitral regurgitation is almost invariably associated with a degree of annular dilatation. Reinforcement of the annulus reduces the tension on leaflet repairs and prevents subsequent dilation of the annulus. Routine annuloplasty, with either band or ring support, is therefore important in providing a durable mitral valve repair. In functional mitral regurgitation due to ischaemia or dilated cardiomyopathy, it also serves to restore the normal size and shape of the mitral annulus. For a small cohort of patients mitral annuloplasty may be used in isolation.

Band Annuloplasty

In most cases of degenerative mitral valve disease our preferred approach is to use band annuloplasty (Fig. 8.5). Band annuloplasty, where only the posterior annulus is reinforced, maintains the native 3-dimensional dynamics of the mitral valve, which are at least partially restricted when a complete ring is used. During systole, the

Fig. 8.5 (**a, b, c**) Band Annuloplasty

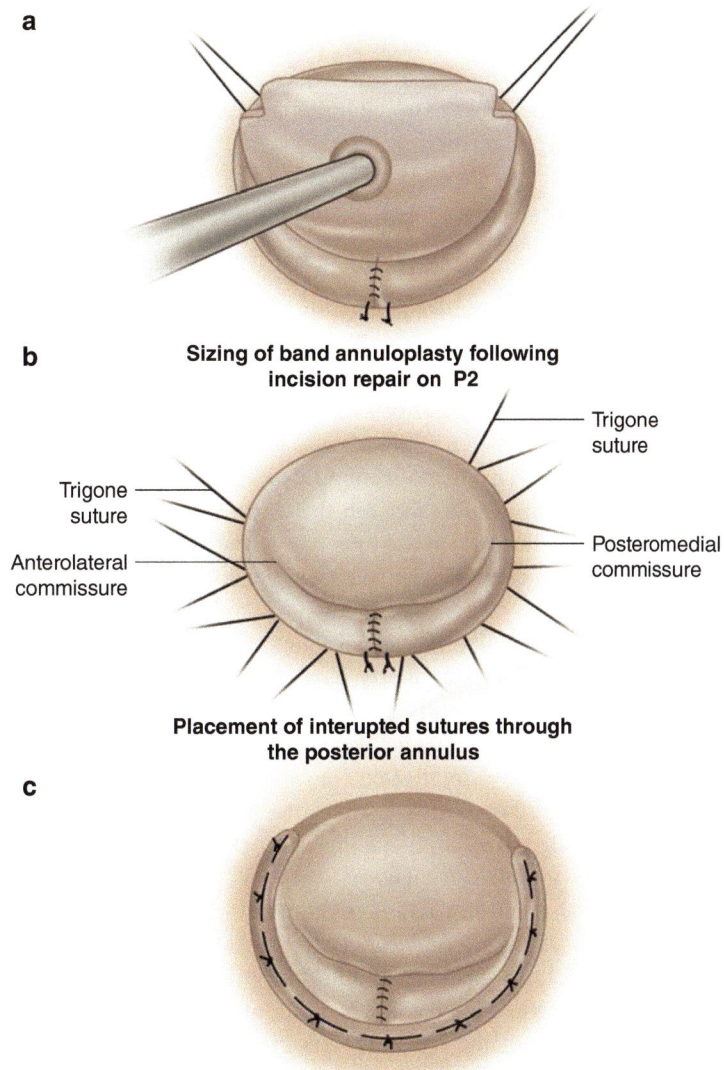

a

Sizing of band annuloplasty following incision repair on P2

b

Trigone suture

Trigone suture

Anterolateral commissure

Posteromedial commissure

Placement of interupted sutures through the posterior annulus

c

Incomplete band annuloplasty implant

mitral annulus moves towards the apex of the left ventricle and reduces in size while, during diastole, it recoils back towards the left atrium and increases in size [5]. Pressure from the aortic root also pushes the anterior leaflet posteriorly helping to close the valve during systole, an effect which is lost by the use of ring annuloplasty.

The size of the band is determined using the inter-trigonal distance matched against the supplied manufacturer's sizers. The trigone is located just above the commissures and is seen as a dimple, especially when the anterior leaflet is pulled towards the posterior leaflet (Fig. 8.5a). Interrupted, non-pledgeted sutures are placed around the posterior annulus and through the band, starting at each fibrous trigone (Fig. 8.5b, c). Failure to anchor the band at each trigone will prevent the band appropriately reinforcing the posterior annulus. The band may then be lowered onto the annulus, sutures tied and scaffolding supporting the band removed. If resection of a posterior leaflet segment has been performed sutures are placed either side of the excised leaflet portion, and not across it, to minimise tension across the completed repair.

Ring Annuloplasty

Several types of ring are available with varying degrees of rigidity and corresponding restriction in the movement of the mitral valve annulus. Insertion of a complete rigid or semi-rigid ring annuloplasty fixes the size of the annulus in systole restricting the normal physiological movement of the mitral annulus through the cardiac cycle. Even a flexible ring inhibits the movement of the annulus more than an equivalent band annuloplasty.

However, ring annuloplasty may be appropriate for some patients, particularly those undergoing mitral valve repair surgery due to functional mitral regurgitation, where annular dilatation is directly implicated in valvular incompetence. In these cases, a rigid or semi-rigid ring which is two sizes smaller than the measure inter-trigonal distance is used. For example, if the mitral annulus is sized at 30, a size 28 or 26 ring is used. An undersized ring annuloplasty helps to restore the mitral annular size and leaflet coaptation leading to good long-term performance of the repaired valve. In the case of functional ischaemic mitral regurgitation under sizing the mitral valve annulus additionally helps correct leaflet restriction often seen at P3, or less commonly P2.

The technical steps for placement of a ring are similar to those of a band with the interrupted sutures extended to include the anterior annulus. Careful spacing of sutures is required to account for the different sizes of the ring and native annulus and allow for an equally distributed compressive effect of the annuloplasty.

Assessing the Valve Repair

Following a completed mitral valve repair the line of leaflet coaptation should be symmetrical at least 6-8 mm and follow the curve of the posterior annulus. The competency of the repaired mitral valve is tested with a methylene blue pen. The valve should be able to withstand a reasonable pressure with no more than trace mitral regurgitation. Additionally, the area of leaflet coaptation can be assessed using an 'ink test'. The line of closure between the valve leaflets is marked. Saline is then aspirated from the left ventricle and the leaflet tissue beyond the marked closure line represents the area of coaptation between the leaflets. At least 6 mm of leaflet tissue in coaptation with the opposing leaflet is indicative of a competent mitral valve repair.

Once the patient is weaned from cardiopulmonary bypass physiological assessment of the valve can be performed by trans-oesphageal echocardiography. If significant regurgitation is still evident at this stage a second run on bypass with further repair or replacement of the valve is indicated.

Key Pearls & Pitfalls

- Mitral regurgitation may also occur where the valve is structurally normal but leaflet coaptation is inhibited by abnormalities in the surrounding structures
- Mitral valve repair in this context remains the gold standard treatment and is preferred to valve replacement due to improved mortality, morbidity and post-operative left ventricular function
- Severe symptomatic mitral stenosis is an indication for percutaneous mitral commissurotomy with surgery the preferred option where unsuitable valve anatomy prohibits percutaneous intervention

- In a midline sternotomy incision, the aorta is cannulated directly followed by bicaval venous cannulation
- T 'P' repair is inspect/respect and resect with respect

Comprehension Questions

1. In functional (or secondary) mitral regurgitation abnormalities in which of the following structures may lead to valvular incompetence?
   (a) Subvalvular apparatus
   (b) Valve leaflets
   (c) Trigones
   (d) **Left ventricle**
   (e) Commissures
2. A transeptal approach to the mitral valve may be preferred if which of the following is true?
   (a) Small right atrium
   (b) **Concomitant tricuspid valve surgery is to be performed**
   (c) Difficult arterial cannulation
   (d) Friable atrial tissue
   (e) Difficult venous cannulation
3. Which of the following mitral valve lesions is likely to be present the simplest surgical repair?
   (a) Bi-leaflet prolapse
   (b) Leaflet perforation due to infective endocarditis
   (c) Primary systolic anterior motion
   (d) Leaflet calcification in rheumatic valve disease
   (e) **P2 prolapse**
4. Which of the following statements regarding the use of neochordae is true?

   (a) Provide a less durable repair than the use of native chords
   (b) **Should approximate the length of healthy native chords**
   (c) Are suitable for attachment to ischaemic papillary muscle tissue
   (d) Should not be locked before tying
   (e) Use prolene suture material
5. Which of the following approaches to annuloplasty causes the least restriction in the physiological movement of the mitral valve during the cardiac cycle?
   (a) Semi-rigid ring annuloplasty two sizes smaller than the inter-trigonal distance
   (b) Semi-rigid ring annuloplasty sized by the inter-trigonal distance
   (c) Rigid ring annuloplasty two sizes smaller than the inter-trigonal distance
   (d) Rigid ring annuloplasty sized by the inter-trigonal distance
   (e) **Band annuloplasty**

References

1. Falk V, et al. 2017 ESC/EACTS guidelines for the management of valvular heart disease. Eur J Cardiothorac Surg. 2017;
2. Carpentier A, et al. Reconstructive surgery of mitral valve incompetence: ten-year appraisal. J Thorac Cardiovasc Surg. 1980;79(3):338–48.
3. Punjabi PP, Chan KMJ. Technique for chordae replacement in mitral valve repair. Ann Thorac Surg. 2012;94(6):2139–40.
4. Colli A, et al. Transapical NeoChord mitral valve repair. Ann Cardiothorac Surg. 2018;7(6):812–20.
5. Ormiston JA, Shah PM, Tei C, Wong M, Section C. Size and motion of the mitral valve annulus in man a two-dimensional echocardiographic method and findings in normal subjects. Circulation. 1981 Jul;64(1):113–20.

Surgery for Mitral Valve Disease: Degenerative Replacement

9

Philip Hartley, Panagiotis G. Kyriazis, and Prakash P. Punjabi

Learning Objectives

- Indications for mitral valve replacement.
- Technique for mitral valve replacement.
- Structures at risk and complications of mitral valve replacement.

Indications for Mitral Valve Replacement

Where mitral valve surgery is indicated, valve repair should be preferred to valve replacement in most cases. Valve repair is associated with improved operative survival, post-operative left ventricular function and avoids the complications from a prosthetic valve [1]. Notably prosthetic endocarditis, thromboembolism and increased risk of haemorrhagic events due to long term anti-

P. Hartley
Department of Cardiothoracic Surgery, Hammersmith Hospital, Imperial College Healthcare NHS Trust, London, England, UK
e-mail: philip.hartley1@nhs.net

P. G. Kyriazis · P. P. Punjabi (✉)
Department of Cardiothoracic Surgery, Hammersmith Hospital, Imperial College Healthcare NHS Trust, London, England, UK

National Heart and Lung Institute, Faculty of Medicine, Imperial College London, London, England, UK
e-mail: panagiotis.kyriazis@nhs.net;
p.punjabi@imperial.ac.uk

coagulation. Mitral valve repairs have also been demonstrated to have comparable durability compared to mechanical mitral valve replacement.

Where a durable repair is not possible, however, mitral valve replacement is indicated with preservation of the subvalvular apparatus. The chords and papillary muscles play an important role in supporting the function of the left ventricle and their resection during mitral valve replacement is linked with poorer postoperative left ventricular function. [2] Where surgical replacement is indicated for severe mitral stenosis, typically in rheumatic valve disease, it is not usually possible to preserve the subvalvular apparatus due to extensive calcification.

Choice of Prosthesis

A number of mechanical and biological prostheses are approved for mitral valve replacement. Mechanical valves do not suffer from structural degeneration although pannus formation on the valve occasionally necessitates reintervention. Additionally the use of a mechanical valve requires lifelong anticoagulation with associated risks of bleeding and thromboembolic events. Biological valves avoid the risks of anticoagulation but structural failure of the valve may require reintervention.

The choice of prosthesis should therefore be made following an individualised assessment of

© Springer Nature Switzerland AG 2022
P. P. Punjabi, P. G. Kyriazis (eds.), *Essentials of Operative Cardiac Surgery*,
https://doi.org/10.1007/978-3-031-14557-5_9

the risks and benefits in consultation with the patient. In patients below the age of 65 and without contra-indications for anticoagulation a mechanical prosthesis is a reasonable choice. In specific incidences such as women of child bearing age or where anticoagulation is high risk a biological prosthesis may be preferred.

Technique for Mitral Valve Replacement

Setup and exposure of the mitral valve is the same as described in the preceding chapter.

The mitral valve annulus is sized with the maximum diameter prosthesis chosen that fits loosely into the annulus. Interrupted, everting, pledgeted, horizontal mattress sutures are placed through the annulus from the left atrial side such that the pledgets sit on the atrial side of the annu-

lus (Fig. 9.1). The posterior mitral valve leaflet can usually be retained, together with its subvalvular attachments, by folding the leaflet tissue on to itself as these sutures are taken. This will not interfere with the function of the valve prosthesis and preservation of the chords optimises postoperative left ventricular function.

For the anterior leaflet it is necessary to resect the smooth portion of the leaflet using an elliptical incision to ensure the leaflet does not obstruct the prosthetic valve. Care must be taken to preserve the primary chords at their attachment to the free edge of the leaflet during this step. The resulting rim of tissue at the free edge of the leaflet can be reattached to the anterior annulus using the horizontal mattress sutures and incorporated into the suture line for the valve prosthesis. In cases where the valve leaflets are extensively diseased it may be necessary to resect them together with the subvalvular

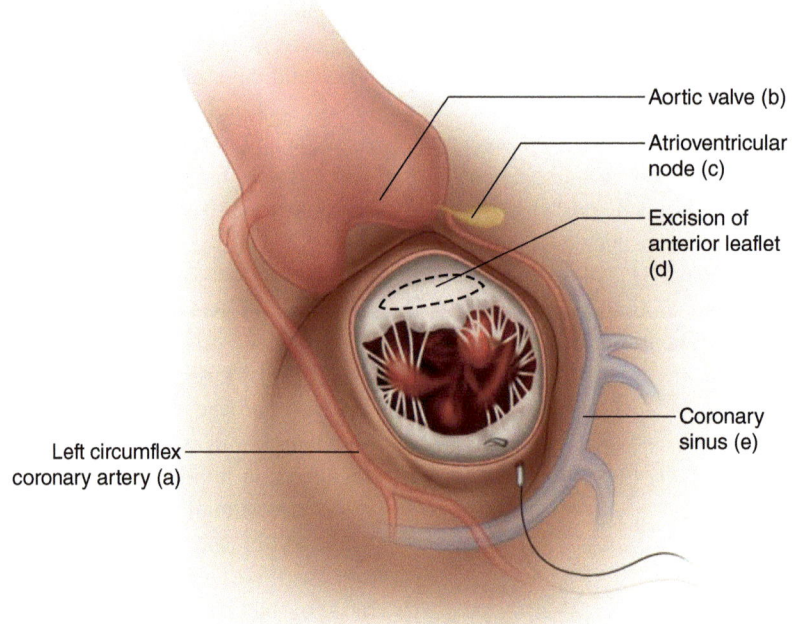

Fig. 9.1 Horizantal/interrupted everting 2.0 ethibond pledgeted sutures placed around the mitral valve annulus avoiding important anatomical structures i.e., (**a**) left circumflex coronary artery, (**b**) aortic valve, (**c**) atrioventricualr node, (**d**) excision of anterior leaflet, (**e**) coronary sinus. (A) Sutures placed around the posterior mitral valveMitral Valve annulus as well as part of the posterior leaflet allowing preservation of the posterior subvalvular apparatus (B) Dotted lines indicate the area of excision of the anterior leaflet of the mitral valve to allow preservation of the anterior subvalvular apparatus minimising the impact of the size of replacementReplacement as well as preserving the subvalvular apparatus

apparatus leaving a healthy rim of leaflet tissue for the placement of sutures.

A number of structures are at risk as sutures are taken through the mitral valve annulus and deep bites risk damaging them. The left circumflex artery passes through the atrioventricular groove adjacent to the mitral valve annulus at 6–9 o'clock. The coronary sinus also follows the course of the posterior mitral valve annulus and is at risk between 4–6 o'clock. At 10–12 o'clock the non-coronary cusp of the aortic valve may be incorporated into sutures taken through the mitral valve annulus. Finally, the atrio-ventricular node and associated artery may be damaged by injudicious sutures taken at 2 o'clock.

Once all the sutures have been placed around the annulus, they are passed through the valve ring from below upwards so that when tied the knots lie on the left atrial side of the valve. The valve is lowered onto the annulus, sutures tied and scaffolding supporting the valve released. The orientation of the prosthesis has a significant effect on the flow dynamics across the valve and in the left ventricle (Fig. 9.2). Bi-leaflet mechanical valves are commonly implanted in the anti-anatomical position (perpendicular to the line of leaflet coaptation of the native valve) and mono-leaflet prosthesis with the larger orifice orientated posteriorly. This helps to minimise disruption to physiological blood flow and maintain left ventricular geometry.

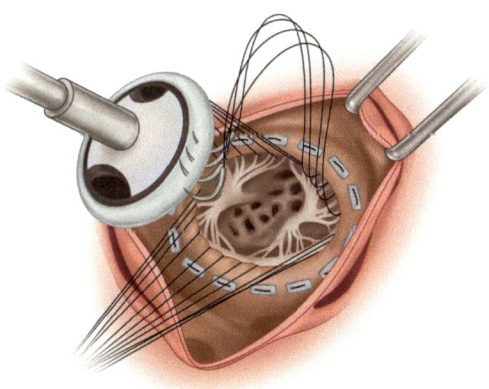

Fig. 9.2 Mitral valve replacement

Calcification of the mitral valve annulus or valve leaflets themselves present a particular hazard during mitral valve replacement. Whilst removing as much calcium as possible allows for the maximum sized prosthesis to be well-seated on the annulus it also risks damaging the annulus, atrioventricular dehiscence, or damage to the left circumflex artery. For this reason, removal of calcium should be performed with care and where an acceptable replacement can be achieved without aggressive decalcification this should be completed.

Injury to the atrioventricular groove may be caused by decalcification of the posterior annulus or forcing too large a sizing ring or prosthesis into the mitral valve annulus. This injury may not be noticed until weaning the patient from bypass and the mediastinum fills with blood. Cardiopulmonary bypass should be reinstituted before cardioplegic arrest. The extent of the injury can then be assessed, and a pericardial patch repair attempted. It may be necessary to remove the prosthetic mitral valve and reimplant a smaller prosthesis during repair.

Key Pearls & Pitfalls

- Valve repair is associated with improved operative survival, post-operative left ventricular function and avoids the complications from a prosthetic valve
- Where a durable repair is not possible, however, mitral valve replacement is indicated with preservation of the subvalvular apparatus
- The choice of prosthesis should therefore be made following an individualised assessment of the risks and benefits in consultation with the patient
- The orientation of the prosthesis has a significant effect on the flow dynamics across the valve and in the left ventricle
- Removal of calcium should be performed with care and where an acceptable replacement can be achieved without aggressive decalcification this should be completed

Comprehension Questions

1. Which of the following is not a reason mitral valve repair is favoured over mechanical valve replacement where technically possible?
   (a) Greater durability following surgery
   (b) Lower operative mortality
   (c) Improved left ventricular function
   (d) **Lower incidence of prosthetic endocarditis**
   (e) Lower incidence of anticoagulation related haemorrhage
2. Which of the following statements is correct regarding the placement of a mitral valve replacement?
   (a) The annulus should be sized with progressively smaller sizing ring
   (b) Pledgeted sutures should be placed through the annulus such that the pledgets lie on the ventricular side of the annulus
   (c) Complete decalcification is always required to result in a well-seated valve prosthesis

   (d) The most common mechanical prosthesis is a trileaflet valve
   (e) **A rim of leaflet tissue is helps to provide a secure attachment for the valve prosthesis**
3. Which of the following structures is not at risk as sutures are taken through the mitral valve annulus?
   (a) Atrioventricular node
   (b) Coronary sinus
   (c) Left circumflex artery
   (d) Non-coronary cusp of the aortic valve
   (e) **Left main stem**

References

1. Thourani VH, et al. Outcomes and long-term survival for patients undergoing mitral valve repair versus replacement: effect of age and concomitant coronary artery bypass grafting. Circulation. 2003;108(3):298–304.
2. Natsuaki M, et al. Importance of preserving the mitral subvalvular apparatus in mitral valve replacement. Ann Thorac Surg. 1996;61(2):585–90.

Post Ischemic Mitral Regurgitation

10

Alessio Giuseppe Vite, Panagiotis G. Kyriazis, and Marco Moscarelli

Abbreviations

aPPM: Papillary muscles approximation
CABG: Coronary artery bypass grafting
IMR: Ischemic mitral regurgitation
LV: Left Ventricular
LVEF: Left ventricular ejection fraction
rPPM: Papillary muscle relocaction

Learning Objectives

- Understand the principles of surgery for mitral valve disease in ischaemic repair
- Understand the pathophysiology leading to mitral valve insufficiency requiring surgery

- Understand the importance of following guidelines in regards to treatment
- Understand the different surgical techniques used in ischemic mitral regurgitation
- Understand the combination of papillary muscle intervention in combination with mitral ring annuloplasty

Introduction

Myocardial infarction is one of the leading causes of death worldwide. Beyond the acute mechanical complications (nowadays reduced with the advent of primary angioplasty), it is clear the pathophysiological evolution that affects the left ventricle which in some cases generates a "new valvulopathy" of the mitral valve. Mitral regurgitation is the second valve disease requiring surgery after the aortic one. The role of left ventricular (LV) longitudinal contraction in ischemic mitral regurgitation (IMR) remains unclear. We hypothesized that reduced longitudinal contraction disrupts normal mitral valve plane displacement during systole and leads to mitral valve tethering, thereby inducing IMR [1]. Mitral valve regurgitation is a major source of morbidity and death worldwide and a frequent cause of heart failure, with complications that include arrhythmia, endocarditis, and sudden cardiac death [2, 3]. Structural deficiencies in the mitral valve and secondary changes induced by abnor-

A. G. Vite (✉)
Papardo Hospital, Messina, Italy

P. G. Kyriazis
Department of Cardiothoracic Surgery, Hammersmith Hospital, Imperial College Healthcare NHS Trust, London, England, UK

National Heart and Lung Institute, Faculty of Medicine, Imperial College London, London, England, UK
e-mail: panagiotis.kyriazis@nhs.net

M. Moscarelli
Anthea Hospital, Bari, Italy
e-mail: m.moscarelli@imperial.ac.uk

mal ventricular size and deformation are implicated in the development of these valvular desease. However, the effect of mitral regurgitation on cardiac function is more than purely mechanical, whereby pump function is maintained at the expense of elevated filling pressures, but extends to impaired contractility and electrical instability. In this chapter we will focus on secondary, post ischemic mitral insufficiency with particular attention to surgical indications and the new repair techniques.

Ischemic Mitral Valve: Pathophysiological Evolution

Mitral regurgitation can occur due to disease of the mitral valve leaflets and/or abnormalities of the mitral valve apparatus or secondary to left ventricular dysfunction. Functionally the mitral valve apparatus consists of several components: [4–6]:

The mitral annulus
The anterior and posterior mitral valve leaflets
The chordal
The anterolateral and posteromedial papillary muscles
The left ventricular myocardium underlying the papillary muscles

Dysfunction or altered anatomy of any of these components can lead to mitral regurgitation. The mechanism of mitral regurgitation may be described as primary or secondary. Primary mitral regurgitation, sometime called degenerative or organic, is due to an intrinsic lesion of the mitral valve apparatus. Secondary mitral regurgitation, sometimes called functional or ischemic, is a disease of the left ventricle; the left ventricular remodeling in dilated cardiomyopathy or the segmental wall motion abnormalities in ischemic cardiomyopathy, can displace the papillary muscles apically and laterally, causing tethering and malcoaptation of the mitral valve leaflets, which leads to secondary mitral regurgitation. The most important scholar of mitral regurgitation (MR) was Carpentier from whom we inherit a schematic and effective classification about MR.

Carpentier type I mitral regurgitation: It is characterized by a normal motility of the leaflets with an associated dilation of the mitral ring; less frequently it is due to a perforation of the flaps in the course of endocarditis. Due to the dilation of the ventricle in the course of dilated myocardiopathy which causes subsequent dilation, especially in the posterior flap, generating a mitral regurgitation characterized by central jet in the echocardiographic examination [7].

Carpentier type II mitral regurgitation: It is characterized by an increased motility of the tendon cords and a consequent increase in the motility of leaflets or leafleats only. The most common cause of primary mitral regurgitation is degenerative mitral valve disease [8, 9].

Carpentier type III mitral regurgitation: It is divided in IIIa type: is characterized by reduced motility of the leafleats during systolic and diastolic excursions. It is usually caused by rheumatic disease or as a result of radiation therapy [10, 11]. III b type: reduced motility during systole, this picture is caused by myocardial ischemia and remodeling of the left ventricle [12, 13] which causes dislocation of the papillary muscles and failure of leafleats. Coaptation. Our interest is focus on type I and type III b; in this chapter we are analyzing mitral regurgitation caused by myocardial ischemic events that cause above all ventricular dysfunction with all the associated pathophysiological mechanism, characterized by: ischemic event, ventricular dilation, mitral annular dilation, displacement of papillary muscles and consequent alteration of coaptation mitral valve leafleats generating mitral regurgitation.

Surgical Indications

Ten years ago as reported in the ESC guidelines, as reported in table 10.1., in course of CABG and LVEF (left venticular eiection fraction) > 30% there is an indication to treat functional mitral valve disease with an **I C** indication only in severe regurgitation. It must always be remembered the functional mitral valve disease is a pathology affecting the left ventricle and the mitral subvalvular apparatus that affects the pap-

Table 10.1. Indications

	Class[a]	Level[b]
Surgery is indicated in patients with severe MR[c] undergoing CABG, and LVEF >30%.	I	C
Surgery should be considered in patients with moderate MR undergoing CABG[d]	IIa	C
Surgery should be considered in symptomatic patients with severe MR, LVEF <30%, option for revascularization, and evidence of viability.	IIa	C
Surgery may be considered in patients with severe MR, LVEF >30%, who remain symptomatic despite optimal medical management (including CRT if indicated) and have low comorbidity, when revascularization is not indicated.	IIb	C

CABG coronary artery bypass grafting; *CRT* cardiac resynchronization therapy; *LVEF* left ventricular ejection fraction; *MR* mitral regurgitation; *SPAP* systolic pulmonary artery pressure
[a]Class of recommendation
[b]Level of evidence
[c]The thresholds for severity (EROA ≥20 mm2; R Vol.30 ml) differ from that of primary MR and are based on the prognostic value of these thresholds to predict poor outcome. d When exercise echocardiography is feasible, the development of dyspnoea and increased severity of MR associated with pulmonary hypertension are further incentives to surgery

illary muscles and the tendon cords, so technically if a timely revascularization of still vital areas of the left ventricle is performed, the performance of the left ventricle and consequentially of the mitral valve apparatus could improve. In light of the above, we were limited to treating only severe mitral valve insufficiencies.

Surgery should be considered in symptomatic patients with severe MR, LVEF <30%, option for revascularization, and evidence of viability, (IIa C).

Surgery may be considered in patients with severe MR, LVEF >30%, who remain symptomatic despite optimal medical management (including CRT Cardiac resynchronization therapy, if indicated) with low comorbidity, when revascularization is not indicated (IIb C).

2012 Guidelines about ischemic mitral regurgitation:

Indications for mitral valve surgery in chronic secondary mitral regurgitation.

The new guidelines 2021 have changed, and the new role of mitral clip.

Colors correspond to Table 10.2. *Chordal-sparing MV replacement may be reasonable to choose over downsized annuloplasty repair. AF indicates atrial fibrillation; CABG, coronary artery bypass graft; ERO, effective regurgitant orifice; GDMT, guideline-directed management and therapy; HF, heart failure; LVEF, left ventricular ejection fraction; LVESD, left ventricular end-systolic dimension; MR, mitral regurgitation; MV, mitral valve; PASP, pulmonary artery systolic pressure; RF, regurgitant fraction; RVol, regurgitant volume; and Rx, medication.

As reported in Table 10.1. is important to evaluate the LVEF, the symptoms and the echocardiographic data of the patient, in addition to the comorbidities from which patient. After a careful evaluation according to guideline-directed management and therapy and the evaluation of heart failure specialists and after diagnosis of mitral regurgitation stage D it is necessary to evaluate: regurgitant volume > 60 ml, the regurgitant fraction>50% with an ERO (effective regurgitant orifice) if these parameters are present and the patient is indicated to CABG for the treatment of valvulopathy and indicated as **II a (as reported in** Table 10.2): Chordal-sparing MV replacement may be reasonable to choose over downsized annuloplasty repair. If we are faced with mitral regurgitation stage D, regurgitant volume > 60 ml, the regurgitant fraction>50% with an ERO > 0.40 cm^2 in patients who have no indication for CABG it will be necessary to evaluate LVEF that: if ≥50% in front of a patient undergoing drug therapy according to guideline-directed management and therapy and the persistence of symptoms and AF (atrial fibrillation) will be indicated for MV surgery with indication **II b**. If we are faced with mitral regurgitation stage D, regurgitant volume > 60 ml, the regurgitant fraction>50% with an ERO > 0.40 cm^2 in a patient who has no indication for CABG and LVEF <50% in front of a patient undergoing drug therapy according to guideline-directed management and therapy and persistent symptoms will be indicated

Table 10.2 Class of recommendation and level of evidence

CLASS (STRENGTH) OF RECOMMENDATION	LEVEL (QUALITY) OF EVIDENCE‡
CLASS 1 (STRONG) Benefit >>> Risk	**LEVEL A**

Suggested phrases for writing recommendations:
• Is recommended
• Is indicated/useful/effective/beneficial
• Should be performed/administered/other
• Comparative-Effectiveness Phrases†:
  – Treatment/strategy A is recommended/indicated in preference to treatment B
  – Treatment A should be chosen over treatment B
	• High-quality evidence‡ from more than 1 RCT
	• Meta-analyses of high-quality RCTs
	• One or more RCTs corroborated by high-quality registry studies

	LEVEL B-R (Randomized)
CLASS 2a (MODERATE) Benefit >>> Risk	• Moderate-quality evidence‡ from 1 or more RCTs • Meta-analyses of moderate-quality RCTs

Suggested phrases for writing recommendations:
• Is reasonable
• Can be useful/effective/beneficial
• Comparative-Effectiveness Phrases†:
  – Treatment/strategy A is probably recommended/indicated in preference to treatment B
  – It is reasonable to choose treatment A over treatment B
	LEVEL B-NR (Nonrandomized)

	• Moderate-quality evidence‡ from 1 or more well-designed, well-\ executed nonrandomized studies, observational studies, or registry studies • Meta-analyses of such studies
	LEVEL C-LD (Limited Data)
CLASS 2b (WEAK) Benefit >>> Risk	• Randomized or nonrandomized observational or registry studies with limitations of design or execution • Meta-analyses of such studies • physiological or mechanistic studies in human subjects
Suggested phrases for writing recommendations: • May/might be reasonable • May/might be reasonable • Usefulness/effectiveness is unknown/unclear/uncertain or not well-established	**LEVEL C-ED** (Expert Opinion)
	• Consensus of expert opinion based on clinical experience
CLASS 3:No Benefit (MODERATE) Benefit >>> Risk (Generally, LOE A or B use only)	COR and LOE are determined independently (any COR may be paired any LOE)
Suggested phrases for writing recommendations: • Is not recommended • Is not indicated/useful/effective/beneficial • Should not be performed/administered/other	A recommendation with LOE C does not imply that the recommendation is weak, Many important clinical questions addressed in guidelines do not lend themselves to clinical trials. Although RCTs are unavailable, there may be a very clear clinical consensus that a particular test or therapy is useful or effective.
CLASS 3: Harm(STRONG) Risk > Benefit	• The outcome or result of the intervention should be specified (an improved clinical outcome or invreased diagnostic accuracy or incremental prognostic information.
Suggested phrases for writing recommendations: • Potentially harmful • Causes harm • Associated with excess morbidity/mortality • Should not be performed/administered/other	† For comparative-effectiveness recommendations (COR 1 and 2a; LOE A and B only), studies that support the use of comparator verbs should involve direct comparisons of the treatments or strategies being evaluated.
	‡ The method of assessing quality is evolving, including the application of standardized, wisely-used, and preferably validation evidence grading tools; and for systematic review, the incorporation of an Evidence Review Committee.
	COR indicates Class of Recommendation; EO, expert opinion; LD, limited; LOE, Level of Evidence; NR, nonrandomized; R randomized; and RCT, randomized controlled trial.

for the edge-to-edge MV repair (mitral clip) trans catheter with indication 2a only if: favorable valve anatomy, if LVEF between 20 and 50%, if LVESD < or = a 70 mm and if PASP < or = 70 mmHg (when exercise echocardiography is feasible, the development of dyspnoea and increased severity of MR associated with pulmonary hypertension are further incentives to surgery). If there is no favorable anatomy with the above data and a severely symptomatic patient, an indication is given to MV surgery with indication 2b.

World Scenario and Surgical Techniques

Ischemic mitral regurgitation is a condition characterized by mitral regurgitation secondary to an ischemic left ventricle. Primarily, the pathology is the result of perturbation of normal regional left ventricular geometry combined with adverse remodeling [14].

Although the surgical treatment of severe chronic ischemic mitral regurgitation (IMR) in patients presenting for CABG is recommended by the American College of Cardiology/American Heart Association guidelines, the surgical approach remains an open issue [15, 16]. Many investigators advocated mitral valve restrictive annuloplasty (RA), meanwhile others have suggested mitral valve replacement [17–19]. Investigators supporting a conservative approach believe that conservation of the continuity between the valve and left ventricle lead to better long-term results and a reverse in left ventricular (LV) remodeling. Nowadays the choice of prosthetic ring is still debated, although there is a global consensus about the use of complete ring instead a band. In contrast, many surgeons prefer mitral valve replacement using a biologic prosthesis with subvalvular apparatus sparing to avoid recurrent MR. In fact, the incidence of recurrent MR after isolated RA was 5% to 30% in several reports [20–22]. A superior repair with decreased recurrence of mitral regurgitation and enhanced reversal of left ventricular remodeling is possible when subvalvular techniques are combined with traditional ring annuloplasty. Further understanding of preoperative parameters that predict disease recurrence and inclusion of concomitant subvalvular techniques in this subset of patients will be the next major advance in this field [23].

Recent techniques of annular (annuloplasty) and subanular mitral valvuloplasty will be reported below. As regards the techniques for preparing the patient using CEC, the choice of the surgical approach and the surgical exposure of the valve, we can say that they are more or less comparable to those reported in the previous chapter (Chap. 5 Mitral valve surgery). In this chapter, in order to avoid unnecessary repetitions, we will limit ourselves to presenting the specific surgical techniques concerning mitral valve plastics with particular attention to subanular techniques.

Prosthetic Ring Choice

During annuloplasty it is important to have a correct surgical exposure both to evaluate the condition of the valve system and to correctly measure the size of the mitral ring. Using a nerve hook, it is recommended to stretch the anterior mitral flap in an antero-posterior direction and compare it to the anterior flap area using the appropriate measuring devices; other surgeons prefer to evaluate the intercommissural distance (between the anterolateral and postero-medial commissures).

There are several types of rings available with differences in materials used, 2D and 3D shape, complete or semi-complete, rigid, semi-rigid, or flexible (Fig. 10.1). For simplicity, these are often referred to as rigid or flexible rings [24].

The rationale for using flexible rings in degenerative MV disease is based on the preservation of the dynamic systolic-diastolic motion of the mitral valve annulus and its role in the contractile performance of the left ventricle. Undersized annuloplasty ring proves to be an effective technique for the treatment of IMR. For K. Fattouch et al semirigid complete annuloplasty ring was related with lower PAPs and mean transvalvular gradient at rest and under stress compared with rigid saddle shape rings [16]. Better tenting parameters were observed in the semirigid ring group that led to better clinical outcomes and lower recurrency of mitral regurgitation. Moreover, lower postoperative posterior angle and coaptation depth were observed.

The standard surgical treatment of chronic IMR is CABG associated with undersized annuloplasty using complete ring. Though, the recurrence of mitral regurgitation remains high (> 30%) because of continous left ventricle remodeling. To get better long term results, in the last decade, several subvalvular procedures in adjunct to mitral anuloplasty have been developed. Among them, surgical papillary muscle relocation represents the most appreciated option

FLEXIBLE E-INCOMPLETE

SEMI-RIGID-COMPLETE

RIGID-COMPLETE

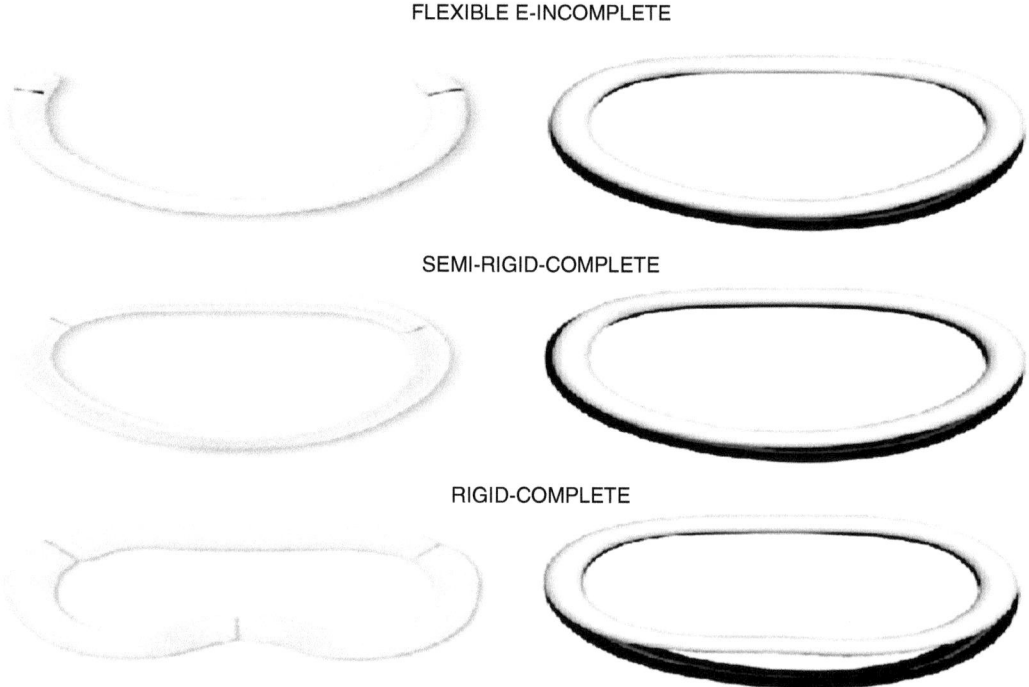

Fig. 10.1 *Different mitral annular ring.* (University of Texas at Austin|UT· Department of Aerospace Engineering & Engineering Mechanics)

capable to restore normal left ventricle geometry. In the next future new preoperative predictors of increased mitral regurgitation recurrence are certainly needed to find an individual time period of treatment in each patient with moderate IMR [25].

Subannular Repair

In the last decade, several investigators proposed different surgical techniques to add to mitral valve annuloplasty to improve the long-term repair results. As previously reported, the ischemic event leads to segmental motility alterations of the left ventricle. The phenomenon of left ventricular remodeling leads to an alteration of the harmonic structure of the left ventricle and consequently of the mitral valve apparatus, which is a constituent part of the left ventricle in a harmonic mechanism of correct systolic-diastolic functioning. The subversion of this harmonic structure leads to the alteration of the mitral valve

functioning, with phenomena of displacement of the papillary muscles, an increase in the tension of the tendon cords and poor coaptation of the mitral flaps which is the basis of post ischemic mitral regurgitation. It is therefore important to integrate the echocardiographic data (width of the ring, length of the tendon cords, position of the papillary muscles) and the anatomical inspection aspect of the mitral valve in order to perform the correct surgical procedure in order to improve the outcome of mitral valve repair. Below we will report the main mitral reparative surgery techniques associated with the most common reparative annuloplasty technique.

Papillary muscle (rPPM) relocation: The main pathophysiological factor of chronic secondary mitral regurgitation (sMR) is the outward displacement of the papillary muscles (PPM) leading to leaflet tethering. For this reason, papillary muscle intervention (PPMi) in combination with mitral ring annuloplasty (RA) has been introduced into clinical practice to correct this displacement, and to reduce the recurrence of mitral regurgitation [24]. Micali et al., showed that MR recurrence in patients undergoing both PPMs intervention and mitral repair annuloplasty was lower than in those who only had mitral repair annuloplasty [24].The group with both PPMi and RA and that with only RA showed a slightly higher reduction in left ventricular diameters. However, in both groups, LV reverse remodelling was <10%. No difference was detected between PPM relocation/repositioning and papillary muscle approximation in terms of LV reverse remodelling [24]. PPM relocation was first reported by Kron et al. [21] and subsequently widely used by our team consist in passing a 3.0 or 4.0 Prolene or Gore-Tex suture twice through the fibrous portion of the posterior papillary muscle tip; usually the anterior and the posterior head of the posterior PPM were both relocated. Each needle of the double-armed suture is then passed up through the adjacent mitral annulus just to the right fibrous trigone or posterior annulus close to P3 segment. In some cases anterior PPM should be relocated and suture then passed to left trigone. Adjustment of the amount of PPM relocation may be performed intra- operatively under LV feeling with saline solution (Fig. 10.2).

As reported by Jensen et al. [26] the relocation of both papillary muscles as adjunct procedure to downsized ring annuloplasty reduces significantly the distance from the posterior papillary muscle to the anterior trigone compared with RA at end-diastole (−7.9% versus 3.8%, P < 0.01) and end- systole (−9.7% versus 2.5%, P = 0.02); accordingly, lateral tethering of the coaptation point was reduced significantly more (P < 0.01). K. Fattouch et al. [27] reported reversal in LV remodeling measured by change in LVEDD (left ventricular end diastolic diameter) and LVESD (left ventricular end systolic diameter) significantly observed in patients treated with PPM relocation (p < 0.05). Postoperative mean tenting area was 1.1 ± 0.2cmq and postoperative mean coaptation depth was 0.5 ± 0.2 cm, with significant reduction respect to patients underwent isolated RA. As regard the follow up data, we report a cumulative survival at 5 years of 91 ± 1.3% after PPMs relocation plus mitral annuloplasty,

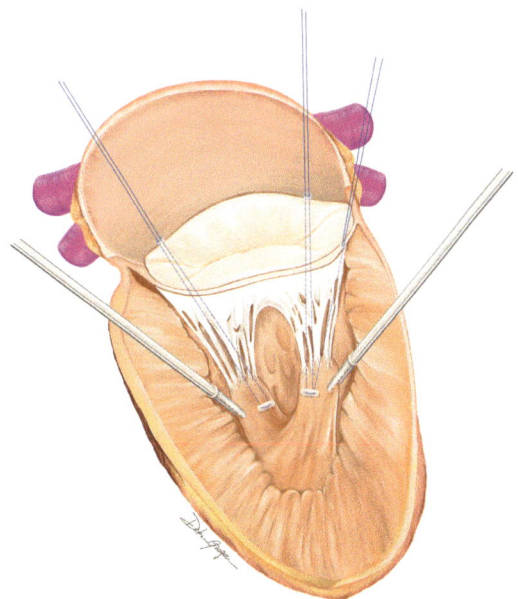

Fig. 10.2 Papillary muscles relocation (rPPM): before placing an annuloplasty ring, the adjunct repair is performed by passing a 3.0 or 4.0 Prolene suture twice through the fibrous portion of the posterior papillary muscle tip; usually the anterior and the posterior head of the posterior PPM were both relocated. Each needle of the double-armed Prolene suture is then passed up through the adjacent mitral annulus just posterior to the right fibrous trigone

five-years freedom from cardiac-related death rate is 91.3 ± 1.6%, five years freedom from cardiac-related events is 84 ± 2.2%, five-years freedom from recurrent MR ≥2 is 97.3 ± 1.1%. Another technique used by our center is the papillary muscle approximation (aPPM) as a variant (Figs. 10.3 and 10.4) where the structural alteration of the left ventricle leads to a dislocation of the papillary muscles, moving away from each other. It is important to calculate the correct approximation distance of the two muscles in order not to generate new thetering phenomena that could cause valve insufficiencies.

Below we report another subanular technique that concerns the tendon cords: in this technique the evaluation of the length and the relationships between the first and second order cords is important.

Chordal cutting: reduced leaflet tethering by chordal cutting in the chronic post-MI setting substantially decreases the progression of LV

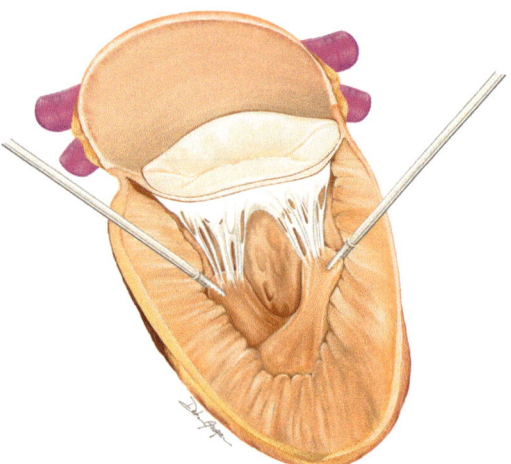

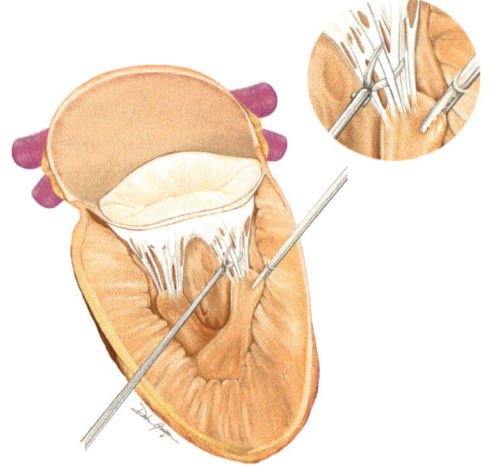

Fig 10.3 Papillary muscle (PPM) approximation: *we can see the dilation of the left ventricle with the consensual displacement of the papillary muscles*

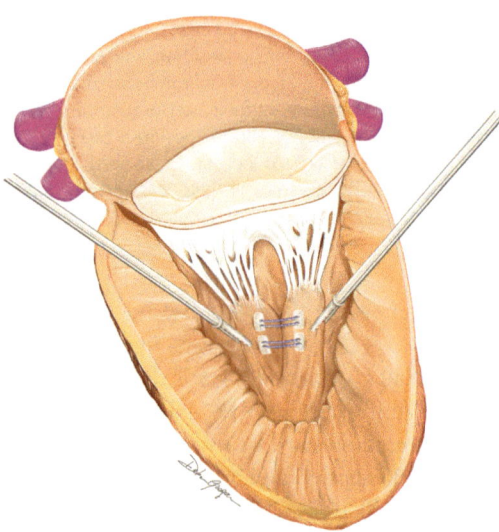

Fig. 10.4 Papillary muscles approximation (aPPM): *two pladjected 4-0 prolene suture are passed into the bodies of both papillary muscles with the aim of bringing the papillary muscles together in the correct position*

Fig. 10.5 chordal cutting technique: *we can see the chordal cutting: cutting a limited number of basal chordae can improve coaptation and reduce leaflets tethering; eliminating secondary chordae in the anterior leaflet can allow the leaflets to assume a more normal and less taut configuration, with more effective coaptation at their free margin*

availability as a strategy to relieve iMR. Quantification of the mitral valve annulus to papillary muscle tip distance may be useful in proper selection of patients for this procedure in the clinical setting [28] Chordal cutting is one such procedure, which has been met with resistance due to the potential for disruption of valvular- ventricular continuity and concern for progressive left ventricular remodeling. However, these procedures target the secondary chordae and leave the basal and marginal chordae intact, thereby preserving valvular-ventricular continuity. In one recent study, addition of bileaflet secondary chordal cutting to reduction annuloplasty resulted in increased leaflet mobility, which significantly decreased the severity of recurrent mitral regurgitation. Importantly, reversal in left ventricular remodeling was observed without adverse effect on left ventricular function [29]; this study showed that concomitant bileaflet secondary chordal cutting (Fig. 10.5) results in decreased severity of recurrent mitral regurgitation and is associated with reversal of remodeling without an adverse impact on left ventricular function. Chordal cut reported by Messas et al.

remodeling with sustained reduction of MR over a chronic follow-up. These benefits have the potential to improve clinical outcomes. Cutting secondary chordae in the chronic post-MI setting does not adversely affect long-term LV remodeling and limits progressive increases in LV volumes. The study of E. Messas et al. [25] confirms the long-term safety of this technique and its

[29]: cutting a limited number of basal chordae can improve coaptation and reduce leaflets tethering; eliminating secondary chordae in the anterior leaflet can allow the leaflets to assume a more normal and less taut configuration, with more effective coaptation at their free margin. In a recent paper from MITRAL Transatlantic Network [30] the authors report as MR progressed to moderate to severe in controls but decreased to trace with ring plus chordal cutting versus trace to mild with chordal cutting alone versus mild to moderate with ring alone (MR vena contracta, 5.9 ± 1.1 mm in controls, 0.5 ± 0.08 with both, 1.0 ± 0.3 with chordal cutting alone, 2.0 ± 0.4 with ring alone; P < 0.01). In addition, LV end-systolic volume increased by 108% in controls versus 28% with ring plus chordal cutting, less than with each intervention alone (P < 0.01); they conclude that combined annular and subvalvular repair improves long-term reduction of both chronic IMR and LV remodeling without decreasing global or segmental LV function.

Cut-and-transfer technique reported by Cappabianca et al [31]: the secondary chordae attached to the central part of the anterior leaflet (usually in the area between A2 and A3) and originating from the PPM, normally 2 or 3 chordae, were cut immediately below their attachment to the leaflet and re-implanted on the free edge of the anterior leaflet with 5-0 Prolene. Authors report at 1 year follow-up, recurrent mitral regurgitation grade 2.9 ± 0.4 versus 0.2 ± 0.4 (p < 0.0001), left ventricular end-systolic volume index (mL/m2) 52.7 ± 13.1 versus 48.2 ± 10.1 (p = 0.07), left ventricular endsystolic index (mL/m2) 92.9 ± 16.5 versus 83.4 ± 15.9 (p <0.005), and ejection fraction (%) 37.8 ± 6.3 versus 44.2 ± 8.1 (p < 0.0001), in the group of patients underwent isolated RA vs RA plus cut-and-transfer.

PPM sling reported by Hvass et al [32]: The technique is performed by insinuating a blunt dissector through the stronger trabeculations at the base of the posterior papillary muscle attachment to the ventricular wall. The base of posterior PPM is separated from LV wall. A 4 mm Gore-Tex tube is used and then placed around the base

of both PPMs. The loop is progressively tightened until the two PPMs are in close contact. The Gore-Tex tube forms an intraventricular ring that is secured with strong sutures. Once tightened there is no residual gap between the bases of the two PPMs. No sutures are placed on the papillary muscles themselves. The author published his results after 10 years in 37 patients [27]: MR is none to trivial in 31 and mild to moderate in 4; follow-up shows stability of all initially successful double-level mitral repairs. Follow-up beyond 1 year shows improvements in ventricular diameters (56 +/- 5 mm), ejection fraction (49 +/- 6), volume (130 +/- 10 mL), and sphericity index (0.55). He concludes that re-approximating the papillary muscles has an immediate effect on mitral leaflet mobility by suppressing the tethering resulting from displacement of the papillary muscles; it has an effect in preventing recurrent mitral regurgitation by avoiding further papillary muscle displacement.

PPM sandwich reported by Ishikawa et al. [33]: the first procedure is the papillary muscle head approximations of the anterior and posterior mitral valve leaflets to achieve coaptation of the two leaflets. At the anterolateral commissural portion, a Teflon pledgeted 3-0 Ticron suture with a double-armed needle is passed through the papillary muscle head of the posterior leaflet and through the papillary muscle head of the anterior leaflet, reinforced with another Teflon pledgets. The same approximation suture is made at the posteromedian commissural portion. They report a postoperative residual mild MR in 4%, without moderate or severe MR was; in the follow-up study, the MR-free rate at 2 years after surgery was 93%.

Key Pearls & Pitfalls

- The effect of mitral regurgitation on cardiac function is more than purely mechanical, pump function is likely maintained at the expense of elevated filling pressures, but inevitably leads to impaired contractility and electrical instability
- Mitral regurgitation occurs due to mitral valve leaflets disease and/or abnormalities of the

mitral valve apparatus or secondary to left ventricular dysfunction
- The most important contribution of MR assessment was from Prof Carpentier who described a schematic and effective classification of MR
- It must always be remembered the functional mitral valve disease is a pathology affecting the left ventricle and the mitral subvalvular apparatus that affects the papillary muscles and the tendon cords
- Ischemic mitral regurgitation is a condition characterized by mitral regurgitation secondary to an ischemic left ventricle; however, primarily, the pathology is the result of perturbation of normal regional left ventricular geometry combined with adverse remodelling

Review QS

1. Is the effect of mitral regurgitation on cardiac function purely mechanical?
   (a) Yes
   (b) **No**
2. Which of the Carpentier MR types best describes the following statement; an increased mobility of tear cords and a consequent prolapse of leaflets;
   (a) Type I
   (b) **Type II**
   (c) Type IIIa
3. Which of the Carpentier MR types best describes the following statement; a reduced motility during systole, this picture is caused by myocardial ischemia and remodeling of the left ventricle [5] which causes dislocation of the papillary muscles and failure of leaflet coaptation
   (a) Type II
   (b) Type IIIa
   (c) **Type IIIb**
4. Which Class best describe the following statement; surgery should be considered in symptomatic patients with severe MR, LVEF <30%, option for revascularisation and evidence of viability
   (a) Class II
   (b) **Class IIa**
   (c) Class IIb
5. What Level of Evidence is the following statement; therapy and persistent symptoms will be indicated for the edge-to-edge MV repair (mitral clip) transcatheter only if favourable valve anatomy, LVEF is between 20 and 50%, LVESD is ≤70 mm and PASP ≤70 mmHg.
   (a) LOE II
   (b) **LOE IIa**
   (c) LOE IIb

References

1. Ishikawa M, Watanabe S, Hammoudi N, Aguero J, Bikou O, Fish K, Hajjar RJ. Reduced longitudinal contraction is associated with ischemic mitral regurgitation after posterior. Am J Physiol Heart Circ Physiol. 2018 Feb 1;314(2):H322–9. https://doi.org/10.1152/ajpheart.00546.2017.
2. Nkomo VT, et al. Burden of valvular heart diseases: a population-based study. Lancet. 2006;368:1005–11.
3. Enriquez-Sarano M, et al. Quantitative determinants of the outcome of asymptomatic mitral regurgitation. N Engl J Med. 2005;352:875–83.
4. Apostolidou E, Maslow AD, Poppas A. Primary mitral valve regurgitation: update and review. Glob Cardiol Sci Pract. 2017;2017(1):e201703. https://doi.org/10.21542/gcsp.2017.3.
5. Otto CM. Textbook of clinical echocardiography. 4th ed. Saunders; 2009. p. 311–2.
6. Enriquez-Sarano M, Freeman W, et al. Functional anatomy of mitral regurgitation: echocardiographic assessment and implications on outcome. J Am Coll Cardiol. 1999;34:1129–36.
7. Olson LJ, Subramanian R, et al. Surgical pathology of the mitral valve: a study of 712 cases spanning 21 years. Mayo Clin Proc. 1987;62:22–34.
8. Griffin BP. Myxomatous mitral valve disease: Valvular heart disease- a companion to Braunwald's heart disease. Philadelphia: Saunders/Elsevier; 2009. p. 243–9.
9. Remenyi B, ElGuindy A, et al. Valvular heart disease 3: Valvular aspects of rheumatic heart disease. Lancet. 2016;387:1335–46.
10. Brand MD, Abadi CA, et al. Radiation- associated valvular heart disease in Hodgkin's disease is associated with characteristic thickening and fibrosis of the aortic- mitral curtain. J Heart Valve Dis. 2001;10(5):681–5.
11. Bursi F, Enriquez-Sarano M, et al. Heart failure and death after myocardial infarction in the community: the emerging role of mitral regurgitation. Circulation. 2005;111(3):295–301.

12. Birsi F, Enriquez-Sarano M, et al. Mitral regurgitation after myocardial infarction: a review. Am J Med. 2006;119:103–12.
13. Nappi F, Singh SSA, Padala M, Attias D, Nejjari M, Mihos CG, Benedetto U, Michler R. The choice of treatment in ischemic mitral regurgitation with reduced left ventricular function. Ann Thorac Surg. Author manuscript; available in PMC 2020 Aug 13. Published in final edited form as:. Ann Thorac Surg. 2019;108(6):1901–12.
14. Bonow RO, Carabello BA, Chatterjee K, de Leon AC, Faxon DP, Freed MD, et al. 2008 focused update incorporated in to the ACC/AHA 2006 guidelines for the Management of Patients with Valvular Heart Disease. A report of the American College of Cardiology/American Heart Association task force on practice guidelines (writing committee to revise the 1998 guidelines for the Management of Patients with Valvular Heart Disease). Circulation. 2008;118:e523–661.
15. Vahanian A, Alfieri O, Andreotti F, Antunes MJ, Baròn-Esquivias G, Baumgartner H, et al. Guidelines on the management of valvular heart disease (version 2012). The joint task force on the Management of Valvular Heart Disease of the European Society of Cardiology (ESC) and the European Association for Cardio-Thoracic Surgery (EACTS). Eur Heart J. 2012(33):2451–96.
16. Fattouch K, Guccione F, Sampognaro R, et al. Efficacy of adding mitral valve restrictive annuloplasty to CABG in patients with moderate ischemic mitral valve regurgitation: a randomised trial. J Thorac Cardiovasc Surg. 2009;138:278–85.
17. Gillinov AM, Wierup PN, Blackstone EH, et al. Is repair preferable to replacement for ischemic mitral regurgitation? J Thorac Cardiovasc Surg. 2001;122:1125–41.
18. Vassileva CM, Boley T, Markwell S, Hazelrigg S. Meta-analysis of short-term and long-term survival following repair versus replacement for ischemic mitral regurgitation. Eur J Cardiothoracic Surg. 2011;39:295–303.
19. Kuwahara E, Otsuji Y, Iguro, et al. Mechanism of recurrent/persistent ischemic/functional mitral regurgitation in chronic phase after surgical Annuloplasty: importance of augmented posterior leaflet tethering. Circulation. 2006;114:I-529–34.
20. Mihaljevic T, Lam BK, Rajeswaran J, et al. Impact of mitral valve Annuloplasty combined with revascularization in patients with functional ischemic mitral regurgitation. JACC. 2007;49:2191–201.
21. Kron IL, Green GR, Cope JT. Surgical relocation of the posterior papillary muscle in chronic ischemic mitral regurgitation. Ann Thorac Surg. 2002;74:600–1.
22. Wagner CE, Irving L. Kron Subvalvular techniques to optimize surgical repair of ischemic regurgitation Curr Opin Cardiol. Author manuscript; available in PMC 2014 Jun 9. Published in final edited form as. Curr Opin Cardiol. 2014 Mar;29(2):140–4.
23. Chang B-C, Youn Y-N, Ha J-W, Lim S-H, Hong Y-S, Chung N. Long-term clinical results of mitral valvuloplasty using flexible and rigid rings: a prospective and randomized study. J Thorac Cardiovasc Surg. 2007;133:995–1003. https://doi.org/10.1016/j.jtcvs.2006.10.023.
24. Micali LR, Qadrouh MN, Parise O, Parise G, Matteucci F, de Jong M, Tetta C, Moula AI, Johnson DM, Gelsomino S. Papillary muscle intervention vs mitral ring annuloplasty in ichemic mitral regurgitation. J Card Surg. 2020;35(3):645–53. https://doi.org/10.1111/jocs.14407.
25. Messas E, Bel A, Szymanski C, Cohen I, Touchot B, Handschumacher MD, Desnos M, Carpentier A, Menasché P, Hagège AA, Levine RA. Relief of mitral leaflet tethering following chronic myocardial infarction by chordal cutting diminishes left ventricular remodeling. Circ Cardiovasc Imaging. 2010 Nov;3(6):679–86. https://doi.org/10.1161/CIRCIMAGING.109.931840.
26. Jensen H, Jensen MO, Smerup MH, et al. Impact of papillary muscle relocation as adjunct procedure to mitral ring annuloplasty in functional ischemic mitral regurgitation. Circulation. 2009 Sep 15;120(11 Suppl):S92–8.
27. Fattouch K, Castrovinci S, Murana G, et al. Papillary muscles relocation and mitral annuloplasty in ischemic mitral valve regurgitation: midterm results. J Thorac Cardiovasc Surg. 2014;
28. Szymanski C, Bel A, Cohen I, et al. Comprehensive annular and subvalvular repair of chronicischemic mitral regurgitation improves long-term results with the least ventricular remodeling. Circulation. 2012;126:2720–7. This study showed that concomitant bileaflet secondary chordal cutting results in decreased severity of recurrent mitral regurgitation and is associated with reversal of remodeling without an adverse impact on left ventricular function
29. Messas E, Guerrero JL, Handschumacher MD, et al. Chordal cutting a new therapeutic approach for ischemic mitral regurgitation. Circulation. 2001;104:1958.
30. Szymanski C, Bel A, Cohen I, et al. Comprehensive annular and subvalvular repair of chronic ischemic mitral regurgitation improves long-term results with the least ventricular remodeling. Circulation. 2012 Dec 4;126(23):2720–7.
31. Cappabianca G, Bichi S, Patrini D, et al. Cut-and-transfer technique for ischemic mitral regurgitation and severe tethering of mitral leaflets. Ann Thorac Surg. 2013;96:1607–13.
32. Hvass U, Tapia M, Baron F, et al. Papillary muscle sling: a new functional approach to mitral repair in patients with ischemic left ventricular dysfunction and functional mitral regurgitation. Ann Thorac Surg. 2003;75:809–11.
33. Ishikawa S, Ueda K, Kawasaki A, et al. Papillary muscle sandwich plasty for ischemic mitral regurgitation: a new simple technique. J Thorac Cardiovasc Surg. 2008;135:1384–6.

Minimally Invasive Mitral Valve Repair/Replacement

11

Daniel Grinberg, Benoît Cosset, Matteo Pozzi, and Jean François Obadia

Abbreviations

MIMVS   Minimally invasive mitral valve surgery
PMR   Primary Mitral Regurgitation
TEE   Transesophageal echocardiogram
TTE   Transthoracic echocardiogram

Learning Objectives

- Understanding the context of the development of minimally invasive approach for the mitral valve, current trends, and the evolution of the technique.
- Understanding the indications for this approach.
- Providing an example of a technique performed in a high-volume European center through a step-by-step description, as well as some helpful "tricks" to perform such procedures.

D. Grinberg (✉) · B. Cosset · M. Pozzi · J. F. Obadia
Department of Cardiovascular Surgery, Hopital Cardiologique Louis Pradel, Lyon Medical School, Bron, Lyon, France
e-mail: benoit.cosset@chu-lyon.fr;
matteo.pozzi@chu-lyon.fr;
jean-francois.obadia@chu-lyon.fr

Review of Current Evidence

During the last three decades, the development of endoscopic operations, first, in general surgery and then, in other surgical specialties, has revolutionized the management of patients by allowing for the growth of minimally invasive access procedures, which decrease operative morbidity and mortality.

In the field of heart surgery, video-assisted minimally invasive mitral valve repair through a mini-thoracotomy was first described by Carpentier and colleagues in 1996 [1]. Technical guidelines were created by the work of "Pioneers" such as Hugo Vanermen (Aalst—Belgium), Freidrich Moor (Leipzig-Germany) and Randall Chitwood (Greenville-USA) [2, 3]. Our department also contributed to the optimization and the propagation of this approach in Primary Mitral Regurgitation (PMR) patients.

The development of dedicated surgical instruments and the standardization of procedures has allowed expert centers to claim <1% 30-day mortality rate for elective mitral cases. Despite a steep learning curve for surgeons, all techniques described for mitral repair through a conventional approach (sternotomy) can be performed by an incision rarely exceeding 4 cm with at least the same success rate.

Unlike the endoscopic approach for lung resection or bowel and gallbladder surgeries, minimally invasive mitral valve surgery

(MIMVS) has been relatively slow to expand as a result of several factors. The outcomes of such procedures are highly affected by the individual surgeon's expertise obtained throughout a long and steep learning curve, as well as the center's volume of cases.

The current trend of recent recommendations towards encouraging surgery early-on in no or barely symptomatic PMR patients (e.g. young patients with severe regurgitation and left ventricular deterioration), however, has promoted the development of the MIMVS approach since less invasive procedures often are more acceptable in such cases. MIMVS also can be preferred in cases with specific challenges (e.g. patients with thoracic deformation, obese patients, parietal decay, prior radiotherapy or prior cardiac surgery in particular with permeable mammary bypass, etc…) while avoiding anterior access and allowing mitral exposure with a minor surgical dissection and heart mobilization.

This approach is considered as the "standard" approach for all mitral valve interventions in our center. In this chapter, we describe our technique, inspired by the original technique described by Hugo Vanermen, and refined through 15 years of practice and around 2000 operations.

Technique/Details/Operative Steps

Preoperative Evaluation

Contraindications for minimal-invasive mitral valve surgery (with regard to conventional strategy) are rare. Specific hurdles must be specifically investigated.

Cardiac Workup
Surgical indication usually relies on a TransThoracic Echocardiogram (TTE) test. Aortic regurgitation must be examined since it jeopardizes the success of an anterograde cardioplegia.

A Transesophageal echocardiogram (TEE) is required in the case of a non-conclusive TTE test. A TEE is required to be performed during the surgery (positioning of the cannulas, assessment of the valvular repair, control of the deairing…) and a contraindication for TEE must be considered as a contraindication for a minimally invasive approach.

If a coronary angiogram is performed within the day prior to surgery, radial access will be preferred in order to preserve the femoral access.

Vascular Workup
The MIMVS approach requires peripheral cannulation through a femoral approach. The vascular workup is mainly driven by the team's preferences. For some surgeons, a full aortic CT-scan is systematically performed and sometimes in conjunction with a coronary CT-scan.

Thoracic Workup
The thoracic workup is driven by the patient's anamnesis and chest-X ray. Severe pleural adhesions can prevent optimal access to the left atrium. The quality of the skin in the incision site must be assessed and the cutaneous incision location is usually drawn the day before the surgery.

Patient's Preparation

Standardization is a key element to ease the coordination of the whole team (anesthetic, nursing, surgical).

Anesthetic Management [4]
Anesthetic management for MIMVS is very similar to "conventional" valvular surgeries. It includes:

- Insertion of a jugular multi-lumen central line.
- Insertion of a right radial arterial catheter for invasive blood pressure measurement.
- A tracheal intubation with a single-lumen endotracheal tube. A double-lumen endobronchial tube insertion with a single-lung ventilation can be avoided for several reasons (their insertion requires a specific training, frequent displacement during patient's mobilization, the necessity to change the double-lumen tube to a single-lumen tube at the end of the proce-

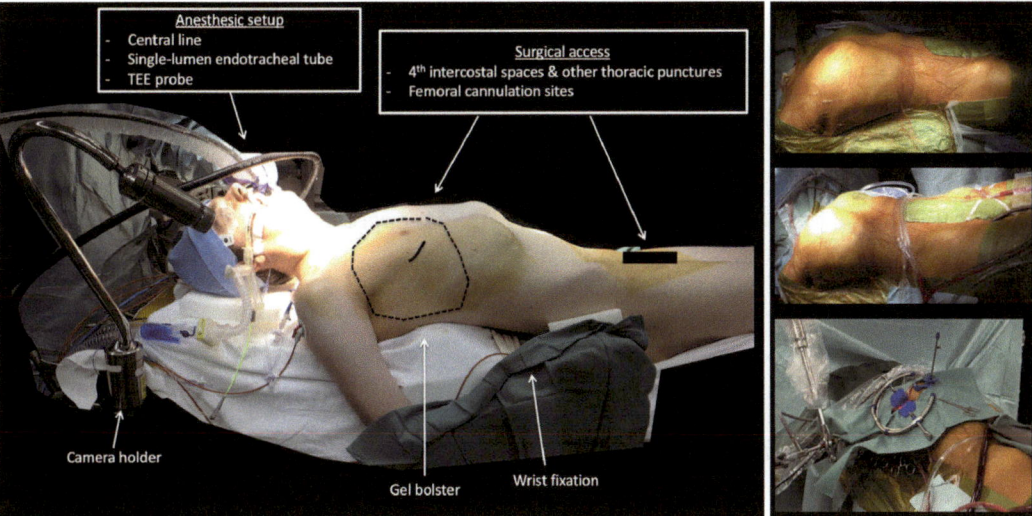

Fig. 11.1 Typical patient's set-up and positioning

dure). In our center, the procedure is started with the peripheral cannulation and the cardiopulmonary bypass (CPB) is initiated as soon as the thorax is open. Thus, mechanical ventilation can be discontinued with the risk of lung injury. Alternatively, a single tracheal lumen associated with an endobronchial blocker can be performed.

– Transcutaneous defibrillation paddles are used since an intra-pericardial defibrillation is impossible through the thoracotomy.

Right Jugular Access

The good quality of the drainage of the right cavities is key for the procedure. A single two-stage venous cannula associated with an active drainage usually provides a sufficient drainage. The quality of the positioning of the cannula prior to the initiation of the CPB is systematically assessed with the TEE.

In some cases, a dual venous cannulation will be preferred (associated tricuspid procedure, large interatrial defect, insufficient drainage, surgeon's preference). Thus, the puncture site must be preserved and included in the operative field.

Patient's Positioning

The patient is placed in supine position at the right edge of the operating table and with a gel

bolster under the shoulders. The right arm is on the right side of the surgical table and slightly folded. The right wrist is maintained along the right hip as the result of a dedicated wrapping.

The optimal patient's positioning, skin prep, and draping must allow access to the surgical working field (right thorax, from the sternum to the midaxillary line as well as the two groins) and free movement of the surgical endoscopic instruments. The sternum must always be kept in the sterile zone in case of an emergency transition to a full sternotomy.

In women, sterile adhesive films are settled in order to pull up the right breast towards the left shoulder in order to lift the inframammary groove in front of the fourth right intercostal space. Thanks to this trick, the scare will be invisible under the breast after the surgery. In male patients, the areola is usually in front of the fourth right intercostal space.

The final steps for the patient set-up are the connection of the thoracoscopic elements (10 mm 30° endoscope maintained by an auto-static camera holder (Endoboy®), CO_2 line) as well as the CPB tubing (Fig. 11.1).

Operative Room Set-Up

In addition to a standard heart surgery setup, MIMVS requires a thoracoscopic tower system (light source, camera hub, CO_2 insufflator) usually placed on the left side of the patients (right side of the principal assistant), fitted with an additional monitor (left side of the principal operator).

Dedicated instrumentation is obviously required, including long-shaft surgical instruments, as well as specific retractors and consumable material.

Surgical Steps

Peripheral Cannulation

General Principles (Fig. 11.2)
In our center, a percutaneous and bilateral femoral cannulation is required to reduce the risk of arteriovenous fistula (ideally the atrial cannula in the left groin and the venous cannula in the right groin). A substantial morbidity rate of MIMVS procedure is directly related to the quality of the cannulation. Failure of the arterial pre-closing

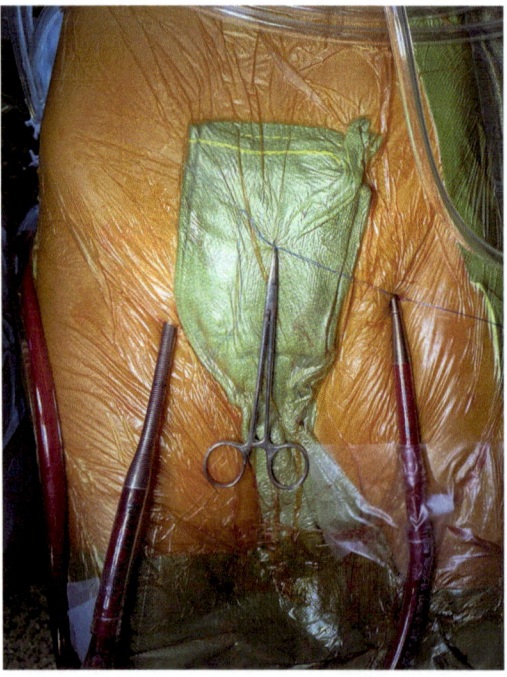

Fig. 11.2 Total percutaneous femoral vessel cannulation technique with the arterial cannula on the left side of the patient and the venous cannula on the right side

system can lead to pseudoaneurysm or stenosis and can require an emergent surgical repair. Misdirection of venous cannula are rare but can be life-threatening (retroperitoneal hemorrhage, large vessel or cardiac perforations).

Two essential principles then always must be carefully respected:

1. Guidewire and cannulas insertion and manipulations must always be guided by Doppler imaging (vascular doppler and TEE).
2. Every vascular penetration site (arterial and venous) must occur under the inguinal ligament in order to avoid insidious retroperitoneal bleeding and to ease potential surgical access.

Arterial Cannulation
Infra-inguinal puncture carefully targets the anterior wall of the mid-common femoral artery before venous cannulation to avoid arterial puncture under systemic heparinization and in order to allow a rapid vascular filling in case of a venous cannulation incident. Trained surgeons often use a pre-closing system such as Prostar® XL or ProGlide® (Abbott Vascular), but a surgical dissection of the anterior wall of the artery can also be performed.

A guidewire is introduced and positioned into descending aorta. After systemic heparinization, an arterial cannula is inserted and safely attached to the surgical draping (in our experience an arterial 17 F cannula fits for a large majority of patients).

Venous Cannulation
The percutaneous venous cannulation is performed on the contralateral side (Fig. 11.2). As previously mentioned, the quality of the venous drainage is paramount. Additionally, venous and right cavity tissue has a thinner thickness. Thus, the position of the guidewire up to the superior vena cava must be continuously monitored all along during the venous cannula insertion with a TEE bicaval view. If a two-stage single cannula is used (e.g. 23/25 Fr Estech Inc., Danville, CA, USA) the tip of the cannula will be pushed a few centimeters into the superior vena cava in order

to avoid the swiping of the distal tip during further atrial retractor insertion. The quality of the venous drainage is assessed after initiation of an active drainage (centrifugal pump or vacuum).

The total percutaneous femoral vessel cannulation technique is particularly suitable for minimally invasive mitral valve surgery with a high success rate and few complications after a short learning curve for surgeons.

Minimally Invasive Access

The surgical access is represented by an anterolateral right mini-thoracotomy (3–5 cm). The choice of thoracic access is essential and drives the valvular access. After the insertion of the atrial retractor, the axis "thoracotomy—atrial opening—mitral valve—apex" must be linear. Usually, the 4th space is preferred (Fig. 11.3). The following "tricks" can be helpful for surgeons to identify the ideal incision site:

- The "Sternal Angle" (or manubriosternal junction) is a useful mark since it corresponds to the attachment of the 2nd pair of costal cartilages.
- The fourth space is also at the mid-height of the rib cage.
- In case of doubt, the videoscope can be inserted through a centimetric thoracic incision in order to assess the optimal height before a full opening. In case of hesitation between two intercostal spaces, the upper-one is preferred since the bottom right quadrant of the atrial opening is often hidden behind an atrial folding.

The use of a rigid intercostal spacer must be avoided since it leads to postoperative pain related to intercostal nerve compression or rib fractures. Soft tissue retractors provide an optimal rib spreading without generating such complications.

Every thoracic penetration orifice generates its own morbidity (bleeding, infection, postoperative pain). Thus, the number and location of these holes must be selected carefully. In our

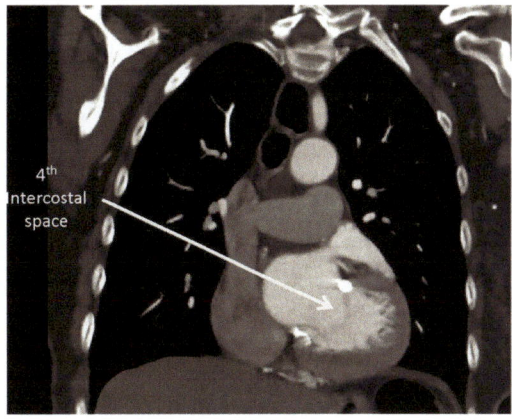

Fig. 11.3 Exposure of the mitral valve through the 4th right intercostal space

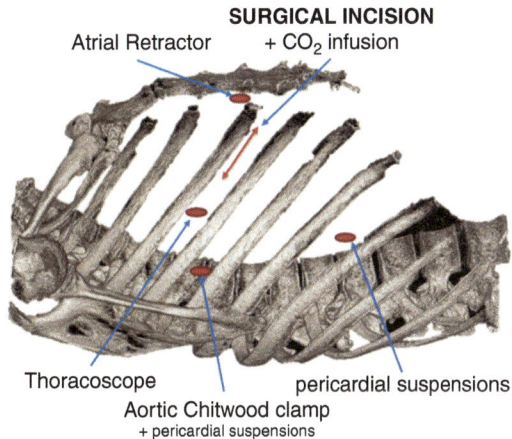

Fig. 11.4 Classical thoracic access for MIMVS

practice, four additional incisions are made (Fig. 11.4):

- The insufflating CO_2 line (flow of approximately 2 l/min without pleural pressure control) is inserted within the thoracotomy and maintained by the soft tissue retractor.
- The thoracoscope is introduced in a dedicated centimetric incision in the fourth intercostal space on the mid-axillary line. This incision will be used for the placement of a thoracic drain at the end of the procedure.
- A rigid transthoracic aortic clamp (Chitwood clamp) is used for every procedure in our department (this position statement is discussed later). The clamp is inserted through a

centimetric incision in the fifth space on the mid-axillary line. This incision will be used for the placement of a second thoracic drain at the end of the procedure.

- A right parasternal punctiform incision is made in the axis of the atrial opening (fourth or fifth space) for the insertion of the atrial retractor. This incision could be used as an outlet port for the epicardial pacing wires
- A punctiform puncture in the 6th space on the mid-axillary line is finally made and is used for the pericardium suspension.

Cardiopulmonary Bypass initiation

As previously mentioned, the CPB is initiated during the thoracic incision and after obtaining of a satisfactory activated clotting time (ACT). The injection pressure must be carefully monitored since it reflects the proper quality of cannulation.

As soon as the CPB outflow reaches the theoretical flow related to the patient's body surface area, the mechanical ventilation can be stopped and the lung deflated in order to get access to the pericardium.

Cardiac Exposure (Fig. 11.5)

The incision of the pericardium is started with the electric scalpel 2 cm under the internal thoracic pedicle (a safe distance from the phrenic nerve)

and horizontally from the diaphragm to the aorta. This high opening provides a large strip of pericardium that is then tightened with two or three stitches, thus covering the lung and pulling the heart upward. A trans-parietal stitch retracting the diaphragm is used only if necessary.

The inferior vena cava is dissected in order to facilitate the subsequent distal extension of atriotomy. The quality of the venous drainage is ultimately assessed before the aortic cross-clamping.

Aortic Cross-Clamping

A purse-string is placed on the anterolateral wall of the aorta prior to the placement of the cardioplegia cannula. This insertion remains the only arterial (high-pressure) opening of the whole intervention. Thus, a specific caution must be taken with respect to a perfect hemostasis after the cannula removal.

Recent studies comparing endoaortic clamps to transthoracic clamps suggested a significantly higher risk of iatrogenic aortic dissection associated with endoaortic balloon occlusion [5]. In our institution, we always use the transthoracic clamp for convenience, financial motivation and the clinical benefit (exceptional clamp related complications). The clamp must be inserted carefully towards the transverse sinus and with continuous sight of the tip of the instrument to avoid any injury to the pulmonary artery or left atrial appendage.

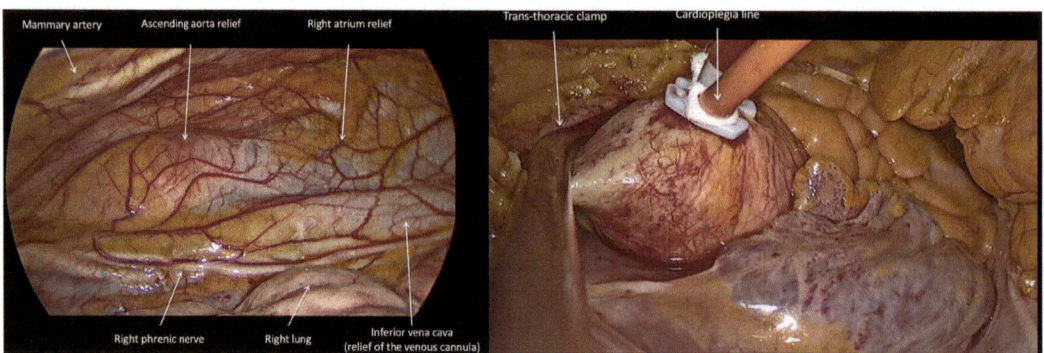

Fig. 11.5 Mediastinal exposure before (left) and after (right) opening of the pericardium

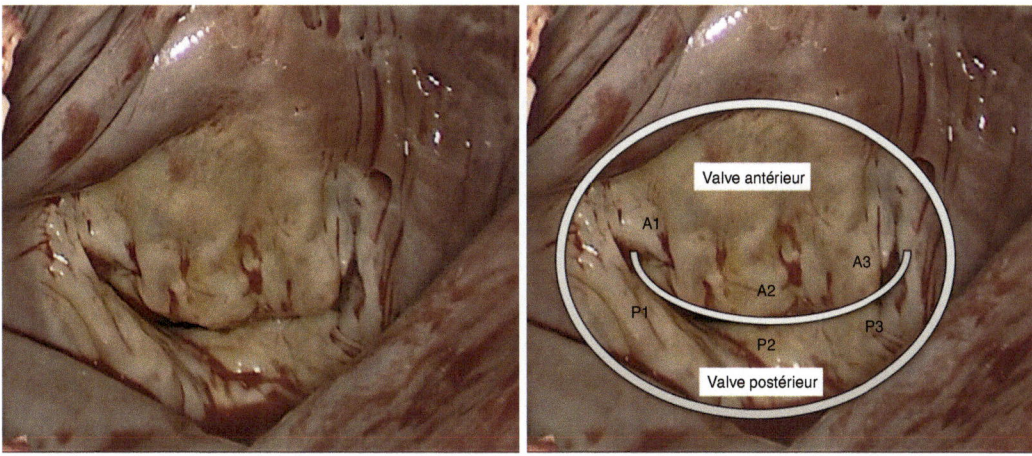

Fig. 11.6 Exposure of the mitral valve after insertion of the atrial retractor

A standard cold crystalloid cardioplegia can be used.

Mitral Valve Exposure (Fig. 11.6)

The dissection of the Syndergaard inter-atrial groove is performed during the cardioplegia installation since it is easily seen in the absence of left atrial venting. The left atrium is then opened behind this line and drained. The superior edge of the atrial opening is pulled toward the sternum as a result of a suture and the incision in prolongated horizontally under the inferior vena cava and toward the left inferior pulmonary vein on top of the incision. A left atrial venting line is introduced in the atriotomy and directed towards the left inferior pulmonary vein. A patent foramen oval is sewn and closed if necessary.

The mitral retractor is inserted and positioned in order to provide optimal valvular exposure.

Mitral Valve Repair

The quality of this video-assisted approach allows for the performance of all types of mitral valve repair techniques as well as prosthetic replacement. The development of MIMVS has led to the description of several dedicated techniques usually grouped under the term "respect techniques" (e.g. subvalvular apparatus reconstruction with Gore-Tex sutures, valvular folding, edge-to-edge suture) in contrast with "resect techniques" describing complexes valvular resection (quadrangular and atypical resection) and chordal plasty.

After several decades of controversy, recent meta-analysis reports similar success rates and long-term outcomes for both types of techniques [6, 7].

End of the Procedure

Closure of the Atriotomy, Deairing, Cross-Clamp Removal, Decannulation

At the end of the mitral valve surgery, the left atrium retractor is removed, and the left atrium is closed by two running sutures. Special caution should be taken while closing both angles since the exposure of these areas are challenging after the aortic-clamp removal.

If a temporary epicardial pacing is required (it is not mandatorily used in our department), the placement of the pacing wire will be done before the aortic-clamp removal with an unloaded right ventricle.

The deairing is performed through the cannula of cardioplegia and the left atrial venting line. Considering the small incision, manual heart manipulation usually performed during a conventional surgery cannot be done. However, the occurrence of cerebral gas embolism is rare as a result of the continuous thoracic CO_2 infusion.

After the aortic-clamp removal, the left atrium is definitively closed.

If a single-lumen endotracheal tube ventilation was selected, the apnea must be kept until the thoracoscope removal as well as a 100% CPB flow rate. The quality of the surgical repair/replacement can be assessed with TEE by filling the ventricle (without lowering the CPB flow). A good result allowed to initiate the closure of the thorax.

The aortic venting is removed and the quality of the hemostasis of this suture is carefully assessed.

Thoracic drainage and closure.

The pericardium is closed loosely with a single suture in order to allow a drainage of pericardial exudate into the right chest.

Two large thoracic drains are inserted through the preexisting thoracic ports into the right pleural cavity and the pericardium. The intrathoracic hemostasis is carefully controlled before the endoscope removal. The mechanical ventilation will resume only at this phase, and a progressive withdrawal from cardiopulmonary bypass is initiated.

Lastly, the intercostal space is narrowed with a large suture to avoid a further pleural hernia,

superficial layers are closed in the habitual manner and local, long-acting anesthesia is infiltrated before dressing the wound.

Decannulation

After weaning from cardiopulmonary bypass, the venous cannula is removed first and a digital compression is initiated. After an ultimate and careful TEE imaging, in the absence of pleural effusion, the systemic protamination is infused. The arterial cannula is removed using the preclosing system. A bilateral vascular compression is applied on both groins for 12 h.

Postoperative Care

Post-operative care following such intervention is usually simple. The standard ICU length-stay rarely exceeds 1 night, and patients are often discharged home within 1 week.

Thoracic bleeding is unusual. Thoracic drains are usually removed after 24 h and transfusion rates are very low. Parietal chest pain generally resolves quickly and patients can be discharged with oral painkillers. Lung complications are uncommon (infection, respiratory failure). We recommend 4 weeks before returning to exercise.

Surgical site infections are also unusual. A clinical inguinal examination should be performed before discharge (Fig. 11.7).

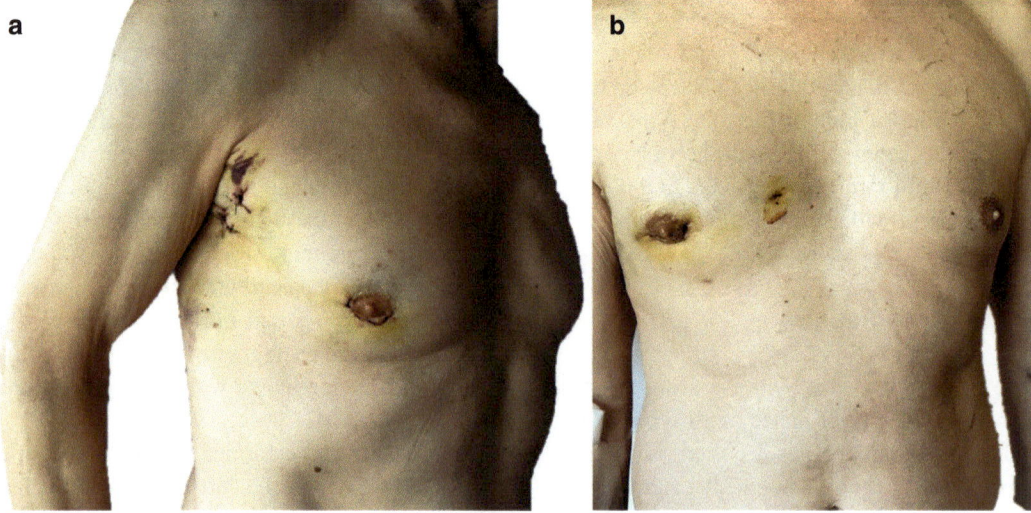

Fig. 11.7 Postoperative photographs showing the esthetical result in a female (**a**) and male (**b**) patient

Results: Outcomes and Data (1/2)

With almost 30 years of history, the minimally-invasive approach has been shown to safely and efficiently treat most mitral lesions similar to the "conventional" approach (sternotomy). Both techniques were widely compared through several large cohort studies and meta-analysis [8–12].

The repair rate for Primary Mitral Regurgitation patients is at least similar regardless of whether MIMVS is used or conventional sternotomy [13]. From an anatomical standpoint, the right mini-thoracotomy gives a logical and direct access to the mitral valve, providing a good opportunity to identify and examine the mitral lesions and to allow for the performance of all kinds of repair techniques.

MIMCS is classically associated with longer CPB duration and operative time, but fewer postoperative bleeding (and thus a lower transfusion rate) and shorter ICU (decreased length of mechanical ventilation) and hospital stay. These findings are largely related to the absence of sternotomy (no sternal retraction, fewer mediastinal dissection, and no high-pressure cavity opening). There is less postoperative pain and parietal infection is infrequent.

Peripheral vascular complications can be easily avoided with meticulous cannulation, the systematic use of Doppler imaging and the mastering of proper use of arterial preclosing devices [13, 14]. Stroke incidence is at least equal to conventional surgery (<2% at 30-day follow-up) as a result of the use of CO_2 and a meticulous deairing protocol. The choice of aortic cross-clamping techniques must be driven by the surgeon's habits.

Rhythmic complications and particularly atrial fibrillation episodes are also infrequent [15, 16].

Decreased transfusions and ancillary needs result in approximately equivalent overall hospital costs [17].

Finally, 30-day all-cause mortality (1.4%) and long-term functional status and mortality are also similar [8, 10].

MIMVS has considerably paved the way of mitral robotic surgery, initially described by the same pioneers previously cited. This technique requires specific training in addition to an expensive set-up. It provides surgeons with a third motion and visual dimension that sometimes is missed in "standard" MIMVS.

Conclusion

Despite initial skepticism as a result of the conviction that smaller incisions lead to poor exposure and inferior outcomes, the minimally invasive approach has progressively demonstrated its safety and efficiency for the treatment of most mitral diseases. Performed in expert centers, MIMVS provides results at least equivalent to those of conventional surgery.

Results still remain dependent on the steep learning curve and initial time and financial investment of the surgeon, which limits the widespread use of this approach. Nowadays, robotic mitral surgery presents an interesting alternative to MIMVS [18, 19].

Finally, the current, massive efforts concerning the development of innovative solutions allowing transapical and trans-vascular treatment of valvular diseases in beating-heart state will probably affect the care of patients with mitral diseases in the decades to come.

Key Pearls and Pitfalls

- MIMVS success resides in the mastering of multiple surgical steps such as the proper patient installation, peripheral cannulation, and valve exposure. A consequent learning-curve is thus necessary to obtain clinical outcomes at least equivalent to those of conventional approaches.
- Protocol standardization is a key element to ease the coordination of different teams and promoting reproducibility and optimal outcomes. An anesthesiologic team trained for Transesophageal imaging is one of the keys for the success of MIMVS program

- A substantial morbidity rate of MIMVS procedure is directly related to the peripheral cannulation.
- Minimally invasive access allows to perform all repair techniques described with a sternotomy, but dedicated repair techniques were developed to ease valvular treatments with such access.
- Starting with a large right lateral thoracotomy is usually recommended for surgeons less experienced with this approach before moving on to decreasing access sizes.

Comprehension questions

General questions regarding minimally invasive mitral valve surgery:

☐ MIMVS is a recent technique that still needs to demonstrate its effectiveness compared to the "conventional" approach

☐ MIMVS only allows for the realization of "respect" repair techniques

☐ training in robotic surgery is recommended before initiating a MIMVS program

☐ dedicated training in an expert center is recommended before initiating a MIMVS program

☐ MIMVS cannot be performed in patients with prior heart surgery with sternotomy

Material and setup

☐ MIMVS must be performed in hybrid surgical rooms

☐ mechanical ventilation with a double-lumen endotracheal tube is mandatory

☐ an intraoperative Transesophageal Echocardiography imaging is required during every procedure

☐ surgical draping always must include the sternum in the operative field

☐ dedicated surgical instruments are highly recommended to perform these procedures

Cannulation

☐ central arterial cannulation can easily be performed during the procedure

☐ a severe peripheral arterial disease could contraindicate a MIMVS approach

☐ a groin incision can be performed as an alternative for the percutaneous cannulation

☐ the position of the guidewire is checked with TEE for both arterial and venous cannulation

☐ the cannulation should be performed only after the thoracotomy

Surgical access

☐ Severe pleural adhesion must contraindicate MIMVS approach

☐ A thoracic CT-scan is always required to be performed before MIMVS

☐ A thoracotomy in the 4th intercostal space usually provides the best access for mitral exposure

☐ Aortic cross-clamping can be performed either with a transthoracic clamp or with endoaortic solutions

☐ The mitral valve is exposed through a transseptal opening

(4–5 quick multiple-choice questions to reinforce the reader's comprehension of the learning objectives)

Disclosure

Daniel Grinberg: N/A
Benoît Cosset: N/A
Matteo Pozzi: N/A
Jean-Francois OBADIA received:

- Research support: Boeringher, Abbott, Medtronic, Edwards
- Consulting Fees/Honoraria: Edwards, Abbott, Medtronic, Servier, Novartis
- Royalty Income: Landanger, Delacroix-Chevalier

References

1. Carpentier A, Loulmet D, Carpentier A, Le Bret E, Haugades B, Dassier P, Guibourt P. [Open heart operation under videosurgery and minithoracotomy. First case (mitral valvuloplasty) operated with success]. C R Acad Sci III 1996;319:219–23.

2. Mohr FW, Falk V, Diegeler A, Walther T, van Son JAM, Autschbach R, Borst HG. Minimally invasive port-access mitral valve surgery. J Thorac Cardiovasc Surg. 1998;115:567–76.
3. Chitwood WR, Wixon CL, Elbeery JR, Francalancia NA, Lust RM. Minimally invasive cardiac operation: adapting cardioprotective strategies. Ann Thorac Surg. 1999;68:1974–7.
4. Ganapathy S. Anaesthesia for minimally invasive cardiac surgery. Best Pract Res Clin Anaesthesiol. 2002;16:63–80.
5. Kowalewski M, Malvindi PG, Suwalski P, Raffa GM, Pawliszak W, Perlinski D, Kowalkowska ME, Kowalewski J, Carrel T, Anisimowicz L. Clinical safety and effectiveness of endoaortic as compared to transthoracic clamp for small thoracotomy mitral valve surgery: meta-analysis of observational studies. Ann Thorac Surg. 2017;103:676–86.
6. Dreyfus GD, Dulguerov F, Marcacci C, Haley SR, Gkouma A, Dommerc C, Albert A. "Respect when you can, resect when you should": a realistic approach to posterior leaflet mitral valve repair. J Thorac Cardiovasc Surg. 2018;156:1856–1866.e3.
7. Mazine A, Friedrich JO, Nedadur R, Verma S, Ouzounian M, Jüni P, Puskas JD, Yanagawa B. Systematic review and meta-analysis of chordal replacement versus leaflet resection for posterior mitral leaflet prolapse. J Thorac Cardiovasc Surg. 2018;155:120–128.e10.
8. Ding C, Jiang D, Tao K, Duan Q. Anterolateral minithoracotomy versus median sternotomy for mitral valve disease: a meta-analysis. J Zhejiang Univ. 2014;15:522–32.
9. Cao C, Wolfenden H, Liou K, Pathan F, Gupta S, Nienaber TA, Chandrakumar D, Indraratna P, Yan TD. A meta-analysis of robotic vs. conventional mitral valve surgery. Ann Cardiothorac Surg. 2015;4:305–14.
10. Sündermann SH, Czerny M, Falk V. Open vs. minimally invasive mitral valve surgery: surgical technique, indications and results. Cardiovasc Eng Technol. 2015;6:160–6.
11. Hickey GL, Grant SW, Hunter S, Zacharias J, Akowuah E, Modi P. Propensity-matched analysis of minimally invasive approach versus sternotomy for mitral valve surgery. Heart. 2018;105(10):783–9.
12. Ding C, Jiang D, Tao K, Duan Q, Li J, Kong M, Shen Z, Dong A. Anterolateral minithoracotomy versus median sternotomy for mitral valve disease: a meta-analysis. J Zhejiang Univ Sci B. 2014;15:522–32.
13. Gammie JS, Zhao Y, Peterson ED, O'Brien SM, Rankin JS, Griffith BP. Less-invasive mitral valve operations: trends and outcomes from the Society of Thoracic Surgeons Adult Cardiac Surgery Database. Ann Thorac Surg. 2010;90:1401–1408, 1410.e1. discussion 1408-10
14. Pozzi M, Henaine R, Grinberg D, Robin J, Saroul C, Delannoy B, Desebbe O, Obadia J-F. Total percutaneous femoral vessels cannulation for minimally invasive mitral valve surgery. Ann Cardiothorac Surg. 2013;2:739–43.
15. Cao C, Gupta S, Chandrakumar D, Nienaber TA, Indraratna P, Ang SC, Phan K, Yan TD. A meta-analysis of minimally invasive versus conventional mitral valve repair for patients with degenerative mitral disease. Ann Cardiothorac Surg. 2013;2:693–703.
16. Cheng DCH, Martin J, Lal A, Diegeler A, Folliguet TA, Nifong LW, Perier P, Raanani E, Smith JM, Seeburger J, Falk V. Minimally invasive versus conventional open mitral valve surgery: a meta-analysis and systematic review. Innovations (Phila). 2011;6:84–103.
17. Hawkins RB, Mehaffey JH, Kessel SM, Dahl JJ, Kron IL, Kern JA, Yarboro LT, Ailawadi G. Minimally invasive mitral valve surgery is associated with excellent resource utilization, cost, and outcomes. J Thorac Cardiovasc Surg. 2018;156(2):611–616.e3.
18. Loulmet DF, Ranganath NK, Neuburger PJ, Nampiaparampil RG, Galloway AC, Grossi EA. Can complex mitral valve repair be performed with robotics? An institution's experience utilizing a dedicated team approach in 500 patients†. Eur J Cardiothoracic Surg. 2019;56:470–8.
19. Hawkins RB, Mehaffey JH, Mullen MM, Nifong WL, Chitwood WR, Katz MR, Quader MA, Kiser AC, Speir AM, Ailawadi G. A propensity matched analysis of robotic, minimally invasive, and conventional mitral valve surgery. Heart. 2018;104(23):1970–5.

Tricuspid Valve Repair/ Replacement

12

Panagiotis G. Kyriazis, Antanas Macys, and Prakash P. Punjabi

Abbreviations

IVC   Inferior vena cava
RA   Right atrium
SVC   Superior vena cava
TR   Tricuspid regurgitation
TV   Tricuspid valve
TVR   Tricuspid valve replacement

P. G. Kyriazis · P. P. Punjabi (✉)
Department of Cardiothoracic Surgery, Hammersmith Hospital, Imperial College Healthcare NHS Trust, London, UK

National Heart and Lung Institute, Faculty of Medicine, Imperial College London, London, England, UK
e-mail: panagiotis.kyriazis@nhs.net;
p.punjabi@imperial.ac.uk

A. Macys
Department of Cardiothoracic Surgery, Hammersmith Hospital, Imperial College Healthcare NHS Trust, London, UK
e-mail: antanas.macys@nhs.net

Learning Objectives

To familiarise with, understand and learn tricuspid valve leading pathology and regurgitation pathophysiology, setup and assessment of tricuspid valve during surgery, decision making and technique for Tricuspid valve repair and replacement.

Introduction

TV Repair

Functional tricuspid regurgitation (TR) is the most common pathology of tricuspid valve (TV), often occurring due to left-sided valve disease and resulting in pulmonary hypertension, right ventricular volume and pressure overload, subsequently right heart side chambers and tricuspid annular dilation, tricuspid leaflet tethering and finally decreased leaflet coaptation. Nevertheless, primary TV pathology affecting tricuspid valvular apparatus can also cause TR. In majority of the cases TR can be successfully treated with TV repair. Preoperative assessment of the TV involves determination of the presence of TR and/or tricuspid annular dilatation. The most common indication for TV repair is the presence of significant TR or tricuspid annular dilatation during mitral valve surgery [1].

TV Replacement

Tricuspid valve replacement (TVR) mostly involves patients with functional tricuspid regurgitation (TR) caused by left heart failure and secondary pulmonary hypertension, though right ventricular infarction or dysfunction, chronic atrial fibrillation, long-standing pulmonary valve disease and atrial septal or ventricular septal defects can also lead to secondary TR. Primary tricuspid valve (TV) disease like TV infective endocarditis, rheumatic disease, congenital tricuspid deformity in Epstein anomaly as well as iatrogenic tricuspid damage from transvenous pacemaker lead implantation or endocardial atrial fibrillation ablation procedure can necessitate TVR. Tricuspid stenosis is a very rare pathology of the TV. Some TVR required patients have had previous cardiac operation and/or failure of tricuspid repair. Preoperative assessment of the tricuspid valve involves determination of the presence of tricuspid regurgitation and/or tricuspid annular dilatation with or without TV apparatus—leaflets and chordae pathological changes which are unlikely to repair and achieve long term TV functional competence [2].

Setup and Approach

TV Repair

The aorta, superior vena cava (SVC) and inferior vena cava (IVC) should be cannulated and tapes passed around the SVC and IVC. These should be snugged prior to opening the right atrium (RA). The TV is approached, either through a vertical or horizontal atriotomy. A vertical atriotomy is performed from the atrial appendage towards the inter-atrial septum while a horizontal atriotomy is performed from the atrial appendage towards the IVC cannula site leaving enough of RA wall to be hooked with atrial retractor for optimal valve exposure (Fig. 12.1).

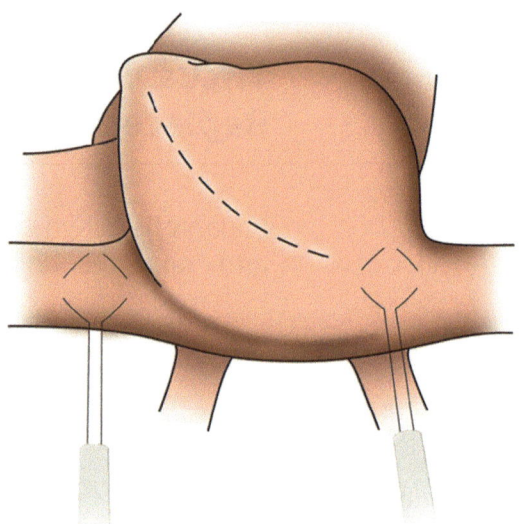

Fig. 12.1 Horizontal right atriotomy (Printed with permission © Gemma Price)

TV Replacement

For sternotomy approach the aorta, superior vena cava (SVC) and inferior vena cava (IVC) should be cannulated and tapes passed around the SVC and IVC. These should be snugged prior to opening the right atrium. For minimal access right anterolateral thoracotomy or redo sternotomy patients peripheral cannulation of the femoral or axillary artery and the femoral vein can be used. The TV is approached, either through a vertical or horizontal right atriotomy (Fig. 12.1).

Assessing the Tricuspid Valve

TV Repair

A systematic analysis of the TV is performed. The TV is first inspected (Fig. 12.2). Note is made of any excessive leaflet tissue, leaflet perforations, ruptured chordae or ruptured papillary muscles. The lesion is then determined using a pair of nerve hooks. Each part of the TV leaflet is lifted up, in turn, to determine the presence of

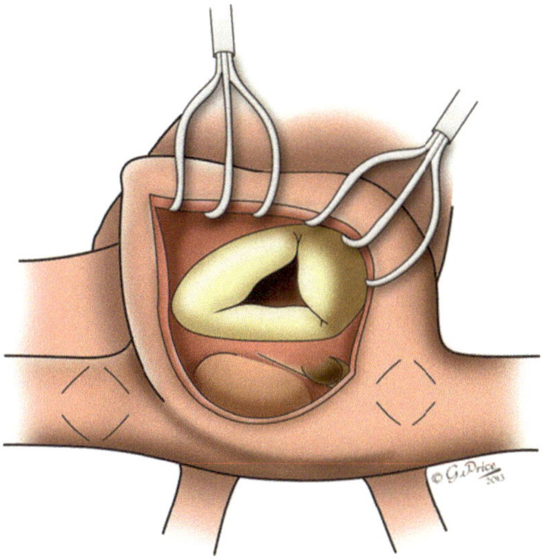

Fig. 12.2 Inspection and assessment of the tricuspid valve (Printed with permission © Gemma Price)

prolapse or tethering. The tricuspid annular diameter is then measured. This is generally taken as the distance between the anteroseptal commissure and the anteroposterior commissure (i.e. the direction of maximal dilatation). It is considered significantly dilated if it is greater than 70 mm when measured intraoperatively. This corresponds to a diameter of 40 mm when measured preoperatively by transthoracic echocardiography in a four chamber view (which measures the distance from the middle of the septal annulus to the middle of the anterior annulus). Majority of functional TRs are related to tricuspid annular dilatation and tricuspid annuloplasty is usually sufficient to address this.

TV Replacement

A full systematic analysis of the TV is performed. The TV inspection involves notice of any excessive or restrictive leaflet tissue, leaflet perforations, ruptured chordae or ruptured papillary muscles. The lesion is determined using a pair of nerve hooks by lifting up each part of the TV leaflet, turning it and identifying the presence of prolapse or tethering. The tricuspid annular

diameter is then measured. After full TV evaluation and when concluded that there is too advanced tricuspid pathology which makes impossible to obtain durable TV repair the decision to replace TV is done.

TV Repair

The Tri-P Repair

Following all other concomitant procedures, the TV is exposed via an oblique incision. Our novel technique of suture annuloplasty involved reduction in tricuspid annular dimension using interrupted pledgeted sutures (Fig. 12.3). Sutures were embedded into the annulus starting at the posteroseptal commissure. A 2-0 Ethibond suture (2.0) within a pledget is passed through the annulus, with an exit pledget emerging 6–8 mm from the first pledget, before being tightened, tied down and cut. This interrupted suture pattern is repeated circumferentially along the annulus up to the anteroseptal commissure, ensuring avoidance of the conduction bundle. On average, eight sutures are embedded along the annular circumference, and each suture is double pledgeted. An on-table water test is performed to test competency of the valve, and if greater competency was required, additional sutures can be implanted crossing the posteroseptal commissure into the septal leaflet annulus.

Ring Annuloplasty

Ring annuloplasty is generally preferred if the tricuspid annular dilatation is severe, particularly if associated with tricuspid leaflet tethering. Most tricuspid rings comprise a short linear segment, corresponding to the septal annulus, and a longer curved segment, corresponding to the posterior and anterior annulus. There is usually a gap between the anterior segment and the septal segment of the ring to avoid suture placement in the region of the conduction system. Annuloplasty can be achieved using different

a b

c

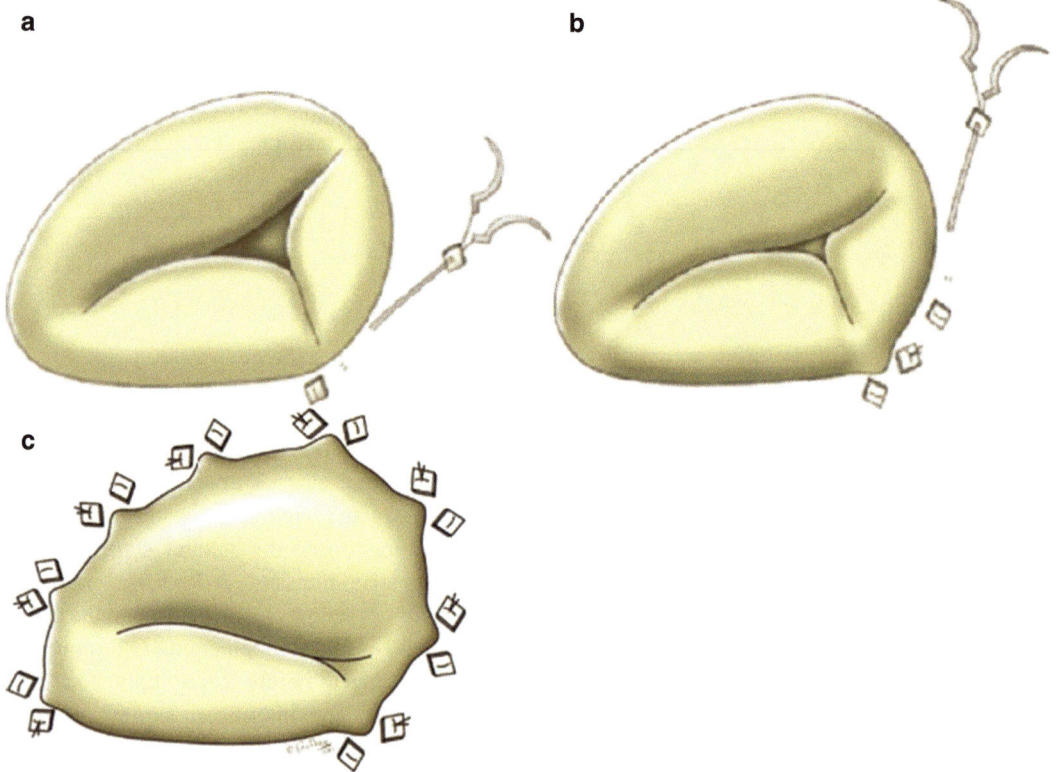

Fig. 12.3 (**a**) Suture annuloplasty of the tricuspid valve (Printed with permission © Gemma Price) (**b**) Suture annuloplasty of the tricuspid valve (Printed with permis-sion © Gemma Price) (**c**) Suture annuloplasty of the tri-cuspid valve (Printed with permission © Gemma Price)

types of annuloplasty devices like flexible ring, standard rigid ring, rigid 3-dimensional ring or pericardial strip [3].

Sizing of the tricuspid annuloplasty ring is performed in several ways. The septal annulus dilates the least in functional TR and, so, mea-surement of its length with a ring sizer can be done to determine the ring size to use. The ring sizer has two notches at its septal segment and a sizer is chosen which aligns, to the anteroseptal and posteroseptal commissures (Fig. 12.4). This should also correspond to the surface area of the anterior and posterior leaflets that are attached to the anterior papillary muscle (Fig. 12.5). Usually, the annuloplasty ring size varies between 30–34 mm for males and 28–32 mm for females [4].

Interrupted, non-pledgeted, 2/0 Ethibond, hor-izontal, mattress sutures are placed around the

tricuspid annulus. The tricuspid leaflet is gently pulled away from the annulus with forceps to visualise its attachment to the annulus. The first septal suture is placed in the middle of the septal annulus, moving round towards the posteroseptal commissure and ending at the anteroseptal com-missure. Sutures are not placed between the anteroseptal commissure and the middle of the septal annulus to avoid damage to the bundle of His. Care should be taken around the region of the anteroseptal commissure to avoid damage to the aortic root.

The sutures are then passed through the sew-ing band of the selected ring. Sutures at the septal annulus are placed through the sewing ring with equal spacing while sutures at the anterior and posterior annulus are passed through the sewing ring with reduced spacing to achieve a reduction annuloplasty.

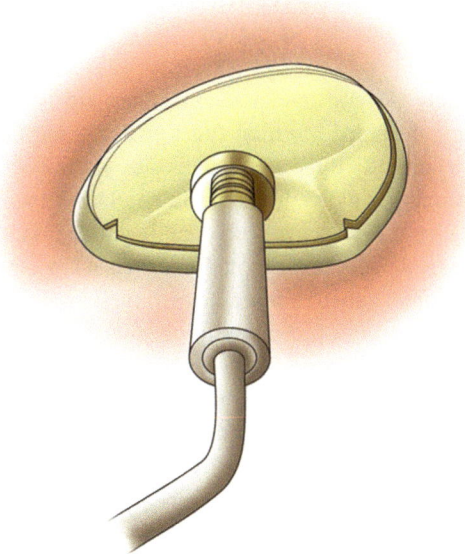

Fig. 12.4 Sizing the tricuspid annulus with reference to the septal annulus (Printed with permission © Gemma Price)

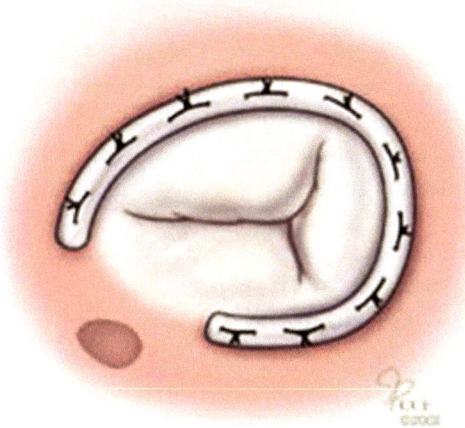

Fig. 12.6 Ring annuloplasty of the tricuspid valve

The annuloplasty ring is then lowered into position and the knots are tied (Fig. 12.6). Valve competency is confirmed by injecting saline through the tricuspid valve into the right ventricle using a 50 ml syringe. The final test of valve competency is done using transoesophageal echocardiography after weaning off cardiopulmonary bypass [5].

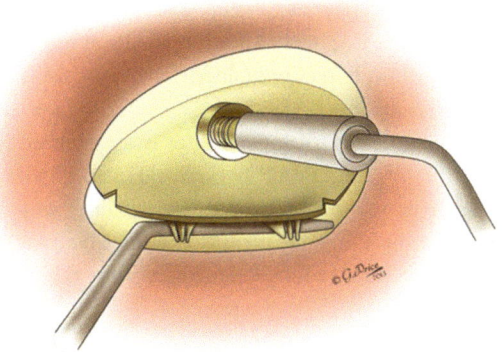

Fig. 12.5 Sizing the tricuspid annulus with reference to the anterior leaflet (Printed with permission © Gemma Price)

Suture Annuloplasty

Satisfactory results can be achieved with suture annuloplasty if the annular dilatation is not severe and there is no associated tricuspid leaflet tethering. A technique which we have used successfully is to plicate the posterior annulus. A pledgeted, 2/0 Ethibond, horizontal, mattress suture is placed either side of the middle of the posterior annulus. This is tightened and tied, reducing the size of the posterior annulus. Further sutures can be placed adjacent to this to further reduce the size of the tricuspid annulus until valve competency is achieved. Other techniques of suture annuloplasty include the De Vega annuloplasty, which comprises a single or double circular suture around the tricuspid annulus, and the Kay annuloplasty, which is applied at the commissural level resulting in bicuspidization of the posterior annulus [6].

Other Repair Techniques

Most techniques described for MV repair can be used in tricuspid valve repair, including leaflet resection and artificial neochord implantation. Also, edge-to-edge "Clover or Alfieri repair" by stitching middle part of the free edge of the leaflets may be used as an adjacent TV repair technique in some cases (Fig. 12.7). In addition, tricuspid leaflet augmentation using autologous pericardium is recommended for use in severely tethered leaflets (Fig. 12.8).

The anterior tricuspid leaflet is augmented by use of an autologous pericardial patch, which increases its size, and hence its surface area of coaptation, allowing increased leaflet coaptation to occur with reduced tension within the right ventricle.

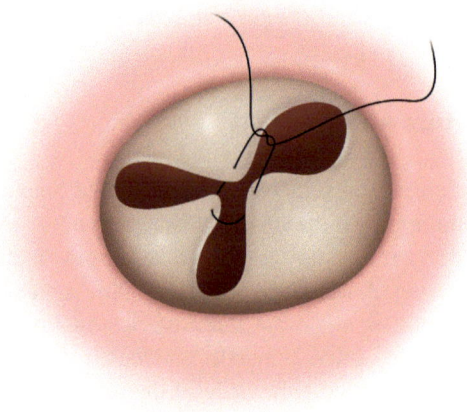

Fig. 12.7 Edge-to-edge "Clover or Alfieri" suture technique

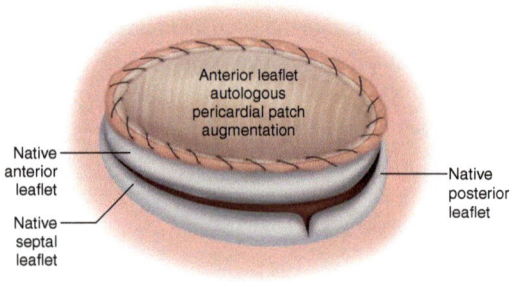

Fig. 12.8 Tricuspid leaflet augmentation using autologous pericardium

Percutaneous Treatment of the Tricuspid Valve

Lately several percutaneous alternatives have been developed to treat functional TR and there are currently three main categories to divided the options for native tricuspid valve disease including heterotopic caval valve implantation, annuloplasty devices and coaptation devices; also, there are reports about transcatheter valve-in-valve and valve-in-ring procedures in patients with tricuspid valve surgery. The standard tricuspid valve surgery is usually performed when the RV is irreversibly dilated and dysfunctional carrying inevitably high risk and mortality rates; hence, there is a clinical need for percutaneous therapies to reduce that high-surgical risk.

Following the success of transcatheter interventions in aortic, pulmonic or mitral valve disease, recent years have witnessed the emergence of numerous percutaneous tricuspid techniques. Three different targets for the current tricuspid transcatheter therapies in the treatment of TR: **implants of transcatheter heart valve** (THV) at the vena cava to reduce reverse backflow, **percutaneous annuloplasty devices** shortening annulus dimension, and **devices improving leafltet coaptation** and reducing the regurgitant orifice.

Transcatheter Therapies for Tricuspid Regurgitation

Unlike aortic and mitral valve disease there is still no specific Transcatheter Tricuspid valve therapy available yet; however, over the last few years several transcatheter advancements specifically targeting treatment of function TR have been TV development. Some devices designed for mitral or aortic disease, such as the MitraClip (Abbott Vascular, Santa Clara, California, United States) or the Edwards SAPIEN valve (Edwards Lifesciences, Irvine, California, United States), and have been successfully adapted for the treatment of TR. There have been a number of studies assessing these devices to evaluate the feasibility, safety and efficacy. In addition, there are reports suggesting a promising novel alternative approach for reintervention on the TV patients with prior tricuspid repair or replacement with bioprosthetic or annuloplasty ring failure, by using a transcatheter aortic or pulmonic valve.

Heterotopic Transcatheter Caval Valve Implantation

The rationale for this intervention is to reduce the regurgitant volume and pressure into the vena cava present in patients with severe TR that leads to hepatic, abdominal and peripheral congestion, thus reducing symptoms of right heart failure.

Caval valve implantation has been performed via specifically designed devices such as the self-expandable TricValve and the balloon-expandable SAPIEN transcatheter aortic valve. The TricValve consists of a pericardial tissue valve on a nitinol stent frame that can be implanted at the inferior vena cava alone or in combination with a specific TricValve for superior vena cava implantation showing acute hemodynamic and clinical improvements in patients. Preoperative inferior and superior vena cava sizing is mandatory and can be an exclusion criterion for this technique if there is a potential risk of valve embolization. The maximum size of this device is 43 mm for the inferior vena cava and 38 mm for the superior vena cava. Before final valve implantation, a peripheral stent is deployed to create a landing zone. The main disadvantage of caval valve implantation is that this therapeutic concept does not reduce TR, only its consequences. No long-term data are available on the safety of the right atrium ventricularization and the persistent right atrium and RV overload due to persistent severe TR.

Three challenges must be taken into account in caval valve implantation procedures: the prox-

imity of hepatic veins just below the diaphragm, the compliance and degree of dilation of the vena cava, and the important anatomic variability of the superior vena cava, making double caval valve implantation a more technically demanding procedure.

Annuloplasty Devices

The pathophysiology of functional TR involves tricuspid annulus dilation. Progressive tricuspid annulus dilation occurs in its anteroposterior plane, which leads to a lack of leaflet coaptation. Tricuspid valve annuloplasty is the basis of current surgical therapy for functional TR and several percutaneous annuloplasty devices have been developed in recent years. These techniques preserve the anatomy of the TV, allowing future treatment options such as THV or percutaneous edge-to-edge repair if necessary.

Various techniques and devices exist for management of functional TR.

Trialign

This device is based on the Kay surgical bicuspidization procedure (conversion of an incompetent TV into a competent bicuspid valve). The Trialign device (Mitralign Inc, Tewksbury, Massachusetts, United States) performs a transcatheter TV repair through the transjugular approach.

TriCinch

The TriCinch (4Tech Cardio, Galway, Ireland) is a transcatheter device designed to reduce functional TR by reducing the annular dimension and restoring leaflet coaptation. It consists of a corkscrew, a Dacron band, and a self-expandable nitinol stent with four available sizes, from 27 to

43 mm. The procedure is usually performed under general anesthesia and with fluoroscopic, TEE and intracardiac echocardiography guidance. However, a successful procedure under conscious sedation and with only fluoroscopic and intracardiac echocardiography guidance was recently reported.

Cardioband

The Cardioband system for the treatment of the TV (Valtech Cardio, Or-Yehuda, Israel) is a percutaneous annuloplasty ring based on the CE-approved Cardioband device for mitral regurgitation. This Dacron adjustable band is fixed in a supra-annular position, similar to a surgical annuloplasty, and allows for bidirectional adjustability (avoiding over-cinching and post-procedural transvalvular gradients) up to a size of a 28-mm surgical ring. The Cardioband delivery system for TR requires a 25-Fr transfemoral introducer sheath. For orientation and safety reasons, a guidewire is placed in the RCA. The procedure is performed under fluoroscopy and 3D TEE guidance. The Cardioband is fastened to the annulus by 17 stainless steel anchors with a length of 6 mm that are implanted from the anterior to the posterior tricuspid annulus. Once the anchors are fixed, the device is cinched and the tricuspid annular dimensions are significantly reduced. Important advantages of this technique include its reversibility and its ability to be adapted to the tricuspid annular geometry, distributing the annular reduction across the annulus, thus reducing the stress on the anchoring sites.

Millipede

The Millipede (Millipede Inc., Santa Rosa, California, United States) annuloplasty device consists of a semirigid, adjustable, complete ring that can be implanted by the surgical or transfemoral approach. It has the advantage of being repositionable and retrievable before deployment and provides a stable annular reduction. It presents an interruption for atrioventricular node in order to reduce the risk of atrioventricular block.

Coaptation Devices

FORMA
The FORMA device (Edwards Lifesciences) is designed to reduce functional TR by occupying the regurgitant orifice and providing a platform for native leaflet coaptation. It consists of a spacer and a rail. The rail tracks the spacer into position and is distally anchored at the RV apex, perpendicular to the tricuspid annulus plane. The spacer is a foam-filled balloon which is positioned in the regurgitant orifice under fluoroscopic and 3D TEE guidance. Two spacer sizes are available: 12 and 15 mm, requiring an introducer sheath of 20 and 24-Fr, respectively, at the left axillary or subclavian vein. The final spacer size is achieved by passive expansion via eight holes in the spacer shaft. Once the spacer is placed in the optimal position to reduce TR, the device is proximally locked and the excess rail length is placed inside a subcutaneous pocket, using a similar technique to a standard pacemaker implantation.

MitraClip in the Tricuspid Valve

Transcatheter TV edge-to-edge repair using the MitraClip (Abbott Vascular) system is a feasible alternative for patients with severe TR. The MitraClip in the tricuspid position mimics the surgical edge-to-edge "clover" technique, which has been validated for the treatment of complex TR, showing satisfactory results at long-term follow-up. The MitraClip device consists of a 4-mm wide cobalt-chromium, polyester-covered implant with two arms that can be opened and closed to grasp the valve leaflets. Tricuspid edge-to-edge repair can be performed by the transjugular or transfemoral approach.

Closure

The RA is closed by a single or double continuous layer of 4/0 polypropylene, starting at either end of the incision.

TV Replacement

Replacement of Tricuspid Valve

Once the decision to replace TV is done, next task is to choose the right type of valve. Most frequently are used biological prostheses as in adults they show mean durability over 15–20 years. Mechanical valves in tricuspid position are uncommon and used mainly in very young patients, but mechanical valves require life-long high anticoagulation. It is also not possible to implant transvenous right ventricular pacing leads in the future; thus, consideration of implantating an epicardial lead is important.

Replacement of TV usually is started by removing all the foreign bodies or infected tissue, but preserving TV subvalvular apparatus as much as possible in order to prevent right ventricular dilatation. Preserved TV leaflets with chordae should be incorporated in suture line while placing annular sutures and not interfere with prosthesis leaflets.

Sizing of the TV for replacement is done in the standard fashion like in mitral valve replacement by putting mitral valve sizes into TV annulus and finding the most optimal size to match the TV annulus. Usually, TVR requires large size prosthetic valve [7].

Placement of suprannular, interrupted, pledged 2/0 Ethibond sutures are usually done with starting suture placement behind the TV annulus, further passing the preserved leaflet edges and leaving pledges on the right atrial side. These sutures are placed into TV annulus everywhere except septal annulus where sutures should be placed at the rim of septal leaflet attachment to the annulus in order to avoid injury to the con-

duction system. Once all the sutures have been placed around the annulus, it is then passed around the chosen prosthetic valve cuff from below upwards so that when the sutures are tied, the knots lie on the right atrial side [8, 9].

During TVR any transvenous pacing wires should be removed and replaced with permanent epicardial wires. Also, permanent epicardial pacing wire implantation should be considered if the new heart block develops during operation.

Closure

After TVR is completed the right atrium is closed by a single continuous layer of 4/0 polypropylene suture, starting at either end of the incision.

Indications

Treatment of secondary TR is targeted at pulmonary hypertension or myocardial disease. Only a selected number of patients with TR receive surgical treatment during surgery for left-sided valve lesions to treat severe TR (Stages C and D) and as a preventative measure for development of severe TR in patients with progressive TR (Stage B). Surgical intervention should be considered for selected patients with isolated TR (either primary TR or secondary TR attributable to annular dilation in the absence of pulmonary hypertension or dilated cardiomyopathy). Severe isolated TR has high mortality rate 8–20%, but most of these interventions were performed after end-organ damage. However, outcomes of patients with severe primary TR are poor with medical management. There is renewed interest in earlier surgery for patients with severe isolated TR before the onset of severe RV dysfunction or end-organ damage. This interest is attributable to (1) an increasing number of patients presenting with right-sided HF from isolated TR, (2) more advanced surgical techniques, and (3) better selection processes, resulting in a lower operative

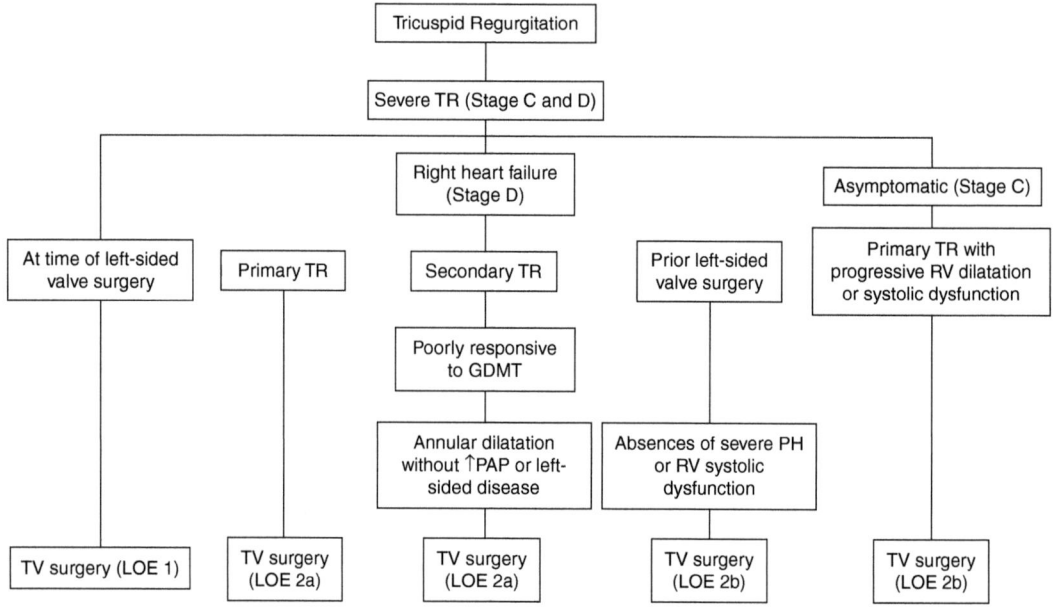

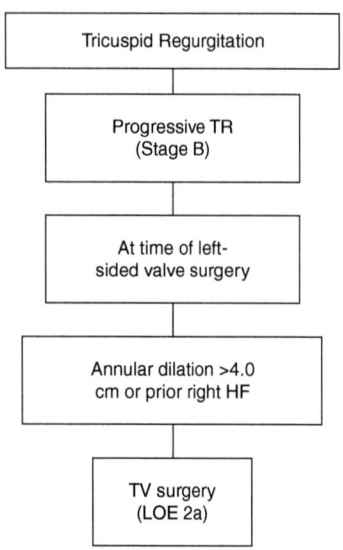

Fig. 12.9 Tricuspid regurgitation: GDMT indicates guideline0directed management and therapy; *HF* heat failure, *PAP* pulmonary artery pressure, *PH* pulmonary hypertension, *RV* right ventricular, *TR* tricuspid regurgitation, *TV* tricuspid regurgitation [10]

risk with documented improvement in symptoms (Fig. 12.9) [10].

There is growing interest in the development of catheter-based therapies for these patients with severe isolated TR.

Both in asymptomatic and minimally symptomatic patients there has been no established optimal time for surgery of tricuspid valve. Evidence from a limited number of cases and data available suggest that serial assessments of

RV size and function might indicate the option of corrective surgery only in selective patients with deteriorating severe primary TR and acceptable surgical risk **Ia**. Healthy patients with no comorbidities, the surgical risk associated with tricuspid valve operation is Low (<1–2% operative mortality rate) in the absence of RV dysfunction or pulmonary hypertension.

It is usually the case that isolated tricuspid valve surgery for severe TR is performed when patients are symptomatic with signs of right-sided HF. Mortality rates for isolated tricuspid valve surgery are more than in isolated aortic or mitral valve surgery and this has been more prominent for re-do tricuspid surgery later after left-sided valve surgery. These rates might be related to the advanced nature of RV failure encountered at the time of the second procedure, residual pulmonary hypertension, LV dysfunction and other valve abnormalities. The risks in place by reoperation have influenced decision-making for initial repair of functional TR at the time of left-sided valve surgery in an attempt to prevent the development of severe TR later after the left-sided valve surgery; however, if there is no significant pulmonary hypertension or severe RV systolic dysfunction, operation for severe symptomatic isolated TR years after surgery for left-sided disease may improve symptoms of right-sided HF, if done before the onset of severe RV dysfunction or end-organ damage with either hepatic or renal dysfunction.

Key Pearls and Pitfalls of Tricuspid Valve Repair

Recently there is more and more emphasis on the importance of addressing secondary TR in clinical practice; hence, the number of Tricuspid Valve interventions is also increasing. So, awareness of pathophysiology of secondary TR and available TV repair techniques are important. In most cases of functional tricuspid regurgitation, tricuspid valve repair is possible by reducing the dilation of the tricuspid annulus. This can be achieved by various techniques including our tri-cuspid 'P' Repair, Tricuspid annuloplasty and/or other techniques. It is important to be aware of important anatomical structures near the tricuspid annulus to avoid any complication.

Comprehension Questions

1. The most common pathology of tricuspid valve is:
   (a) Tricuspid valve infective endocarditis
   (b) Tricuspid stenosis
   (c) **Functional tricuspid regurgitation**
   (d) Congenital tricuspid deformity in Epstein anomaly

2. Which tricuspid annular diameter is considered to be significantly dilated as measured by transthoracic echocardiography in a four chamber view?
   (a) More than 30 mm
   (b) **More than 40 mm**
   (c) More than 60 mm
   (d) More than 70 mm

3. Which is the wrong way to size the tricuspid annuloplasty ring for TV repair?
   (a) Sizing TV septal annulus length between anteroseptal and posteroseptal commissures
   (b) Sizing of surface area of the TV anterior leaflets
   (c) **Sizing of surface area of the TV anterior and posterior leaflets**

4. Where recommended not to place sutures for annuloplasty in order to avoid damage to the bundle of His?
   (a) Between anteroseptal commissure and the middle of the anterior annulus
   (b) **Between anteroseptal commissure and the middle of the septal annulus**
   (c) Between posteroseptal commissure and the middle of the septal annulus
   (d) At the posterior annulus

5. What TV repair technique is most frequently used for functional tricuspid regurgitation?
   (a) Neochord implantation
   (b) Leaflet resection
   (c) **Annuloplasty**
   (d) Tricuspid valve replacement

Key Pearls and Pitfalls of Tricuspid Valve Replacement

Tricuspid valve replacement is performed only when Tricuspid Valve Repair is not possible. The prosthesis of choice in Tricuspid Valve Replacement is a bioprosthesis due to the flow and pressure characteristics of the right heart circulation. It is important to recognise the need for pacemaker after Tricuspid Valve Replacement in view of the proximity of the conduction system to the tricuspid annulus.

Comprehension Questions

1. What is the most frequent tricuspid valve pathology requiring tricuspid valve replacement?
   (a) Functional tricuspid regurgitation
   (b) **Tricuspid valve infective endocarditis**
   (c) Iatrogenic tricuspid valve damage
   (d) Tricuspid stenosis
2. What is the most frequently used prosthesis for tricuspid valve replacement?
   (a) Mechanical aortic prosthesis
   (b) Biological aortic prosthesis
   (c) Mechanical mitral prosthesis
   (d) **Biological mitral prosthesis**
3. What is the mean durability of biological prosthesis in tricuspid valve position?
   (a) Up to 5 years
   (b) 5–10 years
   (c) **10–15 years**
   (d) 15–20 years
4. What are the most frequently used sizes for tricuspid valve replacement? (choose two)
   (a) 19–21 mm
   (b) 23–25 mm
   (c) **27–29 mm**
   (d) **31–33 mm**
5. In which situation should permanent epicardial pacing wires be implanted during tricuspid valve replacement?
   (a) When transvenous pacing wires are present preoperatively and they are removed during operation
   (b) When new heart block develops during operation
   (c) **In both situations**

References

1. McCarthy PM, Bhudia SK, Rajeswaran J, Hoercher KJ, Lytle BW, Cosgrove DM, Blackstone EH. Tricuspid valve repair: durability and risk factors for failure. J Thorac Cardiovasc Surg. 2004;127(3):674–85.
2. Dalrymple-Hay MJ, Leung Y, Ohri SK, Haw MP, Ross JK, Livesey SA, Monro JL. Tricuspid valve replacement: bioprostheses are preferable. J Heart Valve Dis. 1999;8(6):644–8.
3. Tang GH, David TE, Singh SK, Maganti MD, Armstrong S, Borger MA. Tricuspid valve repair with an annuloplasty ring results in improved long-term outcomes. Circulation. 2006;114(1 Suppl):I577–81.
4. Chang BC, Song SW, Lee S, Yoo KJ, Kang MS, Chung N. Eight-year outcomes of tricuspid annuloplasty using autologous pericardial strip for functional tricuspid regurgitation. Ann Thorc Surg. 2008 Nov;86(5):1485–92.
5. Parolari A, Barili F, Pilozzi A, Pacini D. Ring or suture annuloplasty for tricuspid regurgitation? A meta-analysis review. Ann Thorac Surg. 2014;98:2255–63.
6. Shinn SH, Dayan V, Schaff HV, Dearani JA, Joyce LD, Lahr B, Greason KL, Stulak JM, Daly RC. Outcomes of ring versus suture annuloplasty for tricuspid valve repair in patients undergoing mitral valve surgery. J Thorac Cardiovasc Surg. 2016;152(2):406–15.
7. Burri M, Vogt MO, Hörer J, Cleuziou J, Kasnar-Samprec J, Kühn A, Lange R, Schreiber C. Durability of bioprostheses for the tricuspid valve in patients with congenital heart disease. Eur J Cardiothorac Surg. 2016;50(5):988–93.
8. Dhoble A, Zhao Y, Vejpongsa P, Loghin C, Smalling RW, Estrera A, Nguyen TC. National 10-year trends and outcomes of isolated and concomitant tricuspid valve surgery. J Cardiovasc Surg. 2019;60(1):119–27.
9. Alkhouli M, Berzingi C, Kowatli A, Alqahtani F, Badhwar V. Comparative early outcomes of tricuspid Valve repair versus replacement for secondary tricuspid regurgitation. Open Heart. 2018;5(2):e000878.
10. Otto CM, Nishimura RA, Bonow RO, Carabello BA, Erwin JP III, Gentile F, Jneid H, Krieger EV, Mack M, McLeod C, O'Gara PT, Rigolin VH, Sundt TM III, Thompson A, Toly C. 2020 ACC/AHA guideline for the management of patients with valvular heart disease: a report of the American College of Cardiology/American Heart Association Joint Committee on Clinical Practice Guidelines. Circulation. 2021;143:e72–e227.

Cannulation Strategies for Aortic Root Surgery

13

Ourania Preventza and Darrell Wu

Learning Objectives

- Understand the general principles of cannulation in aortic root surgery
- Understand the principles of the different cannulation strategies
- Understand how to select the best cannulation approach for each patient undergoing root surgery
- Understand the advantages and disadvantages of each cannulation strategy
- Understand which patient characteristics should be considered in the decision-making process

The optimal arterial cannulation strategy for proximal aortic surgery with proximal arch involvement remains controversial among large-aortic-volume centers. The most widely used cannulation sites include the femoral, axillary,

innominate, and carotid arteries, as well as the ascending aorta itself. Each cannulation site has advantages and disadvantages. Although to some extent the site of cannulation depends on the type and location of the patient's aortic disease, the choice of cannulation site should be ultimately aimed at facilitating the operation and minimizing complications.

Cannulation Strategies

Central Aortic

Direct central distal aortic cannulation is routine for establishing arterial inflow during cardiopulmonary bypass. For patients with or without distal aortic aneurysmal disease and dissection, epiaortic scanning and intraoperative transesophageal echocardiography can facilitate cannulation of the true lumen (whether directly or through needle puncture) in an area of the aortic wall devoid of atherosclerotic plaque [1]. After a cannulation site is identified, a purse-string suture is placed in that region.

Specifically in cases of ascending dissection, central ascending aortic cannulation has not been historically favored because of the risk of cannulating the false lumen. However, several recent reports describe successful use of central aortic cannulation with good outcomes in patients with acute Type A (or Type I or II) dissection [1, 2]. In

O. Preventza (✉)
Division of Cardiothoracic Surgery, Michael
E. DeBakey Department of Surgery, Baylor College
of Medicine, Houston, TX, USA

Baylor – St. Luke's Medical Center,
Houston, TX, USA

Texas Heart Institute, Houston, TX, USA
e-mail: preventz@bcm.edu

D. Wu
Division of Cardiothoracic Surgery, Michael
E. DeBakey Department of Surgery, Baylor College
of Medicine, Houston, TX, USA

© Springer Nature Switzerland AG 2022
P. P. Punjabi, P. G. Kyriazis (eds.), *Essentials of Operative Cardiac Surgery*,
https://doi.org/10.1007/978-3-031-14557-5_13

cases of acute Type I aortic dissection, trans-esophageal echocardiography is very helpful in guiding wire placement and cannulation of the true lumen.

In cases with only aortic root involvement, central aortic cannulation is the standard of care. In cases of aortic disease involving the proximal or total arch in addition to the aortic root, central aortic cannulation continues to have certain advantages. First, it is technically simple and expeditious, especially in cases of hemodynamic instability. Second, central cannulation can potentially accelerate cooling, which in theory could reduce the cardiopulmonary bypass time. Third, central aortic cannulation avoids the risk of retrograde thromboembolism that is associated with femoral cannulation. One potential disadvantage is that in cases of central aortic cannulation with circulatory arrest, lower levels of hypothermia may be required because removing the cannula when circulatory arrest is initiated results in a period of pure circulatory arrest without antegrade cerebral perfusion (ACP); ACP is initiated after transection of the ascending aorta.

The alternative cannulation sites and techniques described hereafter are mainly used when, in addition to the aortic root, the proximal or total arch must be reconstructed.

Femoral

The femoral artery is the traditional cannulation site for proximal aortic procedures with proximal arch involvement and has been used with excellent results [3]. The main advantages of femoral cannulation are relative ease of access, avoiding direct manipulation of the diseased ascending aorta, and a low incidence of complications. Cannulation is relatively easy in severely obese patients and can be done under direct visualization by using a Seldinger technique or even via an 8-mm graft sutured end-to-side to the femoral artery to avoid prolonged periods of leg ischemia.

A vertical or oblique incision is made in the groin directly over the femoral pulse or by using anatomic landmarks such as the medial edge of the pubic tubercle and anterior superior iliac spine. The common femoral artery is exposed proximal to its bifurcation into the superficial femoral artery and deep femoral artery. After proximal and distal control are obtained, a purse-string suture is placed on the femoral artery at the intended site of cannulation. Heparin is administered, the femoral artery is incised, and an appropriately sized cannula is inserted as the purse string is tightened. The femoral artery can also be cannulated percutaneously: Under ultrasound guidance, a needle is inserted into the artery, followed by passage of wire and dilators and then insertion of the cannula.

Although rare, limb ischemia, nerve injury, and local wound issues are potential complications of femoral cannulation. They are mainly caused by a combination of patient risk factors and technical issues. Failure to recognize the extent of peripheral vascular disease, cannulation below the femoral artery bifurcation, size mismatch between cannula and vessel, and improper closure of the femoral vessel can lead to limb ischemia. Anastomosing an 8-mm graft end-to-side to the femoral artery can prevent prolonged periods of ischemia when a large cannula is inserted directly into the femoral artery. Neuronal damage and wound complications can result from damage caused during surgical dissection or disruption of lymphatic vessels; these complications rarely require surgical intervention.

Despite the relative ease of insertion and low complication rate associated with femoral cannulation, it has several drawbacks that have led to decreasing reliance on it. For instance, femoral artery cannulation in cases of dissection can lead to perfusion of the false lumen, resulting in organ malperfusion and retrograde dissection [4]. In these instances, because these complications can be due to luminal compression or to the dissection itself, it can be difficult to determine whether they result from the disease process or are sequalae of femoral cannulation. It has been suggested that in patients with aneurysmal disease, femoral cannulation can lead to atheroembolism from direct dislodgement of plaque as the cannula is advanced [5]. And in patients with extensive aortoiliac occlusive or aneurysmal disease or with extensive peripheral vascular disease, femoral cannulation is sometimes contraindicated [5].

Additional disadvantages of femoral cannulation include the colder hypothermic temperatures it requires when the arch needs reconstruction, the period of pure circulatory arrest during reconstruction of the arch or the distal aortic anastomosis, and the lack of ACP. Antegrade cerebral perfusion was developed as a way to reduce neurologic complications, and some evidence shows that it improves neurologic outcomes [5, 6]. These complications and the inability to provide direct ACP with femoral cannulation have led to a search for alternative cannulation sites.

Axillary

Axillary cannulation was our preferred technique until almost 10 years ago; now, our initial preference is innominate artery cannulation when the proximal arch needs to be replaced in addition to the aortic root. Cannulating the axillary artery has two key advantages over femoral artery cannulation. First, in patients with severe peripheral vascular disease that makes femoral artery cannulation difficult or impossible, the axillary artery provides a safe alternative site. Second, and more importantly, axillary cannulation makes

it possible to deliver ACP. That said, axillary artery cannulation also carries certain disadvantages. For one, exposing the axillary artery can be time-consuming, especially in obese patients. Also, in some patients, the axillary artery is small, limiting the size of cannula that can be directly inserted into the artery. Finally, axillary cannulation can injure the brachial plexus, complicating postoperative recovery.

The axillary artery is easily exposed through an infraclavicular incision approximately one fingerbreadth beneath the clavicle, extending from the middle to the latter third of the clavicle. The pectoralis major fibers are divided, and through blunt dissection the axillary artery is identified and separated from the brachial plexus and axillary vein (Fig. 13.1a). The axillary artery can be cannulated directly through a purse-string suture after an incision is made, or by the Seldinger technique. The axillary artery can also be cannulated indirectly by anastomosing an 8- or 10-mm graft to it end-to-side with continuous 5-0 or 6-0 polypropylene suture (Fig. 13.1b). The arterial cannula is then secured to the graft with heavy ties and connected. At the end of the operation, the graft is tied with heavy silk ties and large clips, and then trimmed.

Compared with femoral cannulation, direct right axillary artery cannulation seems to be

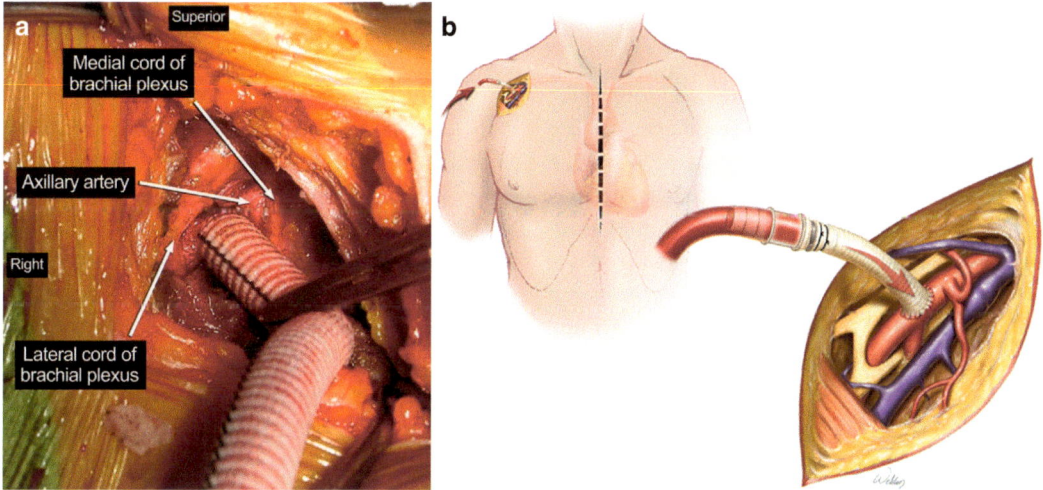

Fig. 13.1 (**a**) Axillary cannulation with a Dacron graft, with the surrounding anatomic structures. (**b**) The Dacron graft can be used as arterial inflow for cardiopulmonary bypass

associated with a higher overall complication rate [7]. However, reports comparing direct and indirect (via a side graft) axillary cannulation show fewer local complications with indirect cannulation but no difference with regard to neurologic outcomes [7].

Innominate

At our institution, innominate artery cannulation has become the standard approach for patients with proximal aortic disease who are undergoing elective and sometimes even emergency surgery [8]. While there are fewer reports about innominate artery cannulation, it appears to have several advantages over femoral and axillary artery cannulation. First, the innominate artery is approached through a traditional median sternotomy, precluding need for an additional incision and decreasing operative time. Second, the cannulation is easier in obese patients. Third, cannulating the innominate artery eliminates the risk of brachial plexus injury, arm ischemia, and arm claudication associated with axillary artery cannulation. Fourth, delivery of ACP eliminates the risk of retrograde cerebral atheroembolism and organ malperfusion associated with femoral artery cannulation. Finally, innominate artery cannulation avoids both the groin incision required for femoral artery cannulation, thereby facilitating postoperative physical therapy and early ambulation.

After median sternotomy, the brachiocephalic vein is encircled and retracted inferiorly. The innominate artery is then exposed and dissected free up to its bifurcation if necessary. Heparin is administered at 1 mg/kg, the near-infrared spectroscopy is carefully monitored, systemic blood pressure is maintained at ≥90 mmHg, a partial occluding clamp is applied, and an 8- or 10-mm graft is anastomosed in end-to-side fashion with a running 5-0 or 6-0 polypropylene suture (Fig. 13.2a, b). The suture line is then reinforced if necessary. The graft is then deaired and connected to the arterial line.

After cannulation, full-dose heparin at 3–4 mg/kg is administered to achieve a target

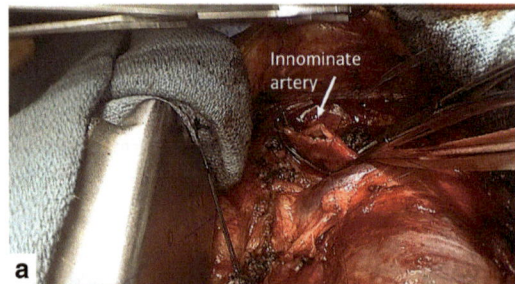

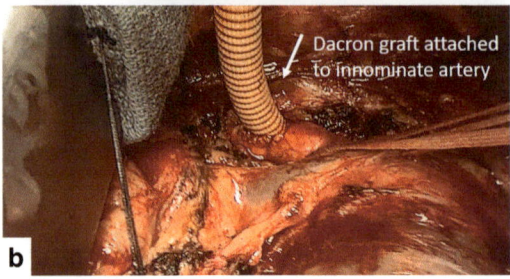

Fig. 13.2 (a) Partial occluding clamp on the innominate artery before arteriotomy. (b) Dacron graft attached to innominate artery end to side to be used as arterial inflow for cardiopulmonary bypass

activated clotting time of 480 s or longer. The patient is then placed on cardiopulmonary bypass and cooled to 23–24 °C. During this time, anesthesia staff places ice around the head and administers mannitol and hydrocortisone to prevent cerebral edema. Any proximal dissection is undertaken during cooling, and once target temperature is reached, flows are reduced, the Rummel tourniquet (or vascular clamp) is cinched down, and selective antegrade perfusion is delivered at a target flow of 10–15 mL/kg/min. The proximal arch is exposed, and a 9F Pruitt catheter is inserted into the left common carotid to deliver left-side perfusion. The left subclavian artery is left open to air, and if there is considerable backbleeding, then a balloon-tip catheter is inserted to inhibit flow. After the distal anastomosis is completed, the occluding clamp is removed from the innominate artery, full flows are resumed, and the graft is deaired and clamped. The NIRS are monitored continuously during this time, and a change of more than 10% from baseline prompts us to increase flow (to >13–15 mL/kg/min) while maintaining an arterial pressure—measured via the right radial arterial line—of 50–70 mmHg. We also use pH-stat blood gas management to increase the arterial partial pressure of CO_2 to maintain cerebral vasodilation. We do not routinely use transcranial Doppler imaging or jugular venous oximetry as a neuromonitoring adjunct.

Similar to femoral and axillary artery cannulation, innominate artery cannulation is not without risks [8]. Inadequate dissection can result in injury of the arterial back wall or of nearby structures such as the trachea. Furthermore, depending on the patient's anatomy, manipulating the innominate artery can injure the phrenic nerve or sympathetic chain. However, in our series [8], we did not encounter any such injuries or any bleeding complications; we therefore consider innominate artery cannulation to be generally safe, and it is our first choice for cannulation.

In cases of prior sternotomy in which the aorta is close to the sternum, our second choice is to cannulate the right axillary artery with a side graft. In patients in extremis, femoral cannulation is preferred if the patient's body habitus is amenable [9].

Cannulation of the innominate artery was first described by Cosgrove in 2000 [10], and we began using innominate artery cannulation in our proximal aortic repairs in 2011. We recently reviewed our experience in 263 patients who underwent innominate artery cannulation with a side graft for proximal aortic repairs involving a combination of aortic root, ascending aorta, and aortic arch along with concomitant valve repair or replacement, CABG, and stent deployment in the descending thoracic aorta [11]. Approximately 10% of our patients had acute or subacute Type A dissection, and 17% had previous sternotomy. The operative mortality was 4.9%, and nine patients (3.4%) had postoperative stroke. We believe that indirectly cannulating the innominate artery with a side graft avoids the "sandblasting" effect that turbulent flow from the catheter tip has on an atheromatous aorta. Other groups have also obtained excellent results by using innominate artery cannulation; in a recent meta-analysis of 1366 operations involving proximal aortic replacement, innominate cannulation was associated with a 4% stroke rate [12].

Femoral Versus Axillary Versus Innominate Artery Versus Central Cannulation

The controversy regarding the optimal arterial cannulation strategy for proximal aortic surgery centers around the greater neuroprotective benefits of ACP alone versus retrograde cerebral perfusion (RCP) with deep hypothermic circulatory arrest versus pure deep hypothermic circulatory arrest with no ACP or RCP. Studies comparing femoral with axillary artery cannulation show a clear trend toward fewer neurologic events with axillary cannulation; however, a detailed meta-analysis of these studies is impossible because of their heterogeneous study designs and populations and the fact that the majority of evidence comes from observational cohort studies [13]. Femoral artery cannulation has historically been used for aortic arch surgery when hypothermic circulatory arrest was needed. Given the acuity and complexity of Type A aortic dissection presentations with different involvement of the proximal aorta, arch, head vessels, and visceral bed, the hemodynamic stability of the patient, and differences in center preferences and experience, the approach to cannulation strategy varies substantially.

We recently reviewed our experience in 938 patients who underwent elective hemiarch or total arch surgery with circulatory arrest between 2006 and 2016 [9]. We performed a multivariable analysis and propensity analysis between right axillary and innominate artery cannulation and found that the two cannulation strategies were associated with equivalent composite adverse event rates, operative mortality, and overall stroke rates, suggesting that these strategies can be used interchangeably. In cases in which no part of the arch is involved and the ascending aorta is not dissected, central cannulation has gained favor when arch reconstruction is needed or the patient has acute Type I aortic dissection.

Overall, cannulation strategies involving any of the four cannulation sites are sound, and the choice among these strategies must take into account the patient's characteristics and aortic disease; thus, it should be tailored to each unique clinical situation to ensure the best outcome.

Key Pearls and Pitfalls

- The optimal arterial cannulation strategy for proximal aortic surgery with proximal arch involvement remains controversial among large-aortic-volume centers
- In cases of ascending dissection, central ascending aortic cannulation has not been historically favored because of the risk of cannulating the false lumen, even though recent reports indicate that this approach has produced favorable results
- In cases with only aortic root involvement, central aortic cannulation is the standard of care; in contrast, in cases of aortic disease involving the proximal or total arch in addition to the aortic root, central aortic cannulation continues to have certain advantages
- While there are fewer reports about innominate artery cannulation, it appears to have several advantages over femoral and axillary artery cannulation
- Cannulation strategies involving any of the four cannulation sites are sound, and the choice among these strategies must take into account the patient's characteristics and aortic disease

Multiple Choice Questions

1. Complications of axillary artery cannulation include
   (a) Phrenic nerve injury
   (b) Sympathetic chain disruption
   (c) Lower-extremity ischemia
   (d) Brachial plexus injury (correct)
2. Innominate artery cannulation has several advantages over femoral and axillary artery cannulation, including
   (a) Requires no additional incision (correct)
   (b) Is the only approach that can deliver ACP
   (c) Can lead to malperfusion and retrograde dissection
   (d) Can lead to brachial plexus injury

References

1. Frederick JR, Yang E, Trubelja A, Desai ND, Szeto WY, Pochettino A, et al. Ascending aortic cannulation in acute type A dissection repair. Ann Thorac Surg. 2013;95:1808–11.
2. Inoue Y, Ueda T, Taguchi S, Kashima I, Koizumi K, Takahashi R, et al. Ascending aorta cannulation in acute type A aortic dissection. Eur J Cardiothorac Surg. 2007;31:976–9. discussion 9–81
3. Harky A, Oo S, Gupta S, Field M. Proximal arterial cannulation in thoracic aortic surgery—literature review. J Card Surg. 2019;34:598–604.
4. Di Eusanio M, Schepens MA, Morshuis WJ, Dossche KM, Di Bartolomeo R, Pacini D, et al. Brain protection using antegrade selective cerebral perfusion: a multicenter study. Ann Thorac Surg. 2003;76:1181–8. discussion 8–9
5. Tsiouris A, Elkinany S, Ziganshin BA, Elefteriades JA. Open Seldinger-guided femoral artery cannulation technique for thoracic aortic surgery. Ann Thorac Surg. 2016;101:2231–5.
6. Benedetto U, Mohamed H, Vitulli P, Petrou M. Axillary versus femoral arterial cannulation in type A acute aortic dissection: evidence from a meta-analysis of comparative studies and adjusted risk estimates. Eur J Cardiothorac Surg. 2015;48:953–9.
7. Sabik JF, Nemeh H, Lytle BW, Blackstone EH, Gillinov AM, Rajeswaran J, et al. Cannulation of the axillary artery with a side graft reduces morbidity. Ann Thorac Surg. 2004;77:1315–20.
8. Preventza O, Bakaeen FG, Stephens EH, Trocciola SM, de la Cruz KI, Coselli JS. Innominate artery cannulation: an alternative to femoral or axillary cannulation for arterial inflow in proximal aortic surgery. J Thorac Cardiovasc Surg. 2013;145:S191–6.
9. Preventza O, Price MD, Spiliotopoulos K, Amarasekara HS, Cornwell LD, Omer S, et al. In elective arch surgery with circulatory arrest, does the arterial cannulation site really matter? A propensity score analysis of right axillary and innominate artery cannulation. J Thorac Cardiovasc Surg. 2018;155:1953–60.e4.
10. Banbury MK, Cosgrove DM 3rd. Arterial cannulation of the innominate artery. Ann Thorac Surg. 2000;69:957.
11. Preventza O, Garcia A, Tuluca A, Henry M, Cooley DA, Simpson K, et al. Innominate artery cannulation for proximal aortic surgery: outcomes and neurological events in 263 patients. Eur J Cardiothorac Surg. 2015;48:937–42. discussion 42
12. Svensson LG, Blackstone EH, Rajeswaran J, Sabik JF 3rd, Lytle BW, Gonzalez-Stawinski G, et al. Does the arterial cannulation site for circulatory arrest influence stroke risk? Ann Thorac Surg. 2004;78:1274–84. discussion-84
13. Gulbins H, Pritisanac A, Ennker J. Axillary versus femoral cannulation for aortic surgery: enough evidence for a general recommendation? Ann Thorac Surg. 2007;83:1219–24.

Ascending Aortic Aneurysm Surgery

14

Edgar Aranda-Michel, Ibrahim Sultan, and Joseph E. Bavaria

Learning Objectives

- Understand the principles of cannulation in aortic root surgery
- Understand the principles of the different cannulation strategies
- Understand how to distinguish the preferred cannulation for each patient
- Understand the advantages and disadvantages for each cannulation strategy
- Understand which are the patient's characteristics involved in the decision making process

E. Aranda-Michel
Division of Cardiac Surgery, Department of Cardiothoracic Surgery, University of Pittsburgh, Pittsburgh, PA, USA

I. Sultan (✉)
Division of Cardiac Surgery, Department of Cardiothoracic Surgery, University of Pittsburgh, Pittsburgh, PA, USA

Heart and Vascular Institute, University of Pittsburgh Medical Center, Pittsburgh, PA, USA
e-mail: sultani@upmc.edu

J. E. Bavaria
Division of Cardiac Surgery, Department of Surgery, University of Pennsylvania, Pittsburgh, PA, USA
e-mail: joseph.bavaria@uphs.upenn.edu

Introduction

Thoracic aortic aneurysms (TAAs) are uncommon and have an incidence of 10 cases per 100,000 patient years [1, 2]. They are most commonly seen in the ascending aorta between the sinotubular junction and the innominate artery. The natural history of aortic aneurysms over time can be continued growth with increased aortic diameter and stresses, ultimately resulting in either dissection or rupture, both of which carry significant morbidity and mortality [3, 4]. However, most aneurysms continue to be asymptomatic and be discovered incidentally [1, 2].

Patient Presentation and Selection

Due to the indolent nature of TAAs, patients typically have other initially presenting pathology warranting imaging which results in the incidental detection of the aneurysm. This can be seen when imaging is performed in patients undergoing valve surgery or non-cardiac thoracic surgery [1, 5]. In patients where the surgical impetus is the TAA, the size and the morphology of the aorta is important. Saccular or large symptomatic aneurysms are typically of greater concern.

Current guidelines recommend prophylactic surgery on isolated TAAs measuring 5.5 cm in patients with no risk factors [2, 6]. In the absence

© Springer Nature Switzerland AG 2022
P. P. Punjabi, P. G. Kyriazis (eds.), *Essentials of Operative Cardiac Surgery*,
https://doi.org/10.1007/978-3-031-14557-5_14

of personal or familial risk factors, imaging surveillance of the aneurysm is recommended to measure growth rate and absolute size of the aneurysm at 6 month or longer intervals [7]. If the growth rate reaches 0.5 cm per year or the size of the aneurysm is 4.5 cm while the patient is undergoing major cardiac surgery, repair of the TAA is indicated [8]. While having a threshold is useful, it does not capture the heterogeneity seen in the TAA population, which is driven by genetic factors. Nearly 20% of TAA cases have a familial history of some sort of aneurysmal formation including a personal of family history of bicuspid aortic valve (BAV) [1]. The most common genetic conditions with connective tissue disorders that predispose patients for TAA development are Marfan syndrome, Loeys-Dietz syndrome, and Ehlers-Danlos syndrome [8]. Patients with connective tissue disorders are likely to dissect or rupture at smaller diameters, reducing the size threshold for these patients to as low as 4–4.5 cm. Each of these conditions affect components of the extra cellular membrane and the vasculature, effectively weakening its mechanical strength. This results in a lower age of TAA presentation as well as size of the TAA at complication in this group compared to non-genetic TAAs [8]. Predicated on these findings, operative indication for familial aortopathy is performed at above 4 or 4.5 cm for Loeys Dietz syndrome and Marfans syndrome respectively [6, 8, 9].

Operative Planning

Preoperative Imaging

As with all patients undergoing cardiac surgery, preoperative imaging is performed which includes coronary angiography, echocardiography, and a CT aortogram. The first two modalities are to assess for other cardiac pathologies that could be surgically intervened on during the aneurysm repair. The CT scan helps to inform operative planning, particularly by understanding the location of the aneurysm. In patients undergoing reoperative surgery, the aneurysm can be concerningly close to the sternum, prohibiting a standard reoperative sternotomy. In such rare cases, peripheral cannulation with deep hypothermic circulatory arrest can be utilized prior to reoperative sternotomy [10].

Cannulation Strategy

Cannulation strategy is predicated on the extent and location of the aneurysm as well as if any concomitant procedures will be performed. For non-aortic surgery, the lesser curve of the aortic arch is cannulated distal to the left carotid artery to minimize cerebral embolic burden. However, in the setting of aneurysmal disease where the ascending aorta is to be resected, and the distal anastomosis is to be performed under circulatory arrest, the distal ascending aorta is cannulated to ensure removal of the cannulation site prior to performing the distal anastomosis. Alternative cannulation sites include the axillary and femoral arteries; both of which are rarely utilized by us.

Circulatory Arrest and Cerebral Protection

Frequently, aneurysmal tissue may terminate proximal to the brachiocephalic arteries which may allow for the distal anastomosis to be performed with the cross clamp in place. This is more common in patients with bicuspid aortic valve. However, to eliminate all aneurysmal tissue, circulatory arrest is typically utilized for hemiarch replacements. To achieve this, systemic hypothermia is employed with an adjunct such as retrograde or antegrade cerebral perfusion (RCP or ACP). RCP is utilized for hemiarch replacements while ACP is used for total arch replacements to adequately perfuse the brain during extended period of circulatory arrest. While RCP does not necessarily 'perfuse' the brain, it allows for uniform cooling of the brain while flushing debris which can be invaluable to prevent cerebral emboli. ACP has the distinct advantage of perfusing the brain but may present with increased risk of embolism [11]. Intraoperative EEG allows for objective measurement of cerebral silence with systemic hypo-thermia and circulatory arrest is initiated once EEG is silent and the bladder temperature reaches 20 °C or lower. Some groups have uti-lized moderate hypothermia as well but there are no conclusive data to support its superiority over deep hypothermia [12].

Surgical Variations

As previously mentioned, thoracic aortic aneu-rysms can present with other aortic pathologies, such as annular or Sinus of Valsalva dilation and/or aortic valve pathology. While not the focus of this chapter, a brief discussion of aortic root and valve procedures is warranted. In the absence of cusp calcification, the aortic valve can generally be preserved with either a remodeling or reim-plantation technique. We prefer the latter in most patients [13]. The sinus segments are resected leaving a 3–5 mm of tissue behind at the level of the annulus. Both coronary arteries are fashioned as buttons and annuloplasty sutures are utilized to seat a Valsalva graft. This is followed by the sec-ondary suture line which has to be hemostatic. The coronary arteries are subsequently reim-planted back on to the polyester graft in an ortho-topic fashion. With advance cusp disease that is not amenable to repair, a modified Bentall proce-dure is performed.

The Surgery

Setup and Cannulation

Most ascending aortic operations are performed via a full sternotomy using a limited skin incision for cosmesis. A full sternotomy is preferable due to the high incidence of aortic root surgery or other additional cardiac operation in this patient population. A standard sternal retractor is used, and the pericardium is suspended for optimal exposure of the heart. It is not uncommon for the heart to be shifted into the left chest because of large aneurysms. Most if not all patients are can-nulated centrally in the ascending aorta, just above

the aortic reflection. We adjust our cannulation site according to the innominate take off while keeping in mind if the patient needs any complex arch work done at the same time. The lesser curve of the aorta is used as a cannulation site since this directs the cannula tip away from the left ventric-ular outflow tract and has the least direct impact, potentially decreasing risk of an iatrogenic aortic dissection. Pursestrings are placed in the aorta prior to systemic heparinization. This is particu-larly important in patients with bicuspid aortic valves and connective tissue disorders who have thin walled aortas as one can easily cause a sig-nificant hematoma in a heparinized patient if the pursestring sutures are not placed partial thick-ness. After the aorta is cannulated, a plane is cre-ated posterior to the superior vena cava (SVC) while being careful not to injure the right pulmo-nary artery. An umbilical tape is passed and a rummel tourniquet is placed lose. The SVC is cannulated with a right-angle cannula (26–28 French) and this is subsequently used for retro-grade cerebral perfusion (RCP) during circulatory arrest (Fig. 14.1). The right atrium is cannulated with a two/three stage cannula. Both these can-nulas are connected with a Y connector to the venous drainage circuit. This Y connector has a three-way stopcock that will then be connected to the cardioplegia line which is what we use for RCP (Fig. 14.2). A retrograde sinus catheter is used on all these cases. Cardiopulmonary bypass (CPB) is then commenced and a left ventricular (LV) vent is placed via the right superior pulmo-nary vein (RSPV).

It is uncommon for us to cannulate the axillary artery for elective aneurysm surgery. However, if needed, a right axillary incision is utilized and after preservation of nerves and the subclavian vein, the patient is given 5000 units of heparin, the inflow and outflow of the artery clamped and an 8–10 mm graft is sewn to the subclavian artery and utilized as the arterial inflow conduit. It is important to have bilateral radial arterial lines in such a situation because after unclamping the axillary artery, the right radial arterial line wave-form and pressure should return to normal and correlate with the left. Moreover, during CPB, the right radial artery is unlikely to be reliable as

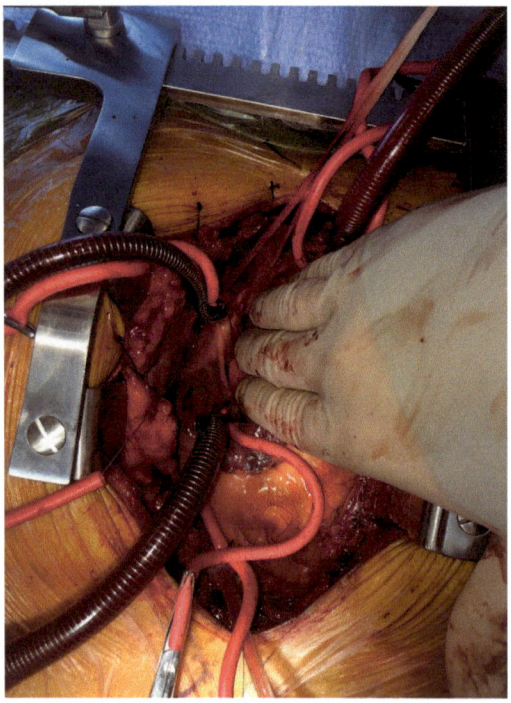

Fig. 14.1 Cannulation strategy depicting aortic arterial cannulation, right atrial cannulation, and superior venous cannulation for retrograde cerebral perfusion

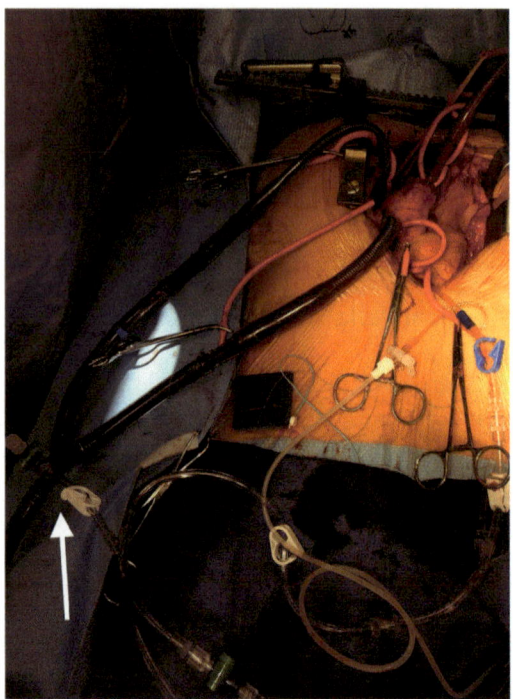

Fig. 14.2 Expanded view of venous cannulation demonstrating the Y connection with the cardioplegia circuit connected to a three-way stop cock (white arrow)

this will invariably have a higher pressure than systemic pressure.

Myocardial Protection and Circulatory Arrest

Most distal anastomoses are performed under circulatory arrest. A 'clamped' distal anastomosis is occasionally performed when it is possible to resect all the aneurysmal aorta with an aortic cross clamp in place and sew it to a graft safely [14].

Once the patient is on cardiopulmonary bypass, a left ventricular vent is placed, the aorto-pulmonary window is dissected, and the patient is systemically cooled to hypothermia. If there is severe aortic regurgitation (AR), the patient is cooled until the arterial inflow is approximately 28 °C before cross clamp is applied. Once the cross clamp is applied, the heart is arrested with high potassium based blood cardioplegia instilled

via the aortic root in the absence of AR or via the coronary sinus in the presence of significant AR. Intermittent antegrade and retrograde cardioplegia is given throughout the operation. The patient is systemically cooled to a core temperature of 18–20 °C. A temperature probe is used to measure myocardial temperature, which is maintained below 13° throughout the operation.

Exposure and Proximal Aortic Surgery

The operating table is placed in a 'back up' position to fully inspect the aortic root. The right atrial cannula is tacked to the skin and two sutures are placed on the anterior wall of the RV just anterior to the aorta to distract the RV away from the proximal aorta.

The aorta is opened approximately 2–3 cm above the sinotubular junction and close to the clamp site. This allows inspection of the entire aortic root before committing to a 'definitive operation'. The aorta is transected in its entirety and the proximal aorta is dissected off the pulmonary artery, the right ventricle and the right atrium. This is all done while carefully looking for any coronary artery anomalies [15]. This is particularly important in patients with bicuspid aortic valves who have a higher incidence of abnormal coronary take off. The aortic valve is then assessed and either repaired if possible or replaced with a tissue or mechanical valve. Once this is done an intra-annular sizer is used to measure the optimal graft size. This is brought into the field. Three equidistant lines are marked on the graft to simulate the three commissures. The graft is then sewn to the proximal aorta with a running 4-0 prolene. Once the anastomosis is complete, an angiocatheter is placed inside the graft and the graft is tested with cardioplegia is being given. This accomplishes two objectives. One can test for hemostasis as well as the competency of the valve. Any repair sutures are placed in the proximal suture line if necessary at this point.

If the sinus of valsalva needs to be resected for aneurysmal disease, a valve sparing root replacement with a valsalva graft or a composite root is sewn in. The details of both are briefly touched earlier in this chapter but the surgical methods are beyond the scope of this chapter.

The Distal Anastomosis

As mentioned earlier in the chapter, most distal anastomoses are performed under circulatory arrest. While the patient is being systemically cooled to a core temperature of 18 °C and iso-electric EEG, proximal aortic surgery is performed to maintain efficient conduct of the operation. Once target core temperature is reached and cerebral silence is observed, our attention is directed towards the arch. The cardioplegia line to the Y circuit/SVC cannula is flushed to deair the circuit. The patient is then placed in deep Trendelenburg to avoid any significant air emboli. This also helps with exposure of the arch. Once the team is ready, the pump is turned off and the arterial line, the right atrial cannula, and the venous line is clamped. The cross clamp is removed. The umbilical tape around the SVC is snared and we begin RCP from the cardioplegia line via the SVC. The arterial cannula is removed, and the arterial cannulation site is resected to healthy tissue. The arch is inspected carefully, and aorta is transected to base of the innominate artery in order to ensure all aneurysmal tissue is removed. At this point, return of blood flow is noted from the arch (Fig. 14.3). It is important to dissect the aorta circumferentially while leaving adventitia behind. This allows for a tension free suture line and provides us ease to place repair sutures if necessary.

The distal aorta is sized using an intra annular valve sizer. The graft is beveled if needed to match and accommodate the curvature of the arch. The graft is then sewn to the hemiarch with a running 4-0 polypropylene. It is critical to intussuscept the graft inside the aorta (Fig. 14.4). This is done to ensure the anastomosis is hemostatic as any increase in the blood pressure would affect the graft prior to the aorta at the anastomosis. In general, felt or glue is not used for the anastomoses. Once the anastomosis is complete, the graft is recannulated and the arch is deaired. CPB is commenced and the patient is rewarmed to normothermia. At this stage the distal anastomosis is inspected for hemostasis and repair sutures are placed if needed.

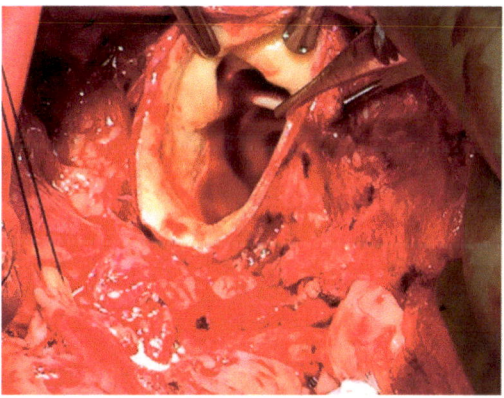

Fig. 14.3 Ascending and aortic arch view illustrating retrograde flow from the RCP circuit through the brachiocephalic vessels

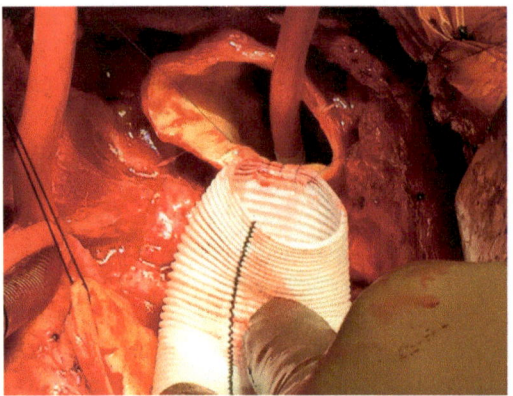

Fig. 14.4 Illustration of distal anastomosis technique with the posterior aspect performed first while intussuscepting the woven polyester graft into the native aorta

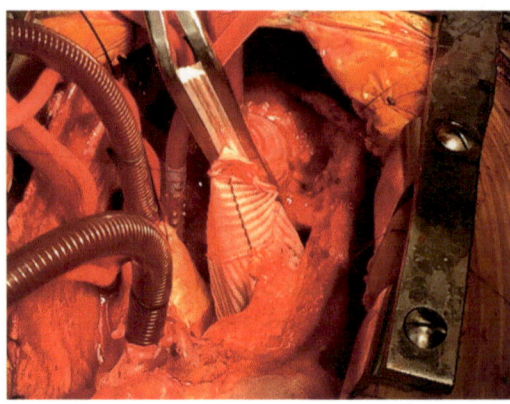

Fig. 14.5 Graft to graft anastomosis to ensure appropriate curvature of the neoaorta

Graft to Graft

It is the view of the authors that a graft-to-graft anastomosis is helpful to ensure normal curvature of the neo aorta as opposed to using a single graft for the operation. For this reason, these operations involve a graft-to-graft anastomosis. This of course is mandatory if root or aggressive arch work is done in order to ensure there is no tension on the aortic root or the arch. Both ends of the graft are trimmed sufficiently to ensure that there is no kink in the graft after taking the cross clamp off. It is important to appreciate that once the heart fills the aortic root will be much more superior in the chest than it is in a flaccid heart. The graft-to-graft anastomosis is performed with 2-0 or 3-0 polypropylene (Fig. 14.5). Usual deairing maneuvers are then employed and the cross clamp is removed. The heart is reperfused and decannulated once successfully weaned off CPB.

Outcomes

Surgical methods and outcomes have improved significantly since the first use of a woven polyester graft to replace an ascending aneurysm by Drs. DeBakey and Cooley in 1956 [16]. If the aneurysm dissects or ruptures, operative mortality can reach as high as 25–40% depending on the patient's condition [17–19]. However, with better understanding of the disease process as well as thresholds for surgical intervention, timely elective surgical interventions are commonplace. This is ideal as the incidence of TAAs have been increasing in recent years which may be a consequence of increase in imaging utilization [20]. Survival has improved significantly over time reflecting on the advances made in the surgical and perioperative management of ascending aortic aneurysms [21, 22].

Key Pearls and Pitfalls

- The optimal arterial cannulation strategy for proximal aortic surgery with proximal arch involvement remains controversial among large-aortic-volume centers
- In cases of ascending dissection, central ascending aortic cannulation has not been historically favoured because of the risk of cannulating the false lumen
- In cases with only aortic root involvement, central aortic cannulation is the standard of care; however, in cases of aortic disease involving the proximal or total arch in addition to the aortic root, central aortic cannulation continues to have certain advantages
- While there are fewer reports about innominate artery cannulation, it appears to have several advantages over femoral and axillary artery cannulation
- Cannulation strategies involving any of the four cannulation sites are sound, and the choice among these strategies must take into account the patient's characteristics and aortic disease

Review Qs

1. Complications of axillary artery cannulation include
   (a) Phrenic nerve injury
   (b) Sympathetic chain disruption
   (c) Lower-extremity ischemia
   (d) **Brachial plexus injury**
2. Innominate artery cannulation has several advantages over femoral and axillary artery cannulation, including
   (a) **Requires no additional incision**
   (b) Is the only approach that can deliver ACP
   (c) Can lead to malperfusion and retrograde dissection
   (d) Can lead to brachial plexus injury
3. Which of the following is not an advantage of femoral cannulation
   (a) Relative ease of access
   (b) Avoid direct manipulation of the diseased ascending aorta

(c) Low incidence of complications
(d) **Lack of Antegrade Cerebral Perfusion**
4. Which are the two key advantages of cannulating axillary artery over femoral artery
   (a) **A safe alternative site**
   (b) Time-consuming process
   (c) **Possible to deliver Antegrade Cerebral Perfusion**
   (d) Size
5. What graft sizes can be used to cannulate indirectly the axillary artery by anastomosis
   (a) **An 8- or 10-mm graft**
   (b) A 7- or 10-mm graft
   (c) An 8- or 9-mm graft
   (d) A 7- or 9-mm graft

References

1. Kuzmik GA, Sang AX, Elefteriades JA. Natural history of thoracic aortic aneurysms. J Vasc Surg. 2012;56(2):565–71. https://doi.org/10.1016/j.jvs.2012.04.053.
2. Mathur A, Mohan V, Ameta D, Gaurav B, Haranahalli P. Aortic aneurysm. J Transl Int Med. 2016;4(1):35–41. https://doi.org/10.1515/jtim-2016-0008.
3. Oladokun D, Patterson BO, Sobocinski J, et al. Systematic review of the growth rates and influencing factors in thoracic aortic aneurysms. Eur J Vasc Endovasc Surg. 2016;51(5):674–81. https://doi.org/10.1016/j.ejvs.2016.01.017.
4. Cheung K, Boodhwani M, Chan K-L, Beauchesne L, Dick A, Coutinho T. Thoracic aortic aneurysm growth: role of sex and aneurysm etiology. J Am Heart Assoc. 2017;6(2):e003792. https://doi.org/10.1161/JAHA.116.003792.
5. Isselbacher EM. Thoracic and abdominal aortic aneurysms. Circulation. 2005;111(6):816–28. https://doi.org/10.1161/01.CIR.0000154569.08857.7A.
6. Hiratzka LF, Bakris GL, Beckman JA, et al. 2010 ACCF/AHA/AATS/ACR/ASA/SCA/SCAI/SIR/STS/SVM guidelines for the diagnosis and management of patients with thoracic aortic disease: executive summary: a report of the American college of cardiology foundation/American heart association task force on practice guidelines, American association for thoracic surgery, American College of Radiology, American Stroke Association, Society of Cardiovascular Anesthesiologists, Society for Cardiovascular Angiography and Interventions, Society of Interventional Radiology, Society of Thoracic Surgeons, and Society for Vascular Medicine. Circulation. 2010;111(2):279–315. https://doi.org/10.1213/ANE.0b013e3181dd869b.

7. Chaikof EL, Brewster DC, Dalman RL, et al. SVS practice guidelines for the care of patients with an abdominal aortic aneurysm: executive summary. J Vasc Surg. 2009;50(4):880–96. https://doi.org/10.1016/j.jvs.2009.07.001.

8. Saliba E, Sia Y. The ascending aortic aneurysm: when to intervene? IJC Hear Vasc. 2015;6:91–100. https://doi.org/10.1016/j.ijcha.2015.01.009.

9. Pape LA, Tsai TT, Isselbacher EM, et al. Aortic diameter >or = 5.5 cm is not a good predictor of type A aortic dissection: observations from the International Registry of Acute Aortic Dissection (IRAD). Circulation. 2007;116(10):1120–7. https://doi.org/10.1161/CIRCULATIONAHA.107.702720.

10. El Oumeiri B, Louagie Y, Buche M. Reoperation for ascending aorta false aneurysm using deep hypothermia and circulatory arrest. Interact Cardiovasc Thorac Surg. 2011;12(4):605–8. https://doi.org/10.1510/icvts.2010.262378.

11. Leshnower BG, Rangaraju S, Allen JW, Stringer AY, Gleason TG, Chen EP. Deep hypothermia with retrograde cerebral perfusion versus moderate hypothermia with antegrade cerebral perfusion for arch surgery. Ann Thorac Surg. 2019;107(4):1104–10. https://doi.org/10.1016/j.athoracsur.2018.10.008.

12. Arnaoutakis GJ, Vallabhajosyula P, Bavaria JE, et al. The impact of deep versus moderate hypothermia on postoperative kidney function after elective aortic hemiarch repair. Ann Thorac Surg. 2016;102(4):1313–21. https://doi.org/10.1016/j.athoracsur.2016.04.007.

13. Sultan I, Komlo CM, Bavaria JE. How I teach a valve-sparing root replacement. Ann Thorac Surg. 2016;101(2):422–5. https://doi.org/10.1016/j.athoracsur.2015.12.035.

14. Sultan I, Bianco V, Yazji I, et al. Hemiarch reconstruction versus clamped aortic anastomosis for concomitant ascending aortic aneurysm. Ann Thorac Surg. 2018;106(3):750–6. https://doi.org/10.1016/j.athoracsur.2018.03.078.

15. Kilic A, Kilic A, Sultan I. Anomalous origin of the left main coronary artery from the right coronary artery. Circ Cardiovasc Imag. 2018;11(12):e008452. https://doi.org/10.1161/CIRCIMAGING.118.008452.

16. Cooley DA. A brief history of aortic aneurysm surgery. Aorta. 2013;1(1):1–3. https://doi.org/10.12945/j.aorta.2013.12.006.

17. Sultan I, Habertheuer A, Wallen T, et al. The role of extracorporeal membrane oxygenator therapy in the setting of Type A aortic dissection. J Card Surg. 2017;32(12):822–5. https://doi.org/10.1111/jocs.13245.

18. Vallabhajosyula P, Gottret JP, Menon R, et al. Central repair with antegrade TEVAR for malperfusion syndromes in acute DeBakey I aortic dissection. Ann Thorac Surg. 2017;103(3):748–55. https://doi.org/10.1016/j.athoracsur.2016.06.097.

19. Sultan I, Szeto WY. Decision making in acute DeBakey I aortic dissection: balancing extensive arch reconstruction versus mortality. J Thorac Cardiovasc Surg. 2016;151(2):349–50. https://doi.org/10.1016/j.jtcvs.2015.10.044.

20. Olsson C, Thelin S, Ståhle E, Ekbom A, Granath F. Thoracic aortic aneurysm and dissection: increasing prevalence and improved outcomes reported in a nationwide population-based study of more than 14,000 cases from 1987 to 2002. Circulation. 2006;114(24):2611–8. https://doi.org/10.1161/CIRCULATIONAHA.106.630400.

21. Sultan I, Bavaria JE, Szeto W. Hybrid techniques for aortic arch aneurysm repair. Semin Cardiothorac Vasc Anesth. 2016;20(4):327–32. https://doi.org/10.1177/1089253216659701.

22. Kilic A, Arnaoutakis GJ, Bavaria JE, et al. Outcomes of elective aortic hemiarch reconstruction for aneurysmal disease in the elderly. Ann Thorac Surg. 2017;104(5):1522–30. https://doi.org/10.1016/j.athoracsur.2017.03.067.

Ascending Aortic Dissection Surgery

15

Ourania Preventza and Darrell Wu

Learning Objectives

- Understand the principles of thoracic aortic aneurysm
- Cerebral protection strategies in patients undergoing circulatory arrest for ascending aortic aneurysm repair
- Understanding the guidelines for surgical management of ascending aortic aneurysms
- Understand the inflection and conduct of operation to replace ascending aortic aneurysms
- Understand the pre-surgery assessment and preparation process as well as during surgery protocol

O. Preventza (✉)
Division of Cardiothoracic Surgery, Michael
E. DeBakey Department of Surgery, Baylor College
of Medicine, Houston, TX, USA

Baylor – St. Luke's Medical Center,
Houston, TX, USA

Texas Heart Institute, Houston, TX, USA
e-mail: preventz@bcm.edu

D. Wu
Division of Cardiothoracic Surgery, Michael
E. DeBakey Department of Surgery, Baylor College
of Medicine, Houston, TX, USA

Acute Type A Aortic Dissection

Acute Type A dissection is a true surgical emergency: Contemporary series report 17–26% perioperative mortality at even the best and most experienced centers [1]. Operative mortality specifically reported by North American centers varies from 5 to 17% [2]. Patients can present with cardiac tamponade, stroke, myocardial infarction, acute aortic insufficiency, visceral malperfusion, lower-extremity malperfusion, or cerebral malperfusion, depending on the extent and location of dissection. The key principle of surgical management of ascending aortic dissection is to resect the intimal tear and reestablish flow into the true lumen. However, several guiding principles must be considered when deciding which operation to perform for acute Type A dissection. Critical questions include the patient's hemodynamic status, the location of the entry tear, the presence and location of malperfusion, the size of the ascending aorta, the size of the aortic arch, the presence of genetic tissue disorder, the presence of aortic insufficiency, and the patient's comorbidities.

Because of the possible complications, acute dissection can be highly lethal, with a mortality rate of approximately 1% per hour [1]. Generally, prompt surgical intervention is key for patient survival, but it may be wise to delay surgery in cases of significant cerebral malperfusion, such as extensive stroke, and visceral malperfusion

© Springer Nature Switzerland AG 2022
P. P. Punjabi, P. G. Kyriazis (eds.), *Essentials of Operative Cardiac Surgery*,
https://doi.org/10.1007/978-3-031-14557-5_15

requiring revascularization followed by correction of metabolic derangement before the ascending dissection is addressed [1]. Sometimes, patients who present with stroke will have received thrombolytics before acute dissection is diagnosed, which makes performing the operation urgently less appealing. Unlike paraplegia from spinal cord impairment, hemispheric impairment warrants delaying or reconsidering surgery. For these reasons, certain patients with acute ascending aortic dissection are medically managed and have delayed surgery. Chiu and Miller [3] from Stanford reported that cerebral injury has not been routinely used as an exclusion criterion for operative intervention at their institution. In addition, they mentioned that patients undergoing operative repair within 5–8 h of symptom onset have a much better prognosis and greater resolution of their symptoms than patients with a longer duration of symptoms. In patients with devastating neurological injury, no benefit of surgical intervention was seen.

The hemodynamically unstable patient often presents in extremis due to pericardial tamponade, stroke, myocardial infarction, or acute aortic insufficiency. Invasive monitoring through an arterial line and establishing a central line for intravenous infusions are essential for these patients. In this circumstance, some suggest cannulating the femoral vessels in the operating room, either by the Seldinger technique or through open cutdown. If the patient is not in extremis, we prefer right axillary or innominate artery cannulation (if the innominate artery is not dissected) with a Dacron graft to be used for arterial inflow. A Y-branch from the arterial line can provide alternate arterial inflow if it is needed after the aortic reconstruction (Fig. 15.1); likewise, a Y-branch off the venous line allows additional drainage of the heart, if necessary, and facilitates cooling. Direct ascending aortic cannulation in acute Type A dissection is also an option and has been used with good results [4].

In cases of aortic rupture, the pericardium will be tense. In this instance, it is better to initiate cardiopulmonary bypass—to avoid a hypertensive crisis after the tamponade is released—and to start cooling. Inserting a left ventricular vent into the right superior pulmonary vein is imperative, as is inserting a coronary sinus catheter for retrograde cardioplegia. If there is massive aortic insufficiency and the heart distends, the aorta is clamped and the left ventricular vent is inserted so the heart can be decompressed. Clamping the aorta is not advisable because it can pressurize the false lumen, thereby increasing the extent of dissection and leading to malperfusion. Nonetheless, aortic clamping is necessary if the heart distends because of massive aortic insufficiency. If the heart is not distending because the aortic valve is competent, then there is no need to clamp the ascending aorta. In both instances, after the target temperature of moderate hypothermia (around 24 °C; lower levels of moderate hypothermia are preferred in cases of femoral or direct aortic cannulation) is reached, the pump is stopped and circulation is arrested. The anterior wall of the ascending aorta then can be transected and incised up toward the innominate artery. An additional (9F Pruitt) perfusion catheter can be used to provide antegrade cerebral flow through the left common carotid artery (Fig. 15.1). In such cases, we prefer to use bilateral cerebral perfusion (via the innominate or right axillary artery and the 9F Pruitt catheter in the left common carotid artery), especially when the reconstruction is expected to take more than 30 min [5].

The aortic lumen is examined to find the intimal tear, and the aorta is resected proximally and distally. The aortic false lumen can be obliterated with approximation of the intima and adventitia with interrupted 6-0 polypropylene suture. BioGlue is sometimes used to appose the layers of the aortic wall. Then the distal anastomosis is constructed, usually with a 24–28-mm Dacron graft and a double-armed 3-0 or 4-0 polypropylene suture, followed by a second layer of interrupted pledgeted or running 3-0 or 4-0 suture to reinforce the anastomosis. Some centers routinely use a layer of felt to reinforce the anastomosis. Next, if the initial cannulation site was the femoral artery, then the side arm of the Dacron graft used for the distal reconstruction is connected to the Y-branch of the arterial line off the femoral cannula, the Dacron graft is deaired, and flow is resumed through the graft, establishing antegrade flow and full cardiopulmonary bypass.

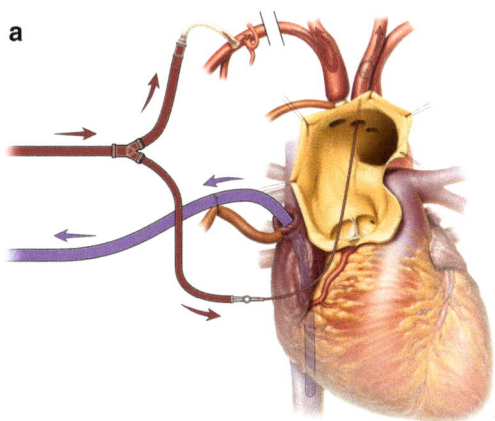

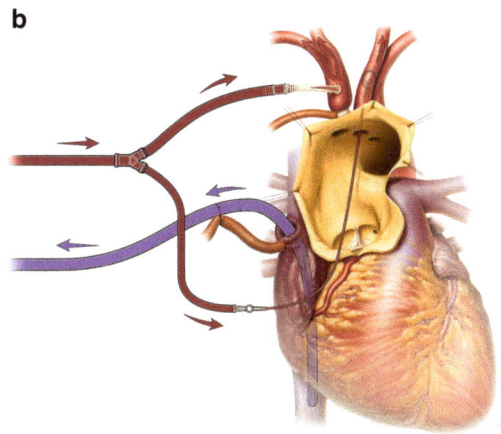

Fig. 15.1 A Y-branch from the arterial line connected to the Dacron graft off the axillary artery (**a**) or off the innominate artery (**b**) can provide alternate arterial inflow during cardiopulmonary bypass. Also, it can be used to provide bilateral antegrade cerebral perfusion during circulatory arrest

After the distal anastomosis is complete, attention is turned to the aortic valve and aortic root, and the ascending graft is clamped. At that point, rewarming is started. If no valve repair is required and a tube graft alone is sufficient, rewarming to 36.5 °C is initiated. Otherwise, if more work is required on the aortic valve or root, then partial rewarming to 28 °C is initiated. In patients with healthy leaflets and without any connective tissue disorder, the aortic valve can usually be preserved with leaflet resuspension or commissural plication.

Decision-making regarding the aortic root is generally based on the presence or absence of genetic tissue disorder, aneurysmal involvement,

degree of dissection, and involvement of coronaries. In patients with connective tissue disorders such as Marfan or Loeys-Dietz syndrome, we replace the aortic root. The choice of mechanical valve versus bioprosthesis depends on the patient's age and indications for or contraindications to anticoagulation. Valve-sparing operations have been also performed [6]. In our practice, we usually avoid performing valve-sparing procedures in emergency cases such as cases of Type A or Type I aortic dissection. If there is no aortic root aneurysm and only the aortic valve cusps are significantly diseased, with some degree of aortic insufficiency, then the aortic valve is replaced and a supracoronary graft is attached without replacement of the root. If there is no root aneurysm, the aortic valve cusps are not diseased, and there is some degree of aortic insufficiency, then the aortic valve can be saved and commissural plication can be performed. Finally, in our practice, we perform coronary bypasses in patients with evidence of segmental wall motion abnormalities, inability to separate from bypass, or extensive involvement of the intimal orifice of the main coronary arteries.

In general, we perform the least extensive operation that will result in patient survival and durable repair. If the aortic arch requires more than just hemiarch replacement, the distal aortic anastomosis is constructed, with or without an elephant trunk technique. The head vessels can be reimplanted by an island technique or variations of the Y graft technique.

Many authors have provided excellent descriptions of their repair techniques for Type A dissection, with the principal aims of establishing flow into the true lumen and protecting against aortic rupture, aortic regurgitation, and coronary ischemia [2, 6–8]. However, according to International Registry of Acute Aortic Dissection (IRAD) data, the mortality associated with repairing acute Type A dissection remains 17–26% [1]. The prevailing thinking is that treating Type A aortic dissection with a hemiarch technique carries lower operative risk than replacing the full arch. It does not necessarily entail subsequent aortic intervention, and the operative risk is mitigated in the future. When and if reintervention is necessary, it can be referred to experienced aortic centers where repairs and replacements are performed with respectable morbidity and mortality risk. In contrast, performing a total arch replacement under emergency circumstances incurs a greater early morbidity and mortality risk due to longer bypass and surgery times and a higher risk of stroke. Fleischman et al. [9] recently analyzed their experience regarding selective arch and root replacement over a 10-year period in 195 cases of acute Type A dissection. The authors replaced the arch or root only if there was intimal tear extending into these regions. They found that ascending aorta– and hemiarch-replacement patients had similar survival to patients who underwent arch replacement, and their reintervention rate was only 8%. Omura et al. [10], who also compared total and non-total arch replacement for patients with acute Type A dissection, reported in-hospital mortality of only 12.5% and an incidence of neurologic deficits of only 7%. They also found no significant difference in survival or need for reintervention between the two surgical approaches.

However, some unanswered questions remain regarding total arch replacement, such as which patients should undergo it and risk needing additional aortic surgery later, and whether there is a survival benefit. The Malantis group [11] has attempted to answer some of these questions by advocating an aggressive approach of performing a branched total arch repair first, followed by thoracoabdominal stenting and balloon rupture of the septum. This second procedure is performed either during the same hospital stay after the patients have been discharged from the intensive care unit, or after they have been discharged from the hospital and readmitted soon thereafter. Indications for this approach include malperfusion, enlarging false lumen, or collapsed true lumen. The group's results are outstanding, with no early deaths and a low rate of neurologic complications.

The frozen elephant trunk technique was introduced in an attempt to enable remodeling of the descending and thoracoabdominal aorta and potentially minimize future intervention in these segments of the aorta (descending and thoracoabdominal), depressurize the false lumen, and expand the true lumen [12]. If these patients need future intervention, the frozen elephant trunk provides a good platform for further endovascular intervention. The frozen elephant trunk technique entails total arch replacement, and it is recommended when the arch is dilated more than 4–4.5 cm and there is a tear in the arch that cannot be repaired otherwise. The frozen elephant trunk technique is associated with higher overall adverse event rates than standard techniques when used to repair acute Type A aortic dissection [13].

Another evolving approach is antegrade stent delivery to the descending thoracic aorta under direct vision, in an effort to minimize subsequent operations in the thoracoabdominal aorta and, ultimately, to promote thoracoabdominal aortic remodeling. This procedure is commonly confused with or referred to as the frozen elephant trunk procedure—which is not, as it does not entail a total arch operation with manipulation of the arch vessels. When we perform hemiarch replacement and antegrade stent delivery, we leave little of the native aortic tissue in place (Fig. 15.2). We have recently published our results with this technique [14]; we found that in the short term, the patients with antegrade stent delivery had lower operative mortality, and in the mid term, remodeling of the false lumen was seen in stented patients, who had better overall midterm survival than patients who underwent traditional hemiarch replacement.

A few technical points bear mentioning. Because the tissue is inflamed and fragile, the aim is to obtain a secure and hemostatic anastomosis. We routinely reapproximate the layers in the proximal aorta with interrupted 6-0 polypropylene suture, which we sometimes reinforce with BioGlue. In the area of the noncoronary sinus, a small piece of felt is used to obliterate the space between the false and true lumen. Similarly, we reapproximate the distal aortic layers, and occasionally we use BioGlue. The distal anastomosis is constructed as described previously; this is done under circulatory arrest to keep tension

a

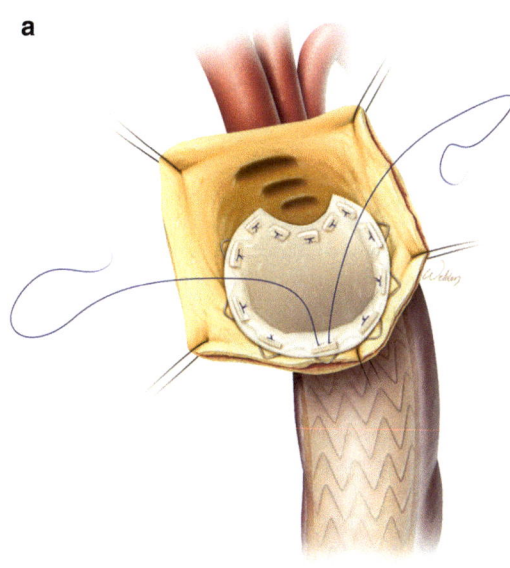

b

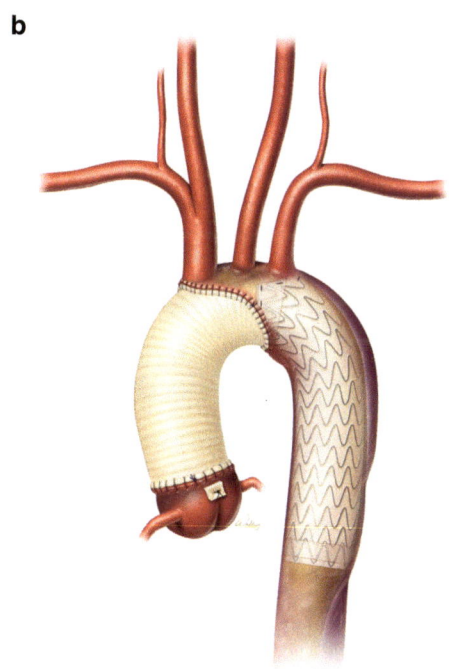

Fig. 15.2 (**a**) The stent is delivered below the left subclavian artery. The arch vessels stay intact. (**b**) Ascending and proximal arch replacement with antegrade stent delivery in a patient with Type I aortic dissection

off the anastomosis until it is completed. Cross-clamping the dissected aorta before circulatory arrest is avoided, as previously mentioned.

Chronic Ascending Aortic Dissection

Medical management with antihypertensive medication is the first-line therapy for chronic dissection. Surgery is indicated when the ascending aorta becomes aneurysmal or when the dissection becomes symptomatic. There are several issues to consider when operating on chronic dissections that become aneurysmal, and the steps are similar to those of ascending aortic aneurysm surgery. Not uncommonly, chronic dissecting aneurysmal arches that require replacement are seen in patients with prior repair of isolated ascending aortic dissection [15].

Key Pearls and Pitfalls

- Due to the indolent nature of TAAs, patients typically have other initially presenting pathology warranting imaging which result in the incidental detection of the aneurysm
- Current guidelines recommend prophylactic surgery on isolated TAAs measuring 5.5 cm in patients with no risk factors
- In the setting of aneurysmal disease where the ascending aorta is to be resected, and the distal anastomosis is to be performed under circulatory arrest, the distal ascending aorta is cannulated to ensure removal of the cannulation site prior to performing the distal anastomosis
- Retrograde Cerebral Perfusion is utilized for hemiarch replacements while Antegrade Cerebral Perfusion is used for total arch replacements to adequately perfuse the brain during extended period of circulatory arrest
- A full sternotomy is preferable due to the high incidence of aortic root surgery or other additional cardiac operation in this patient population

Questions

1. The key principle of the surgical management of acute Type A dissection is
   (a) Replacing the aortic root in all cases

(b) Ensuring flow into true lumen, and replacing the ascending aorta and the proximal arch (correct)

(c) Repairing the descending aorta first

(d) Replacing the aortic arch in all cases

2. If the dissection involves the aortic root and the root is aneurysmal, optimal management in addition to the ascending and hemiarch replacement is

(a) Root repair/replacement (correct)

(b) Replacing the aortic valve with a supra-coronary graft

(c) Ascending and hemiarch replacement with aortic valve resuspension

(d) Total arch replacement with aortic valve replacement

References

1. Berretta P, Patel HJ, Gleason TG, Sundt TM, Myrmel T, Desai N, et al. IRAD experience on surgical type A acute dissection patients: results and predictors of mortality. Ann Cardiothorac Surg. 2016;5:346–51.

2. Preventza O, Coselli JS. Differential aspects of ascending thoracic aortic dissection and its treatment: the North American experience. Ann Cardiothorac Surg. 2016;5:352–9.

3. Chiu P, Miller DC. Evolution of surgical therapy for Stanford acute type A aortic dissection. Ann Cardiothorac Surg. 2016;5:275–95.

4. Kamiya H, Kallenbach K, Halmer D, Ozsoz M, Ilg K, Lichtenberg A, et al. Comparison of ascending aorta versus femoral artery cannulation for acute aortic dissection type A. Circulation. 2009;120:S282–6.

5. Preventza O, Simpson KH, Cooley DA, Cornwell L, Bakaeen FG, Omer S, et al. Unilateral versus bilateral cerebral perfusion for acute type A aortic dissection. Ann Thorac Surg. 2015;99:80–7.

6. David TE. Surgery for acute type A aortic dissection. J Thorac Cardiovasc Surg. 2015;150:279–83.

7. Cohen RG, Hackmann AE, Fleischman F, Baker CJ, Cunningham MJ, Starnes VA, et al. Type A aortic dissection repair: how I teach it. Ann Thorac Surg. 2017;103:14–7.

8. Hussain ST, Svensson LG. Surgical techniques in type A dissection. Ann Cardiothorac Surg. 2016;5:233–5.

9. Fleischman F, Elsayed RS, Cohen RG, Tatum JM, Kumar SR, Kazerouni K, et al. Selective aortic arch and root replacement in repair of acute type A aortic dissection. Ann Thorac Surg. 2018;105:505–12.

10. Omura A, Miyahara S, Yamanaka K, Sakamoto T, Matsumori M, Okada K, et al. Early and late outcomes of repaired acute DeBakey type I aortic dissection after graft replacement. J Thorac Cardiovasc Surg. 2016;151:341–8.

11. Matalanis G, Ip S. A new paradigm in the management of acute type A aortic dissection: total aortic repair. J Thorac Cardiovasc Surg. 2019;157:3–11.

12. Preventza O, Coselli JS, Mayor J, Simpson K, Carillo J, Price MD, et al. The stent is not to blame: lessons learned with a simplified US version of the frozen elephant trunk. Ann Thorac Surg. 2017;104:1456–63.

13. Preventza O, Liao JL, Olive JK, Simpson K, Critsinelis AC, Price MD, et al. Neurologic complications after the frozen elephant trunk procedure: a meta-analysis of more than 3,000 patients. J Thorac Cardiovasc Surg. 2020;160(1):20–33.e4.

14. Preventza O, Olive JK, Liao JL, Orozco-Sevilla V, Simpson K, Rodriguez MR, et al. Acute type I aortic dissection with or without antegrade stent delivery: mid-term outcomes. J Thorac Cardiovasc Surg. 2019;158:1273–81.

15. Preventza O, Price MD, Simpson KH, Cooley DA, Pocock E, de la Cruz KI, et al. Hemiarch and total arch surgery in patients with previous repair of acute type I aortic dissection. Ann Thorac Surg. 2015;100:833–8.

Valve Sparing Aortic Root Procedure: Yacoub's Procedure

16

Gopal Soppa, Rajdeep Bilkhu, Marjan Jahangiri, and Magdi Yacoub

Abbreviations

CPB	Cardiopulmonary bypass
LVOT	Left ventricular outflow tract
RSPV	Right superior pulmonary vein vent
RVOT	Right ventricular outflow tract
STJ	Sino-tubular junction
TOE	Transoesophageal echocardiography
VSRR	Valve sparing root replacement

Learning Objectives

- To define the morphology and physiological properties of the aortic root
- Describe the indications and requirements for valve sparing aortic root replacement

G. Soppa
Barts Heart Hospital, London, UK
e-mail: Gopal.soppa@nhs.net

R. Bilkhu
London, UK

M. Jahangiri (✉)
Cardiac Surgery, Department of Cardiothoracic Surgery, St. George's Healthcare NHS Trust, London, UK
e-mail: marjan.jahangiri@stgeorges.nhs.uk

M. Yacoub
Imperial College London, London, UK
e-mail: M.Yacoub@imperial.ac.uk

- Describe the echocardiographic measurements required to perform valve sparing aortic root replacement using the remodelling technique
- Describe the operative steps of the remodelling technique
- Understanding of the advantages of the remodelling technique over the reimplantation technique

Morphology and Physiology of the Aortic Root

The aortic root not only channels blood but also supports the aortic valve leaflets. Anatomically, the aortic root consists of the aortic valve leaflets, the sinuses of Valsalva, the interleaflet triangles, the sino tubular junction and the aortic annulus. Whilst the term annulus implies a circular structure, there is no histological or anatomical structure that directly fits with its description, rather, the annulus is often considered to be formed of a circular 'ring' defined by the nadirs of the aortic valve leaflet attachments or the ventriculo-aortic junction [1].

The morphology of the sinuses of Valsalva is crucial to create appropriate currents in the supravalvular region and are important for initiating and coordinating aortic valve closure and promoting coronary artery blood flow (Fig. 16.1a, b). The morphology of the root allows blood to be ejected in a laminar flow pattern, with little stress on the aortic leaflets and aortic wall [2].

Background and Indications for Surgery

Aortic root replacement is performed for pathology of the aortic root, including aneurysm, dissection, connective tissue disease and in some cases, endo-carditis of the aortic valve. Valve-sparing aortic root replacement (VSRR) is performed for aortic aneurysm when the aortic valve leaflets are normal and the aortic valve annulus is not dilated. Annular size greater than 28 mm, have a higher rate of late aortic incompetence due to progressive annular dilation [3, 4], hence a full root replacement may be the preferred option depending upon the patient's comorbidities. Operations of the aortic root carry significant risks and morbidity [5]. Given the interplay of the aortic root components already described, the main aim of the Yacoub technique of VSRR is to restore and maintain the form and functional integrity of the aortic root. We describe in detail our preferred technique for VSRR for aortic root aneurysms (Fig. 16.3).

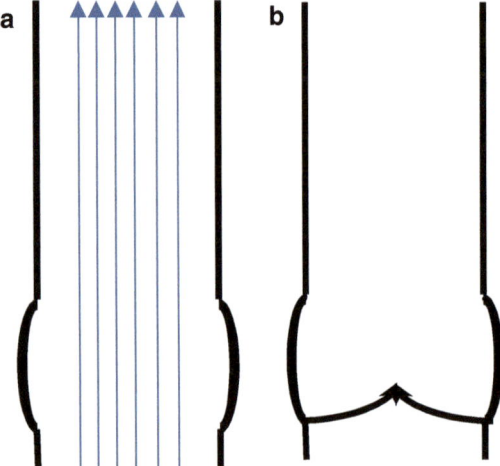

Fig. 16.1 (**a**) Laminar flow through the aortic valve during systole. (**b**) Currents formed within the aortic sinus in diastole, helping to initiate aortic valve closure and assist with coronary flow [1]

Intra-operative Transoesophageal Echocardiography (TOE) Measurements

Intra-operative TOE assessment of the aortic valve for incompetence due to leaflet prolapse or annular dilatation is carefully assessed and the measurements, shown in Fig. 16.2a, b, are recorded. These measurements, taken in the mid-oesophageal aortic valve long axis view, are the following: (1) Diameter of the LVOT, just below the leaflet attach-

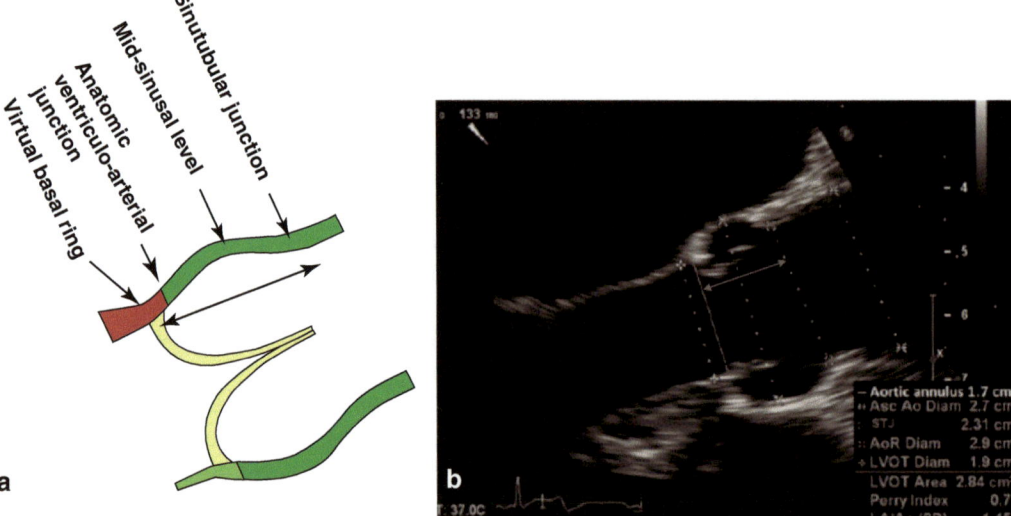

Fig. 16.2 (**a**, **b**) Aortic root measurement at various levels required for planning VSRR procedure. Double-ended arrow provides height of commissures

ment, (2) Diameter at the level of the leaflet attachments, (3) Diameter of the sinuses, (4) Diameter of the sinotubular junction (STJ), (5) Diameter of the aneurysm above the STJ and (6) Commissural height, measured as the distance from imaginary lines between measurements (2) and (4).

Operative Technique

Cannulation Strategy

Following median sternotomy, cardiopulmonary bypass (CPB) is established at 35 °C through central (distal ascending aorta or proximal aortic arch) or peripheral (femoral or axillary) cannulation if concomitant aortic arch surgery is required or to maximise the excision of the ascending aorta. Venous return is achieved usually by right atrial (or bicaval) cannulation depending on the need for concomitant procedures (Fig. 16.3b). Myocardial protection is achieved using antegrade cold blood-based cardioplegic solution with topical cooling of the myocardium. A left ventricular vent is inserted via the right superior pulmonary vein (RSPV) (Fig. 16.3c). Subsequent maintenance cardioplegia is instituted via the coronary ostia. The aortic cross clamp is applied distally as possible, ensuring the entire width of the aorta is safely within the clamp. Prior to this,

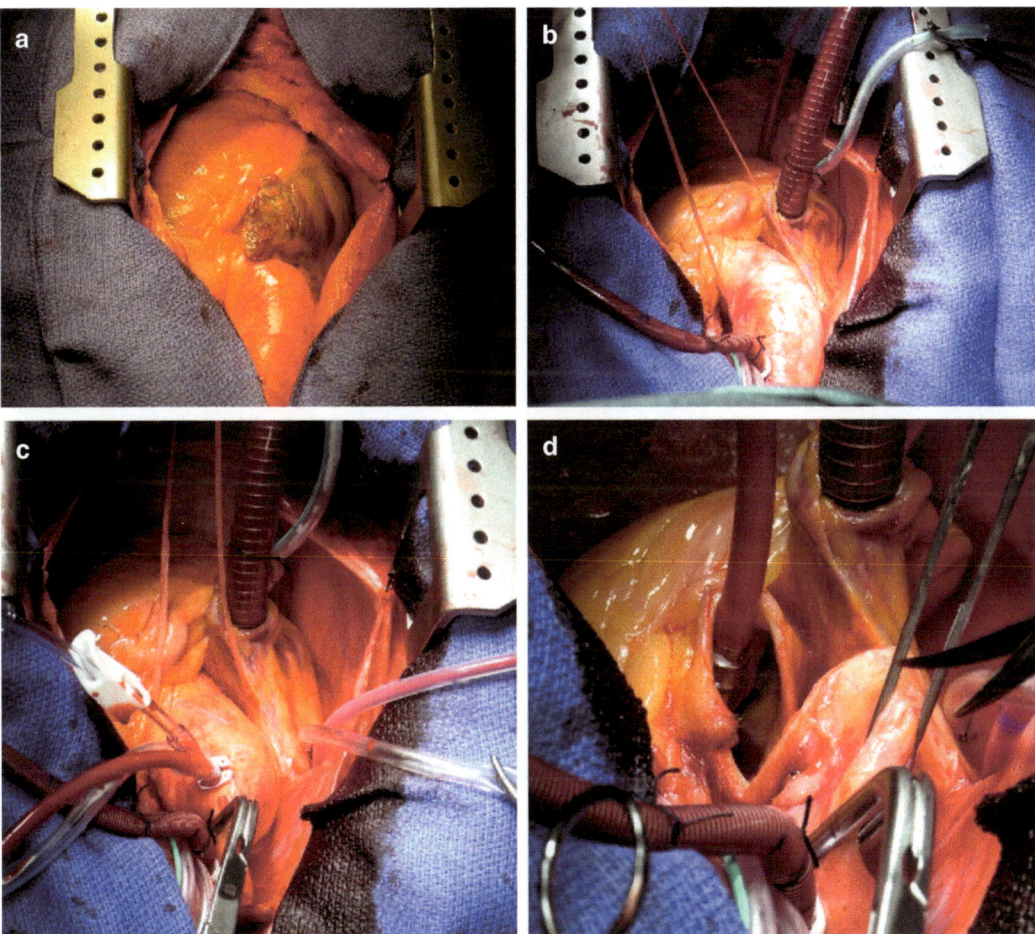

Fig. 16.3 Aortic root aneurysm (**a**) with right atrial to distal ascending aorta CPB and isolation of aorta from main pulmonary artery (**b**). Cross-clamp applied and ante-grade cold blood cardioplegia delivery and insertion of RSPV vent (**c**). The aorta is transected well above the ST junction (**d**)

to facilitate clamping of the entire aorta when the ascending aorta is dilated, the aorta is dissected away from the main pulmonary artery using diathermy and a tape is passed around the aorta.

Valve Assessment

The ascending aorta is opened transversely after administration of cardioplegia. Care is taken to perform the aortotomy well above the STJ and valve commissures (Fig. 16.3d).

The integrity of the aortic valve is inspected to determine if it can be repaired (Fig. 16.4a). This involves an assessment of the morphology of the aortic valve and root systematically, i.e. valve leaflets, coronary ostia, aortic annulus and ventriculoaortic junction. The leaflets are inspected for symmetry, fenestrations, cusp fusion or prolapse. Cusp plication is performed if there is evidence of

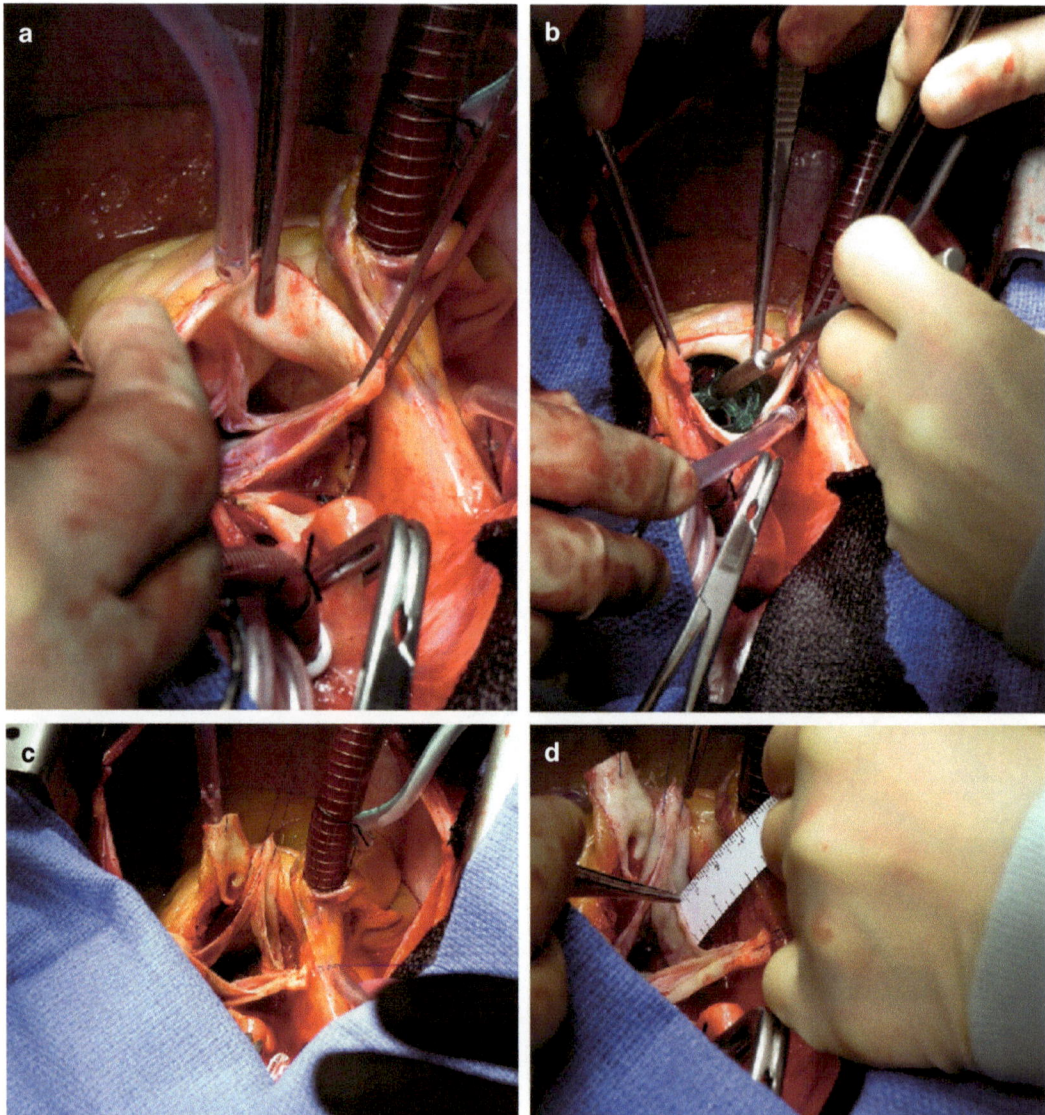

Fig. 16.4 Aortic valve inspection (**a**) and sizing of the annulus (**b**). Excision of root aneurysm and isolation of coronary buttons (**c**) and measurement of leaflet height (**d**)

cusp prolapse. The depth of each sinus is measured. Commissural height is measured (Fig. 16.4d). The leaflet cusps should be normal and the aortic annulus should not be dilated or the leaflets should not appear stretched with little coaptation. The position of the coronary ostia, their proximity to the valve commissures and nadir of the relevant sinus and annulus, as well as intramural course is noted. If there is a single coronary ostium, great care must be ensured in mobilising the coronary button. Differences in the depth of each sinus must be appreciated in the remodelling procedure as this impacts on how the prosthetic graft is tailored. Mild aortic regurgitation is usually caused by separation of the commissures at the STJ level due to the aortic aneurysm if no leaflet prolapse exists. This can usually be corrected by re-suspending the commissures.

Preparation of the Aortic Root

If the valve is deemed to be suitable for VSRR, the annulus is sized using an aortic valve sizer. The diseased aorta is excised, leaving a 3–5 mm rim of tissue above the aortic annulus and around the coronary buttons which are partially mobilised (Fig. 16.4c). Care must be taken to ensure enough remnant aortic sinus to sew the graft. The extent of coronary button mobilisation is dependent on the aneurysm size and degree of freedom required to reach the prosthetic graft without kinking of the coronary artery. If the coronary artery follows an intramural course, careful dissection to maintain the integrity and position of the coronary ostium must be maintained without disturbing the commissures. Haemostasis around the coronary buttons and RVOT muscle is secured at this stage with low power cautery.

Customising the Graft

A prosthetic graft 3 mm larger than the measured annular size is selected. This avoids inducing aortic stenosis or cusp prolapse. Teflon-buttressed 4/0 polypropylene stay sutures are placed on each of the commissures and traction applied upwards

until optimum coaptation of the cusps is achieved, with the Teflon pledget being placed on the outside of the commissure. The distance between the commissures at this position is measured. This is roughly one-third the circumference of the required graft. The graft is cut at three points to match the commissures of the aortic valve and shaped to match the aortic sinuses of Valsalva in depth and width (Fig. 16.5a–d). The cut on the graft usually extends at least nine rings into the graft or at least one and a half times the height of the commissures. It can be further trimmed later, as required. The three commissures are sutured to the corresponding apices of the cuts on the graft, using 4/0 polypropylene, with the suture passing from inside the graft to the outside. Care is taken to ensure that the orientation is exactly in the long axis of the graft, with no distortion, ensuring symmetry (Fig. 16.5e). The graft is then lowered into position and the sutures tied, with the knots on the outside. The excess graft at the sinuses can be trimmed at this stage (Fig. 16.5f).

After securing the middle of the graft neo-sinus to the nadir of the remaining sinus, a continuous 4/0 polypropylene is used to suture the graft to the remaining aortic sinus tissue (Fig. 16.6a). This step ensures symmetry of the sinuses and commissures which must be a key aim of the VSRR remodelling technique. The needle is passed outside the graft on reaching the commissure and the suture tied to the commissure-fixing sutures. This suture line needs to be haemostatic and, so, care is taken to ensure that there is good apposition between the annulus and the graft, without any irregularities. Needle entry into the tissues at 90° degrees with minimum torqueing of the needle will aid in reducing needle hole size and therefore improve haemostasis. This process is repeated for each neo-sinus. Following formation of all neo-sinuses, additional interrupted sutures are used, if necessary, to close any potential leakage areas as this is inaccessible after the cross clamp is released (Fig. 16.6b). The graft is filled with saline and competence of the aortic valve is checked (Fig. 16.6c). The left coronary ostia is then fully mobilised and an opening made in the graft opposite the coronary button, using thermal cautery. It is anastomosed to the opening

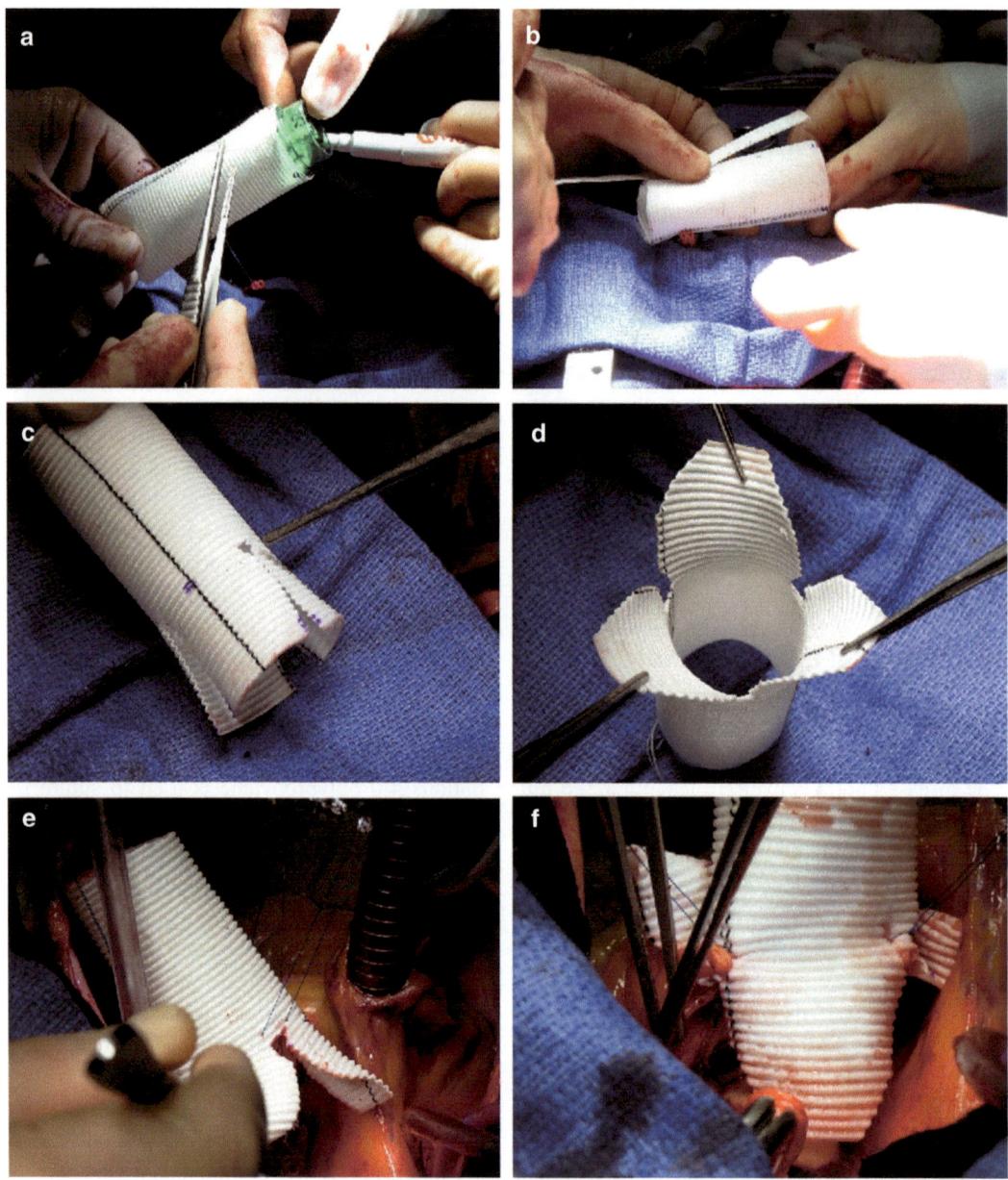

Fig. 16.5 Steps of fashioning the prosthetic graft (**a–d**) and fixing the commissures (**e, f**)

in the graft, using continuous 5/0 polypropylene (Fig. 16.6d). This is repeated for the right coronary ostia. We do not use strips or rings of Teflon to ensure further haemostasis of the coronary anastomosis. We believe this can complicate the procedure and its need is obviated by accurate suturing. Furthermore, if future surgery is needed, Teflon can cause severe adhesions and thus mak-

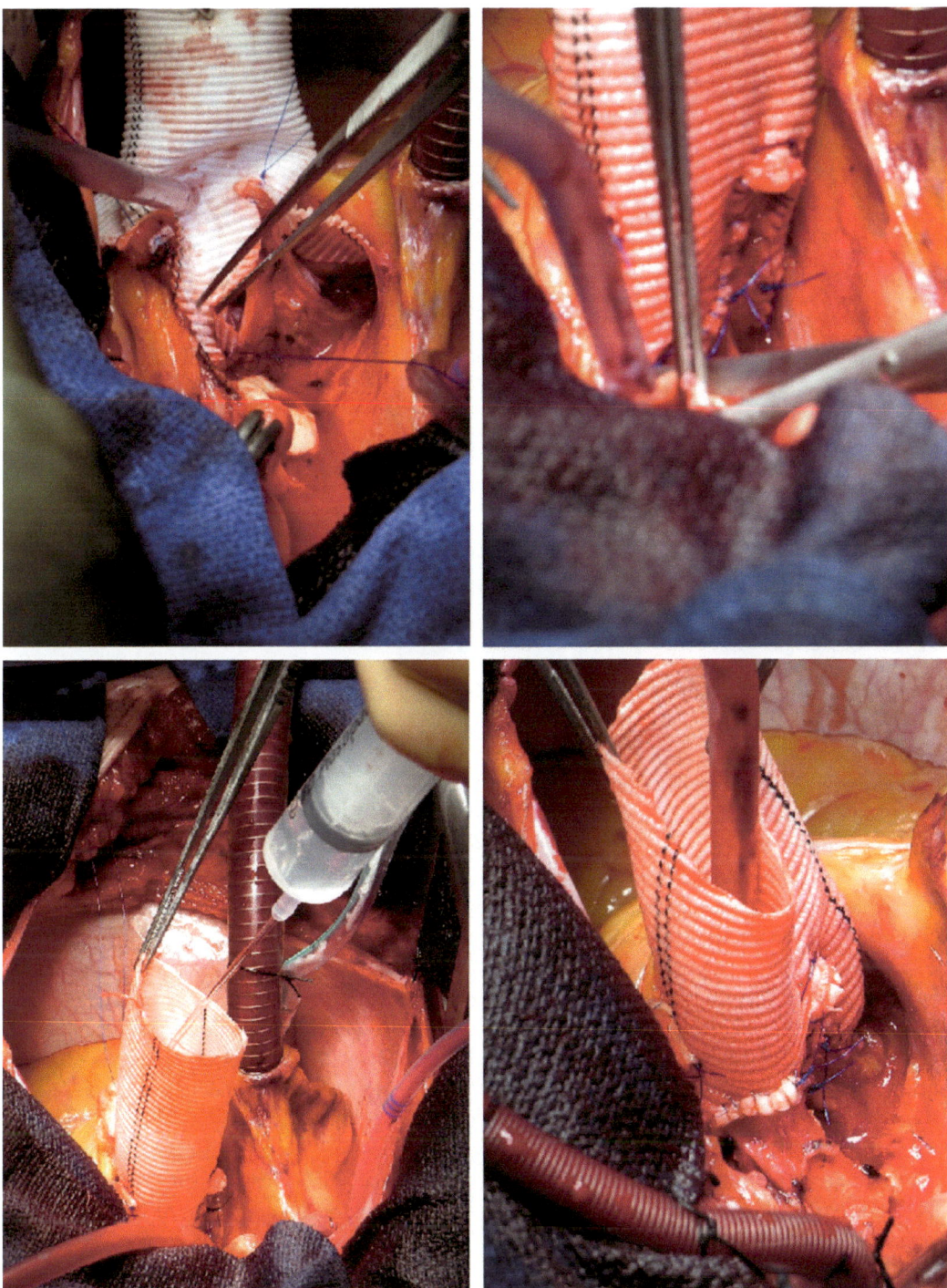

Fig. 16.6 Steps of completing the proximal suture line and re-implantation of the coronary buttons

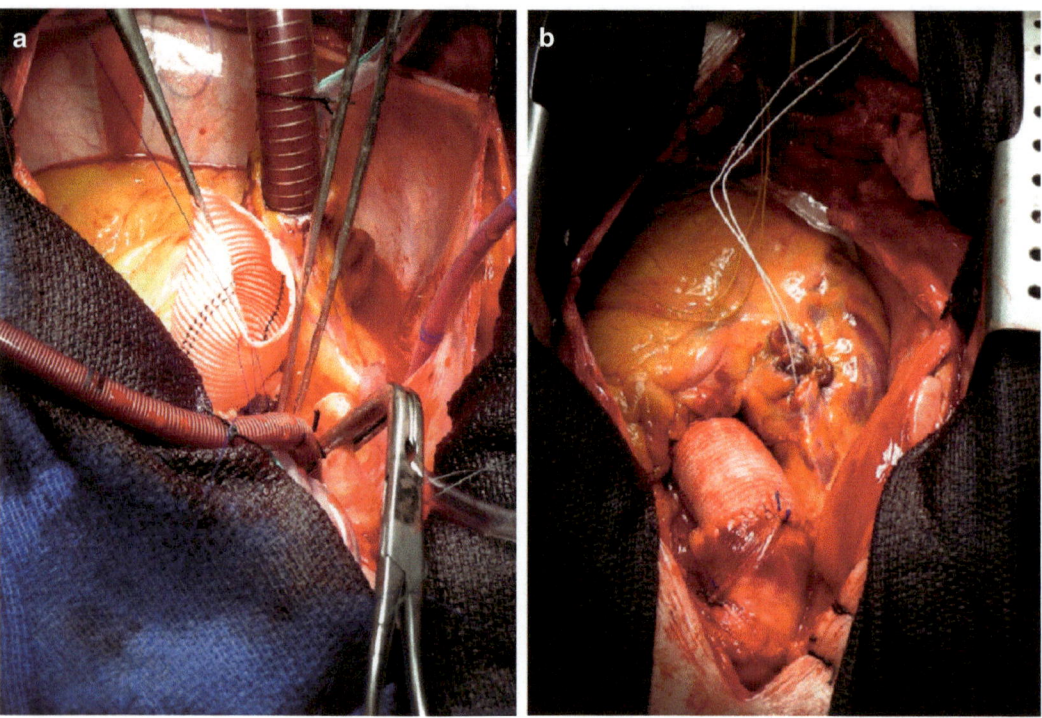

Fig. 16.7 Completion of a 'closed' distal anastomosis (**a**) and final result (**b**)

ing redo surgery complex. The graft is then trimmed to the required length distally and anastomosed to the distal ascending aorta, using continuous 4/0 polypropylene (Fig. 16.7a). If the remaining ascending aorta is larger than the graft, but does not require replacement, then the graft can be trimmed and cut more obliquely to match the size of the remaining aorta. The cross clamp is then released after a thorough, TOE-guided, de-airing procedure. The competence of the aortic valve is assessed on TOE with a suitable afterload and coaptation length of the aortic valve leaflets noted (ideally 7–9 mm). When possible, flow in both coronary arteries is confirmed on colour-Doppler imaging. Following confirmation of satisfactory valvular function, CPB is discontinued and haemostasis secured (Fig. 16.7b).

Remodelling vs. Reimplantation

Both methods of VSRR have been widely debated over the years. There has been a suggestion that the remodelling technique, as originally described, does not stabilise the aortic annulus and therefore, the annulus may dilate over time and result in aortic regurgitation, particularly in patients with Marfan Syndrome.

A number of modifications of both the remodelling technique and reimplantation technique have been described. In 2006, Lansac and colleagues described the addition of a subvalvar prosthetic annuloplasty ring to the remodelling technique and reported a lower reoperation rate for patients with annuloplasty ring as opposed to those undergoing the standard technique (13 vs. 4.2%) [6].

In addition, Schäfers and colleagues have emphasized that measurement of valve cusp effective height and correction of valve cusp prolapse, result in good mid and long-term outcomes. In their series, 173 of 274 patients with significant pre-operative aortic regurgitation underwent valve cusp repair. Freedom from aortic regurgitation of grade 2 or more was 91% and 87% at 10 years for bicuspid and tricuspid aortic valves respectively. Freedom from reoperation was 96% at 5 and 10 years, and freedom from valve replacement was 98% at 5 and 10 years [7]. David's reimplantation series demonstrated slightly improved freedom from moderate to severe aortic regurgitation of 98.3% and 92.9% at 5 years and 10 years respectively. Overall freedom from reoperation was 94.8%, with 296 of 374 patients undergoing reimplantation and the rest undergoing remodelling [8]. However, remodelling of the aortic root was associated with non-significant higher risk of reoperation (hazard ratio = 3.37; CI: 0.88–12.82; P = 0.07) [8].

A criticism of the originally described reimplantation technique was the non-physiological reconstruction of the aortic root and what impact implanting the aortic valve within a straight tube graft had on the native valve cusp leaflets. Schäfers and colleagues reported their in vitro comparison of valve cusp motion in a remodelling and reimplantation techniques using porcine models. They identified that valve cusp opening in the reimplantation technique was significantly faster with frequent systolic contact of the valve leaflets with the aortic wall than the remodelling technique, which was seen to demonstrate smoother valve mobility given the presence of neo-sinuses of Valsalva [9]. This may be explained by the reduced physiological distensibility of the aortic root after reimplantation. It has been noted in vivo and there is suggestion that the valve opening pattern demonstrated in the remodelling technique may impact durability of the valve. Yacoub and colleagues have demonstrated that the remodelling technique also maintains and preserves normal geometry as well as dynamic function of the root [10]. A modification of the original reimplantation technique was to utilise a graft with 'in-built' neo-sinuses and this was described by De Paulis and colleagues in 2000. Long term results from this group have demonstrated freedom from moderate to severe aortic regurgitation of 94% at 5 years and 87% at 10 and 13 years, with 6 patients requiring reoperation (1 for endocarditis and 5 for severe aortic regurgitation) [11].

Given the lack of a specific recommendation of which technique to use, a recent systematic review and meta-analysis aimed to provide consensus on which technique should be used [12].

This study looked at 4777 patients between 1988 and 2012. The mean age was 51 and 71% were male with 46% of patients having severe aortic regurgitation (varying between 6.4 and 100% in the included papers). Mean follow up time was 4.4 years. Analysis revealed that there was no difference in terms of survival or reoperation rates based on the operative technique employed (reimplantation or remodelling, or modification of these). The presence of severe pre-operative aortic regurgitation was the only factor associated with increased risk of reoperation. The authors conclude that to improve the results of valve sparing root replacement, maintaining aortic valve cusp effective height and using techniques to reduce the size of a dilated aortic annulus will help to restore valve coaptation and maintain function.

In light of the results of this review the choice of valve sparing procedure should be based on the technical expertise of team as well as the pre-operative characteristics of the patient, i.e. if annular reduction is required prior to restore and maintain valve function or if the patient is suitable to have valve preserving surgery.

Key Pearls and Pitfalls

1. Consider VSRR using remodelling technique where annulus is not dilated and there is no significant aortic regurgitation
2. Careful inspection of aortic valve leaflets and address any leaflet prolapse prior to root repair
3. Ensure maintenance of symmetry of the root during repair
4. Avoid excessive mobilisation of the coronary buttons during dissection

Comprehension Questions

1. Above what aortic annular dimension has been shown to increase risk of reoperation following VSRR? **Answer = C**
   (a) 24 mm
   (b) 26 mm
   (c) 28 mm
   (d) 30 mm

2. A vascular graft of what size should be selected when performing remodelling VSRR? **Answer = D**
   (a) Annulus diameter + 5 mm
   (b) Annulus diameter + 1 mm
   (c) Annulus diameter
   (d) Annulus diameter + 3 mm
3. When suturing the scallops of the vascular graft to the remaining sinus tissue, where should suturing start? **Answer = C**
   (a) From the commissure towards the nadir of the sinus
   (b) Midway between the top of the commissure and the nadir of the sinus
   (c) From the nadir of the sinus
   (d) Suturing can begin from any point in the sinus
4. Cusp motion has been shown to be same in both the originally described reimplantation technique versus the remodelling technique (T/F) **Answer = False**

References

1. Charitos EI, Sievers H-H. Anatomy of the aortic root: implications for valve-sparing surgery. Ann Cardiothorac Surg. 2013;2(1):53–536.
2. Moscarelli M, De Paulis R. The golden perfection of the aortic valve. Int J Cardiol. 2016;205:165–6.
3. Erasmi AW, Sievers HH, Bechtel JFM, Hanke T, Stierle U, Misfeld M. Remodeling or reimplantation for valve-sparing aortic root surgery? Ann Thorac Surg. 2007;83:S752–6.
4. Patel ND, Weiss ES, Alejo DE, Nwakanma LU, Williams JA, Dietz HC, et al. Aortic root operations for Marfan syndrome: a comparison of the Bentall and valve-sparing procedures. Ann Thorac Surg. 2008;85:2003–10.
5. Stamou SC, Williams ML, Gunn TM, Hagberg RC, Lobdell KW, Kouchoukos NT. Aortic root surgery in the United States: a report from the society of thoracic surgeons database. J Thorac Cardiovasc Surg. 2014;149(1):116–22.
6. Lansac E, Di Centa I, Bonnet N, Leprince P, Rama A, Acar C, et al. Aortic prosthetic ring annuloplasty: a useful adjunct to a standardized aortic valve-sparing procedure? Eur J Cardiothorac Surg. 2006;29:537–44.
7. Aicher D, Langer F, Lausberg H, Bierbach B, Schäfers HJ. Aortic root remodeling: ten-year experience with 274 patients. J Thorac Cardiovasc Surg. 2007;134:909–15.
8. David TE. Current readings: aortic valve-sparing operations. Semin Thorac Cardiovasc Surg. 2014;26(3):231–8.
9. Fries R, Graeter T, Aicher D, Reul H, Schmitz C, Böhm M, et al. In vitro comparison of aortic valve movement after valve-preserving aortic replacement. J Thorac Cardiovasc Surg. 2006;132(1):32–7.
10. Yacoub MH, Aguib H, Gamrah MA, Shehata N, Nagy M, Donia M, et al. Aortic root dynamism, geometry, and function after the remodeling operation: clinical relevance. J Thorac Cardiovasc Surg. 2018;156(3):951–962.e2.
11. De Paulis R, Chirichilli I, Scaffa R, Weltert L, Maselli D, Salica A, et al. Long-term results of the valve reimplantation technique using a graft with sinuses. J Thorac Cardiovasc Surg. 2016;151(1):112–9.
12. Arabkhani B, Mookhoek A, Di Centa I, Lansac E, Bekkers JA, De Lind Van Wijngaarden R, et al. Reported outcome after valve-sparing aortic root replacement for aortic root aneurysm: a systematic review and meta-analysis. Ann Thorac Surg. 2015;100(3):1126–31.

Valve-Sparing Aortic Root Surgery by the Reimplantation Technique

17

Maral Ouzounian, Malak Elbatarny, and Tirone David

Abbreviations

AD	Aortic dissection
AI	Aortic insufficiency
AS	Aortic stenosis
AV	Aortic valve
AVS	Aortic valve sparing
BAV	Bicuspid aortic valve
Bio-CVG	Bioprosthetic composite valve grafting
CI	Confidence interval
CVG	Composite valve grafting
HR	Hazard ratio
HTAD	Hereditary thoracic aortic disorders
IRR	Incident rate ratio
LV	Left ventricle
LVOT	Left ventricular outflow tract
M-CVG	Mechanical composite valve grafting
OR	Odds ratio
RCT	Randomized control trial
STJ	Sinotubular junction
TAAD	Thoracic aortic aneurysmal disease
TAV	Tricuspid aortic valve
TEE	Transesophageal echocardiography
TTE	Transthoracic echocardiography

M. Ouzounian (✉) · M. Elbatarny · T. David
Division of Cardiovascular Surgery, Peter Munk
Cardiac Centre, University Health Network,
Toronto, ON, Canada

University of Toronto, Toronto, ON, Canada
e-mail: Maral.Ouzounian@uhn.ca;
m.elbatarny@mail.utoronto.ca; tirone.david@uhn.ca

Learning Objectives

1. Provide an overview of the rationale for AVS with the reimplantation technique with review of current evidence.
2. Describe patient selection and define ideal patient candidates for reimplantation in the context of underlying pathology.
3. Describe the step-by-step operative technique including intraoperative assessment to assess candidacy and quality of repair.
4. Highlight principles of perioperative management to facilitate success of reimplantation AVS.
5. Discuss outcomes of AVS by the reimplantation technique including:
   (a) Comparison with CVG procedures
   (b) Outcomes in special populations: BAV, Marfan Syndrome, Dissection
   (c) Recent insights from hemodynamic flow studies of post-AVS patients

© Springer Nature Switzerland AG 2022
P. P. Punjabi, P. G. Kyriazis (eds.), *Essentials of Operative Cardiac Surgery*,
https://doi.org/10.1007/978-3-031-14557-5_17

Introduction

In a large subset of patients with aortic root pathology, aortic valve cusps are morphologically normal. AVS operations were thus developed to treat aortic root aneurysms while preserving the native aortic valve and have become established alternatives to CVG procedures for patients with favorable cusp morphology. Although AVS techniques have been available for over 30 years [1, 2], the proportion of AVS operations among patients undergoing root replacement in the United States has remained approximately 15% and is not increasing [3]. Reluctance to perform AVS may be due in part to concerns regarding the durability of these procedures and the lack of comparative data regarding the long-term safety and effectiveness of AVS compared to traditional Bentall procedures.

Although AVS operations have undergone several technical modifications, all developed with a common objective of avoiding the thromboembolic complications associated with mechanical valves and structural valve deterioration associated with biological prostheses. AVS, most commonly by the reimplantation technique, has replaced CVG as standard of care in selected patients. The reimplantation technique (also known as the David procedure) is the focus of this chapter.

Choice of Procedure in the Context of Pathology

Ideal Patient Candidates for the Reimplantation Procedure

Ideal candidates for AVS operations are patients with aortic root aneurysms and morphologically and functionally normal trileaflet aortic valves. In this context, AVS operations have proven to be durable and associated with reduced valve-related morbidities [4, 5] compared to CVG procedures [6–8]. Over the years however, AVS techniques have been extended to include patients with Aortic Insufficiency (AI), cusp prolapse, Bicuspid Aortic Valve (BAV), and acute Aortic Dissection (AD.) Even in the presence of these aforementioned conditions, patients with thin and pliable cusps of adequate cusp height are good candidates for AVS operations.

Aortic Pathology and Mechanism of AI

Understanding the mechanism of AI, as assessed by Transthoracic or Transesophageal Echocardiography (TTE or TEE), is a crucial step in deciding candidacy for reimplantation or any AVS procedure. AI is associated with a wide spectrum of cusp pathology ranging from none or minimal (such as in isolated Sinotubular Junction (STJ) dilation), to severe and unrepairable (such as severely calcified or stenotic cusps). Significant echocardiographic morphological features include geometry and dimensions of each component of the aortic root: the aortic annulus; sinuses of Valsalva; STJ; cusp number, thickness, and mobility; and resultant hemodynamics (Fig. 17.1). These have been classified by El Khoury and colleagues (Fig. 17.2) [9]. Repair of valves with restricted cusps or those that are calcified or stenotic is generally not advisable, therefore these conditions should usually not be treated with AVS, except perhaps in children.

Reimplantation may be undertaken in carefully selected patients with BAV. Aortic root dilation in these individuals is theorized to be a direct result of underlying genetic aortopathy and/or secondarily as a result of valvular dysfunction. The mechanism of AI associated with BAV can include various pathologies: restrictive or calcified conjoint cusp, cusp prolapse, or fenestrations, a severely dilated annulus, or a combination of the above. Often, the conjoint cusp is large and prolapsing with a median raphe. The jet is often eccentrically directed and there may be asymmetrical root dilation, especially with greatest dilation in the posterior sinus. Of note, if only the posterior sinus is aneurysmal, complete root replacement may not be necessary. BAV repair strategies must similarly address each of the pathological components of the root in an effort

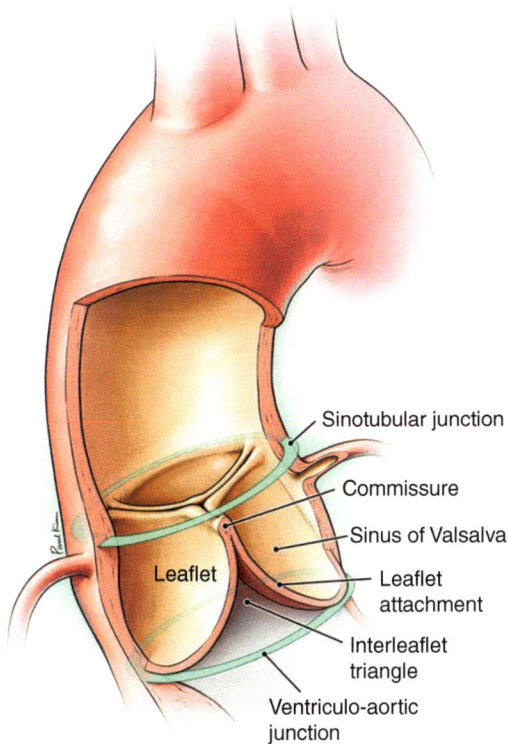

Fig. 17.1 Echocardiographic morphological features of the aortic root

to restore functional root geometry, and may include free-margin plication, free-margin resuspension, raphe resection or shaving, and various techniques of annular downsizing.

In addition to cusp morphology, underlying disease pathology can aid in the decision to undertake AVS and choice of AVS technique. For example, patients with degenerative ascending aortic aneurysms have central AI secondary to STJ dilation for whom repair would entail STJ remodeling. Older patients without annuloaortic ectasia and hypertensive root aneurysms are amenable to AVS with the remodeling procedure. Those with heritable thoracic aortic disorders (HTAD) such as Marfan Syndrome, Loeys-Dietz Syndrome, and Familial Thoracic Aortic Aneurysm most often have annuloaortic ectasia and root aneurysms. These conditions predispose patients to much higher risk for long term annular dilation but generally have normal valve cusps. Therefore they are frequently best treated with an AVS technique that stabilizes the aortic annulus. As such, reimplantation, as opposed to remodeling, is the procedure of choice in this group. Proponents of the remodeling procedure have

AI Class	Type I Normal cusp motion with annular dilation or cusp perforation				Type II Cusp prolapse	Type III Cusp restriction
	1a	1b	1c	1d		
Mechanism	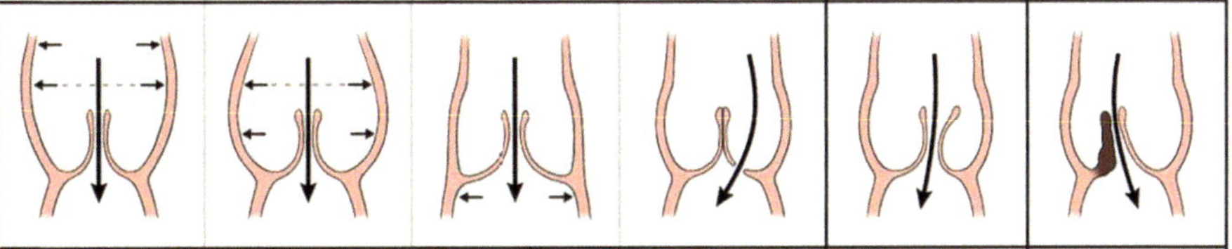					
Repair Technique Primary	STJ remodeling *Ascending aortic graft*	Aortic valve sparing: *Ascending aortic graft*	SCA	Patch repair *Autologous or bovine pericardium*	Prolapse repair *Free margin plication* *Triangular resection* *Free margin resuspension*	Leaflet repair *Shaving declacification patch*
Secondary	SCA		STJ annuloplasty	SCA	SCA	SCA

Fig. 17.2 Repair-oriented functional classification of aortic insufficiency (AI) with description of disease mechanisms and repair techniques used

suggested that remodeling with annuloplasty may also be a viable option, however, long-term durability data in this specific patient population is lacking. Less commonly, patients with HTAD may have myxomatous cusps leading to prolapse and eccentric AI. These individuals may still undergo AVS combined with cusp repair techniques.

Optimal root management in the context of acute type A dissection remains controversial. Despite known advantages in elective patients, concerns of the immediate safety of a more complex operation and the risk of late secondary AI, lead to limited uptake of AVS in of acute AD patients (<10%). Although the technical details of aortic valve reconstruction do not differ, additional time required and the challenge of dealing with extensive hematoma and dissected tissues are such that this approach should be undertaken by surgeons facile with the techniques in the elective setting. Therefore a combination of factors including: extent of root pathology, patient condition, and surgeon experience with AVS must be taken into account to ensure successful management of this challenging clinical condition. Furthermore, longer-term multicenter follow-up is necessary to confirm the favorable long-term outcomes that have been reported in well-selected patients in preliminary single center studies.

Finally, aneurysm size or duration of onset of aortic pathology impacts candidacy. Patients who present with larger aortic diameters (>6 cm) or with long standing AI often have damage to the cusp tissue (commissural stress fenestrations or furled and restricted leaflet edges). The larger the root aneurysm, the more likely that the cusps have been damaged by chronic AI and are not appropriate substrates for a durable repair.

Techniques for aortic cusp repair are detailed in Chap. 7. While preoperative assessment is critical to the decision to proceed with AVS, intraoperative cusp assessment is essential for confirming candidacy for reimplantation. The approach to intraoperative decision making is detailed in the subsequent "Operative Technique" subsection of this Chapter.

Operative Technique

Overview and Principles of the Technique

AVS procedures have undergone several technical modifications over the years. This chapter describes the original David procedure, that involves reimplanating the aortic valve into a straight Dacron graft [10]. Reimplantation of the AV firmly anchors the aortic graft proximally below the annulus along the Left Ventricular Outflow Tract (LVOT). All components of the aortic root are suspended inside a tubular graft, thus fixing the diameter and shape of the aortic annulus and STJ (Fig. 17.3) [11, 12]. As such, reimplantation, in contrast to remodeling, reduces the diameter of the aortic annulus and prevents late dilatation of the aortic annulus. We believe

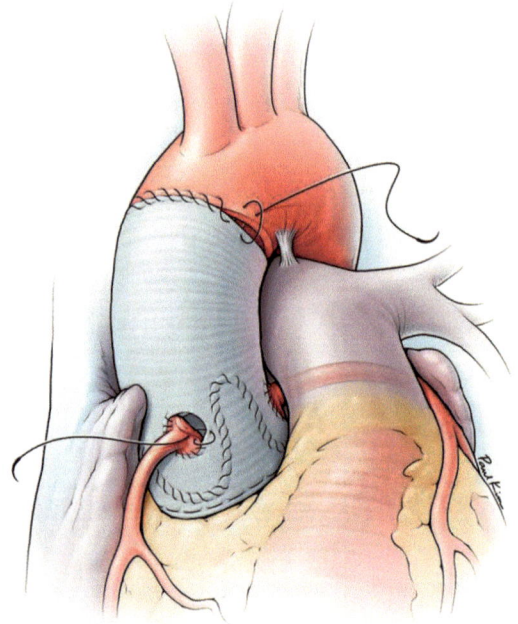

Fig. 17.3 Reimplantation of the aortic valve. Sutures are passed below the aortic annulus in a single horizontal plane along the fibrous portion of the left ventricular outflow tract and following the scalloped shape of the aortic annulus along the muscular interventricular septum. These sutures are also passed from the inside to the outside of a tubular Dacron graft. The commissures and the aortic annulus are sutured inside the graft and the coronary arteries reimplanted

that the LVOT suture with multiple pledgeted sutures is crucial in reducing and stabilizing the annular diameter, particularly in patients with connective tissue disorders. Although the root hemodynamics within a tubular Dacron graft are less physiological than in the remodeling procedure, these differences have not translated into worse long-term durability.

Several modifications of the technique have been utilized including creation of neo-aortic sinuses or the use of the Valsalva graft [13], however the effects of these specific modifications have been difficult to quantify. We have modified our practice to return to the original description of the reimplantation procedure and presently reimplant the valve into a straight Dacron graft.

Cannulation and Myocardial Protection

We perform arterial cannulation in the distal ascending aorta or arch and single two-stage venous cannulation of the right atrial appendage. Antegrade cardioplegia is delivered using direct ostial cannulation. Ostial cannulae are secured to the ostia using 4-0 prolene in order to deliver cardioplegia throughout the case without interruption. Careful review of the preoperative angiogram is important to detect coronary ostial abnormalities which is not infrequently noted in patients with BAV or other congenital aortopathies.

Intraoperative Preprocedural Assessment

The final decision to undertake a reimplantation procedure hinges on intraoperative assessment with TEE and direct visualization of the native valve. Confirmation of the mechanism of AI from preoperative assessment and inspection of the cusps allows the surgeon to confirm the feasibility of AVS and plan additional reconstruction if needed.

The number of cusps is assessed. In patients with BAV, Sievers type 0 valves are ideal, although type I is not a contraindication if cusps

are relatively symmetrical. If asymmetrical annular enlargement is present, a finding which is common but not exclusive to BAV, commissural position must be adjusted during valve reimplantation for symmetry. This not only ensures valve competence but also equally distributes tension to protect against late failure.

Cusp tissue quality is the main determining factor for a successful AVS operation. Cusps must be pliable (not sclerotic), free of multiple major fenestrations, and free of calcification. Furthermore, adequate cusp height is essential as cusp augmenting procedures have not been durable. An eccentric jet of any severity on intraoperative TEE has 92% sensitivity and 96% specificity for cusp prolapse [14]. Additionally, presence of a fibrous band both on TEE and by visual inspection can help localize prolapsing cusps [14]. In decreasing order of frequency, prolapse affects the right, non-coronary, and left coronary cusps [14]. Prolapse may be induced at the time of repair by constraining the valve inside the graft and the position and height of each cusp must be reassessed after reimplantation of the valve. The cusps should be coapting within the body of the sinus (and not below the annulus) and any residual prolapse should be corrected with either central cusp plication or Gore-Tex reinforcement of the free margin. At minimum, effective cusp height must be 8 mm [14, 15] for successful reimplantation and some authors advocated direct measurement of the effective cusp height after the valve is reimplanted [16, 17]. AV repair techniques are detailed comprehensively in Chap. 7. We liberally use cusp repair techniques in conjunction with AVS to correct cusp prolapse, particularly in patients with BAV or those with cusp asymmetry.

Tissue Dissection (Fig. 17.4)

Once AV cusps have been deemed of adequate quality and quantity for preservation, with any repairs performed as necessary, the coronary arteries are detached from the aortic root as buttons, leaving 4–6 mm around each orifice. Coronary arteries which are too close or encroach-

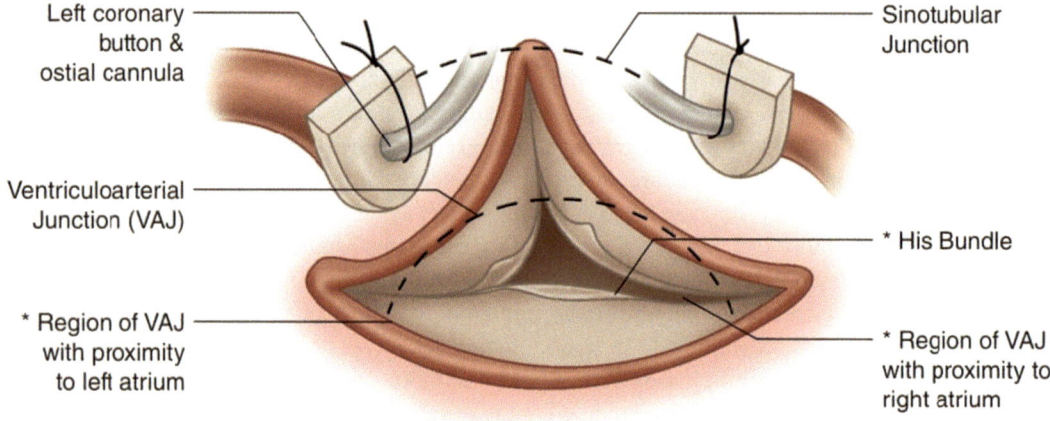

Left coronary
button &
ostial cannula

Sinotubular
Junction

Ventriculoarterial
Junction (VAJ)

* His Bundle

* Region of VAJ
with proximity
to left atrium

* Region of VAJ
with proximity to
right atrium

Fig. 17.4 Surgical dissection to prepare the ventriculoaortic junction with danger areas identified (asterisk). Coronary buttons with ostial cannulae in situ. (Hopefully the illustrator can do a better job of this and the subsequent figures!)

ing upon the aortic annulus should be left attached proximally. This step can be performed simultaneously with delivery of cardioplegia. The aortic sinuses are excised except for a few millimeters that are left attached to the aortic annulus.

Next, the ventriculoaortic junction is prepared by first separating the aortopulmonary window. The dissection is continued to at least 1 cm below the level of the ventriculoaortic junction. External dissection of the aortic root is extended to the anatomical limits of the dissection and care must be taken not to open the surrounding cardiac chambers. Inadequate external dissection is a common pitfall that must be avoided to secure the graft deep into the LVOT circumferentially.

Graft Selection and Sizing

The Dacron graft is sized to facilitate cusp coaptation based on the following measurements: ideal diameter of the STJ, the height of the cusps, or the height of the commissure. Commissural height plus 10–20% or doubled cusp height, undersized by 10–20% result in a graft size with adequate cusp coaptation. A geometric valve sizer may also be used to estimate graft size and assess annuloaortic ectasia. Grafts that we currently use are 26–34 mm in diameter, with most patients receiving a 28 or 30 mm graft. Graft undersizing may lead to cusp prolapse whereas

oversizing results in inadequate cusps coaptation; both conditions create AI and failure of the repair.

Aortic Annuloplasty (LVOT Suture Line)

At this stage, the graft is sutured circumferentially to the outside of the LVOT with multiple [9–12] horizontal mattress sutures. The objective of this layer is to reduce the size of the aortic annulus and facilitate cusp coaptation. This suture line is crucial in patients with annuloaortic ectasia to reduce the size of the annulus and to prevent future dilatation and valve incompetence. Generous plication of a slightly oversized graft is helpful in constructing neo-sinuses.

We routinely use felt pledgets inside the LVOT for patients with connective tissue disorders. Suture position on the graft should match that of the annulus. A 2–4 mm gap is left at the annular position where the membranous septum joins muscular septum to avoid the Bundle of His. Sutures placed in the membranous septum should be slightly higher close to the commissure (and correspondingly higher on the graft).

Once sutures are passed circumferentially through the graft, the graft is lowered to its anatomical limits, far below level of aortic cusps. The AV is then reimplanted inside the graft by suspending the three commissures inside the

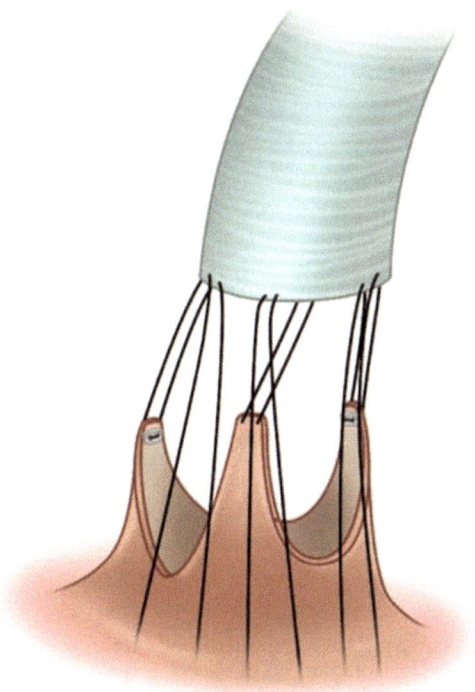

Fig. 17.5 Aortic annuloplasty. 10–12 horizontal mattress sutures are placed to plicate the aortic annulus before parachuting the graft

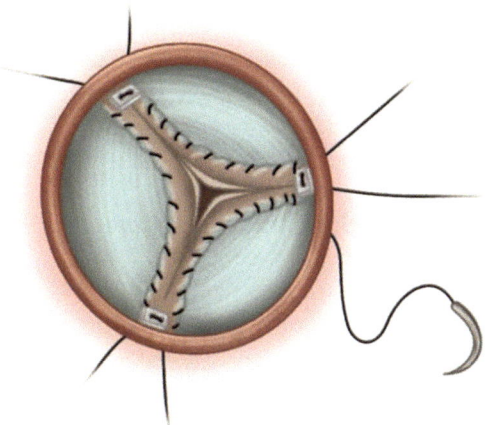

Fig. 17.6 Hemostatic suture line

graft and fixing the remnant aortic sinus tissue to the wall of the graft (Fig. 17.5). Commissural placement is crucial to achieving adequate cusp coaptation height. Pethig et al identified that if the point of coaptation of the valve cusps is ≥2 mm above the lower edge of the prosthesis, there is associated long term stability of the repair [18]. Cusps may be assessed by direct visual inspection; additionally others have suggested caliper-measured cusp height.

Aortic Annuloplasty (Hemostatic Suture Line)

The objective of this running horizontal mattress layer is hemostasis by following the scalloped geometry of the annulus. One bite is taken close to the aortic annulus, one through remnant of aortic sinus. For maximum precision, bites are taken individually in and out of the graft to be certain of suture position (Fig. 17.6).

Coronary Button Reimplantation

At this stage, the coronary buttons are reimplanted into their respective neoaortic sinuses. In most cases, coronary arteries may be reimplanted in the center of the neo-aortic sinuses, although the right coronary button is often closer to the right-non commissure. Mobilizing the aortic tissue and the external root dissection generally provides adequate mobilization of the coronary arteries. As with any root replacement procedure, appropriate positioning of the coronary buttons is crucial to avoid kinking, twisting or other malpositioning that leads to cardiac ischemia. Management of anomalous coronary arteries is challenging and beyond the scope of this chapter.

Reassessment and Secondary Cusp Repair

After coronary reimplantation, the cusps are once again critically re-examined for any prolapse, symmetry, and the height and depth of coaptation. If needed, additional cusp repair is performed as described in detail in Chap. 7 to ensure that all cusps are coapting at the same level and well above the aortic annulus. In our practice, cusp repair by free margin plication is required in approximately 50% of cases. We plicate the Nodule of Arantius with prolene, 3 mm at a time, obliterating the cul-de-sac created by plication, and continually reassessing for symmetry of coaptation height. Alternatively, the free margin is plicated using goretex woven through the cusp edge.

Post-procedural Intraoperative Assessment

Prior to removal of the aortic cross clamp, valve competence may be crudely tested by delivery of a dose of cardioplegia into the neo-aortic root. However it is intraoperative TEE after weaning from cardiopulmonary bypass, which provides the most detailed and definitive intraoperative guidance on the quality of the repair. Mild AI after reimplantation AVS is not uncommon and does not necessarily indicate inadequate repair, but is only acceptable if it is central with no evidence of residual prolapse and adequate coaptation length/height. Evidence suggests that mild AI remains stable or stabilizes over the long term and does not predict late failure [19], although this study investigated pre-discharge TTE not intraoperative TEE. Rather, the following features are the strongest predictors of failure of AV repair over the long term: level of coaptation relative to the annulus, the presence of $\geq$ moderate residual AI, and length of cusp coaptation <4 mm [20]. In our experience, effective height, defined as the distance between the basal ring and top of cusp coaptation, should be $\geq$1 cm and coaptation height, defined as the length of cusp coaptation, should be $\geq$6 mm.

Transvalvular gradients should also be assessed to rule out stenosis (Peak gradient <30 and mean gradient <15 mmHg). Patients with BAV undergoing concomitant cusp repair are most at risk for post-procedural AS [21].

Outcomes of Reimplantation

Reimplantation vs. CVG

Theoretical benefits of AVS procedures include avoiding the complications associated with pros-

thetic valves, specifically, the risks of systemic thromboembolism and lifelong anticoagulation associated with mechanical valves, or the risks of structural valve deterioration and associated with bioprosthetic valves. In the absence of RCTs, observational studies comparing long-term survival and freedom from valve-related complications may inform the relative long-term safety and effectiveness of AVS compared to traditional CVG procedures.

We reported a propensity-matched analysis of 616 patients aged <70 years and without aortic stenosis who underwent elective aortic root replacement surgery (AVS, N = 253; CVG with a bioprosthesis (bio-CVG), N = 180; CVG with a mechanical prosthesis (m-CVG), N = 183) [6]. After adjusting for clinical covariates, both bio-CVG and m-CVG procedures were associated with increased long-term major adverse valve-related events compared to patients undergoing AVS (HR 3.4, p = 0.005; and HR 5.2, p < 0.001, respectively). They were also associated with increased cardiac mortality (HR 7.0, p = 0.001; and HR 6.4, p = 0.003). As expected, bio-CVG procedures were associated with increased risk of reoperations (HR 6.9, p = 0.003), and m-CVG procedures were associated with increased risk of anticoagulant related hemorrhage (HR 5.6, p = 0.008) compared to AVS procedures.

Gaudino et al also reported a propensity-matched analysis of 890 consecutive patients undergoing root replacement with overall operative mortality of 0.2% [7]. When limiting the analysis to patients undergoing Reimplantation AVS, the difference in late reoperation between the AVS and m-CVG becomes non-significant (p = 0.63)

We also reported the largest risk-adjusted systematic review and meta-analysis investigating AVS (primarily by reimplantation) vs. CVG in the general population https://pubmed.ncbi.nlm.nih.gov/31981499/. This consisted of 26 comparative papers (N = 6218) and overall follow-up of 5.8 years. AVS patients had superior late survival (IRR: 0.68, 95%CI: 0.54–0.87), freedom from late bleeding (IRR: 0.21, 95%CI: 0.11–0.42 p < 0.01) and freedom from thromboembolic complications (IRR: 0.36, 95%CI: 0.22–0.60, p < 0.01). Results for survival and bleeding remained significant when considering only propensity-matched or adjusted data. Late freedom from reintervention was equivalent in AVS vs. CVG. Additionally, perioperative outcomes including mortality, MI, re-exploration for bleeding, or stroke were equivalent. Additionally, risk of late thromboembolism/stroke was significantly lower in AVS vs. CVG in the overall (though not adjusted-only) comparison. Late reintervention at 6.1 years of mean follow up were equivalent. Furthermore, AVS procedures appeared to be safe in the perioperative period: there were no differences in perioperative mortality, MI, re-exploration for bleeding, or stroke in propensity-adjusted comparisons.

Patients undergoing reimplantation AVS may also have superior quality of life compared to those undergoing CVG. Franke et al showed significantly better mean scores in the following patient-reported Physical Functioning (78 vs. 63, p = 0.041) and General Health (69 vs. 53, p = 0.004) among other quality of life domains [22].

Although an RCT will likely never be performed, there is evidence that in patients with aortic root aneurysms and normal or nearly normal aortic valve cusps, AVS operations are associated with lower valve-related morbidities compared with CVG root procedures without compromising perioperative safety or late freedom from reintervention. We suggest that potentially AVS-eligible patients be referred to a high-volume aortic center to ensure optimal early and late outcomes, given the strong volume-outcome relationship [23].

Reimplantation in Marfan Syndrome

A recent systematic review and meta-analysis of 23 studies reporting the outcomes of 2976 patients with Marfan syndrome undergoing aortic root surgery were analyzed (CVG, N = 1624 vs. AVS, N = 1352) [8]. When compared to CVG, AVS operations were associated with reduced risk of thromboembolism (OR = 0.32; 95% CI, 0.16–0.62, p = 0.0008), late hemorrhagic complications (OR = 0.18; 95% CI, 0.07–0.45; p = 0.0003) and endocarditis (OR = 0.27; 95%

CI, 0.10–0.68; p = 0.006). Importantly there was no significant difference in reintervention rates between AVS and CVG (OR = 0.89; 95% CI, 0.35–2.24; p = 0.80).

Reimplantation in Dissection

The vast majority of acute dissections involve the aortic root and often require root replacement. Root replacement may offer more definitive management reducing the risk of late reoperation although the evidence for this remains limited. Furthermore it is important to prioritize minimizing early morbidity and mortality in this acute critical circumstance, before considering long term benefit.

Several groups from experienced centres have indicated the safety of performing valve sparing procedures by the reimplantation technique in appropriate patients with acute dissection [24–29]. A recent systematic review and meta-analysis examined the current state of the evidence for root replacement techniques in patients with acute type A dissection [24]. A total of 27 studies with 3058 patients were analysed: in-hospital mortality favored AVS procedures: AVS: 2% vs. CVG: 8%. Survival at midterm also favored AVS procedures: AVS: 98.8% (95%CI 91.7–100%) vs. CVG: 81.3% (95%CI 78.5–83.9%). More recently, Sievers et al. reported their 20-year institutional experience with AVS during acute type A dissection repair [25]. Thirty-day mortality was 14% and was not different between patients undergoing reimplantation, remodeling, or root preservation with commissural resuspension [25]. Mortality and reintervention at 15 years were not different between the three groups. Rosenblum et al. also reported their single center experience with AVS (reimplantation technique) compared to CVG in acute type A aortic dissection repair in 136 cases [29]. Thirty-day mortality was lower for AVS (2/59, 3.4% vs. 11/77, 14.3%, p < 0.01). At 9-years, AVS was associated with improved survival (92 vs. 59%, p < 0.01). The incidence of valve reintervention was low and not different between groups.

In this challenging patient population, an individualized approach that is related to the extent of the root pathology, the patient's condition and the surgeon's experience with AVS is essential. Longer-term multicenter follow-up is necessary to confirm the favorable long-term outcomes that have been reported in well-selected patients in preliminary single center studies.

Reimplantation in BAV

Reimplantation AVS is increasingly undertaken in the BAV population with excellent results. Bavaria et al report no significant difference in 5 year freedom from reintervention between BAV and TAV patients (BAV = 97%; TAV = 100%, p = 0.6). Of note, in this series, all BAV patients underwent concomitant cusp repair which suggests these techniques do not compromise late outcomes [30]. Similarly, our propensity-matched series comparing BAV and TAV showed no significant differences in late reoperation. Freedom from reoperation at 10 years was 98.6% in TAV and 95.8% in BAV (p = 0.42). Cusp repair was performed in 79% of the BAV patients [31].

Hemodynamics of Reimplantation

One of the theoretical advantages of AVS is improved postoperative hemodynamics. Svensson et al demonstrated that LV mass index at 3 years postoperatively was lowest (and close to normal range) among patients undergoing primarily reimplantation AVS versus CVG [32]. One caveat to this finding, however, is that patients undergoing AVS also had lower preoperative LV mass index.

Studies investigating MRI 4D flow have also provided evidence of improvement in eccentric flow of dilated aortic roots, post-AVS by reimplantation [33] and that the hemodynamics post-AVS by reimplantation is superior to that of valved conduits [34]. Furthermore, comparison between post-reimplantation AVS patients and age-matched healthy volunteers showed very similar hemodynamics [35, 36]. Attempts to reduce altered wall shear stress have led to interest in Valsalva grafts and other methods of neo-

sinus construction. One case study demonstrated that cylindrical grafts may result in 90° malrotation of helical flow about the coronary ostia, but with uncertain clinical significance [37]. Furthermore, other studies have failed to show any significant difference between the use of a cylindrical graft and reimplantation with the Stanford modification (two graft technique) [36]. A major criticism of Valsalva grafts is the spherical sinus shape, unlike the physiologic aortic annulus that evolves within a cylinder [38]. We therefore continue to use cylindrical grafts in our practice. Because findings related to vorticity have been conflicting with respect to variation in neo-sinus construction technique, some have suggested pressure differences across the aortic cusps may play a greater role than sinus morphology in vorticity [36].

Hemodynamic 4D flow studies with respect to AVS procedures remain in relative infancy. Further study is warranted to ascertain clinical significance and guide surgical technique optimization.

Key Pearl/Pitfall

At minimum, effective cusp height must be 8 mm

Coronary arteries which are too close or encroaching upon the aortic annulus should be left attached proximally.

Inadequate external dissection is a common pitfall that must be avoided to secure the graft deep into the LVOT circumferentially.

Commissural height plus 10–20% or doubled cusp height, undersized by 10–20% result in a graft size with adequate cusp coaptation.

We routinely use felt pledgets inside the LVOT for patients with connective tissue disorders.

2–4 mm gap is left at the annular position where the membranous septum joins muscular septum to avoid the Bundle of His.

Ensure that all cusps are coapting at the same level and well above the aortic annulus.

cusp repair by free margin plication is required in approximately 50% of cases. We plicate the Nodule of Arantius with prolene, 3 mm at a time, obliterating the cul-de-sac created by plication, and continually reassessing for symmetry of coaptation height.

Mild AI after reimplantation AVS is not uncommon and does not necessarily indicate inadequate repair, but is only acceptable if it is central with no evidence of residual prolapse and adequate coaptation length/height.

In our experience, effective height, defined as the distance between the basal ring and top of cusp coaptation, should be ≥ 1 cm and coaptation height, defined as the length of cusp coaptation, should be ≥ 6 mm.

Comprehension Questions

1. Which of the following is true with regards to BAV in the context of reimplantation AVS procedures?
   (a) Sievers Type 0 morphology valves are generally not good candidates for AVS
   (b) Prolapsing aortic valve cusps are best identified under direct vision on the arrested heart
   (c) Sievers Type I morphology is not a contraindication to AVS
   (d) Five year freedom from reintervention for BAV patients undergoing AVS is >90% but still significantly lower than TAV

Answer: C

2. Which of the following features on post-bypass echo suggest possible need for revision of a reimplantation AVS root replacement?
   (a) Mild aortic insufficiency
   (b) Cusp coaptation at the level of the annulus
   (c) Coaptation height of 7 mm
   (d) Mean gradient of 10 mmHg across the aortic valve

Answer: B

3. Which of the following patients may benefit more from reimplantation vs. remodeling AVS
   (a) 67 year-old male with Bicuspid Aortic Valve presenting with acute Type A dissection
   (b) 60 year old female with Loeys-Dietz, a severely regurgitant trileaflet aortic valve, and mildly prolapsing cusps
   (c) 37 year old male with no known connective tissue disease, undergoing elective

root replacement, found to have thin friable aorta and isolated annuloaortic ectasia as the mechanism of AI
   (d) all of the above

Answer: D

Conflicts of Interest The authors have no conflicts of interest to declare

Funding SourcesNo funding was provided for this work

References

1. David TE, Feindel CM. An aortic-valve sparing operation for patients with aortic incompetence and aneurysm of the ascending aorta. J Thorac Cardiovasc Surg. 1992;103(4):617–22.
2. Sarsam MA, Yacoub M. Remodeling of the aortic valve anulus. J Thorac Cardiovasc Surg. 1993;105(3):435–8. Available from http://www.ncbi.nlm.nih.gov/pubmed/8445922
3. Stamou SC, Williams ML, Gunn TM, Hagberg RC, Lobdell KW, Kouchoukos NT. Aortic root surgery in the United States: a report from the Society of Thoracic Surgeons database. J Thorac Cardiovasc Surg. 2015 [cited 2016 Jun 29];149(1):116–22.e4.. Available from http://www.ncbi.nlm.nih.gov/pubmed/24934089
4. David TE, David CM, Manlhiot C, Colman J, Crean AM, Bradley T. Outcomes of aortic valve-sparing operations in marfan syndrome. J Am Coll Cardiol. 2015;66(13):1445–53. Available from http://ovidsp.ovid.com/ovidweb.cgi?T=JS&PAGE=reference&D=medl&NEWS=N&AN=26403341
5. David TE, Feindel CM, David CM, Manlhiot C. A quarter of a century of experience with aortic valve-sparing operations. J Thorac Cardiovasc Surg. 2014;148(3):872–80. Available from http://ovidsp.ovid.com/ovidweb.cgi?T=JS&PAGE=reference&D=medl&NEWS=N&AN=24930611
6. Ouzounian M, Rao V, Manlhiot C, Abraham N, David C, Feindel CM, et al. Valve-sparing root replacement compared with composite valve graft procedures in patients with aortic root dilation. J Am Coll Cardiol. 2016;68(17):1838–47. Available from https://www.ncbi.nlm.nih.gov/pubmed/27765186
7. Gaudino M, Lau C, Munjal M, Avgerinos D, Girardi LN. Contemporary outcomes of surgery for aortic root aneurysms: a propensity-matched comparison of valve-sparing and composite valve graft replacement. J Thorac Cardiovasc Surg. 2015;150(5):1130–1. Available from https://www.ncbi.nlm.nih.gov/pubmed/26234456
8. Flynn CD, Tian DH, Wilson-Smith A, David T, Matalanis G, Misfeld M, et al. Systematic review

and meta-analysis of surgical outcomes in Marfan patients undergoing aortic root surgery by composite-valve graft or valve sparing root replacement. Ann Cardiothorac Surg. 2017;6(6):570–81. Available from https://www.ncbi.nlm.nih.gov/pubmed/29270369

9. Boodhwani M, de Kerchove L, Glineur D, Poncelet A, Rubay J, Astarci P, et al. Repair-oriented classification of aortic insufficiency: impact on surgical techniques and clinical outcomes. J Thorac Cardiovasc Surg. 2009;137(2):286–94. Available from https://www.ncbi.nlm.nih.gov/pubmed/19185138

10. David T. The David procedure in 10 steps. In: AATS aortic symposium. New York, NY; 2018.

11. David TE, Maganti M, Armstrong S. Aortic root aneurysm: principles of repair and long-term follow-up. J Thorac Cardiovasc Surg. 2010;140(6 Suppl):S14–9. discussion S45–51. Available from https://www.ncbi.nlm.nih.gov/pubmed/21092781

12. de Kerchove L, Mosala Nezhad Z, Boodhwani M, El Khoury G. How to perform valve sparing reimplantation in a tricuspid aortic valve. Ann Cardiothorac Surg. 2013;2(1):105–12. Available from http://ovidsp.ovid.com/ovidweb.cgi?T=JS&PAGE=reference&D=prem&NEWS=N&AN=23977566

13. De Paulis R, Chirichilli I, Scaffa R, Weltert L, Maselli D, Salica A, et al. Long-term results of the valve reimplantation technique using a graft with sinuses. J Thorac Cardiovasc Surg. 2016;151(1):112–9. Available from https://www.ncbi.nlm.nih.gov/pubmed/26349596

14. Boodhwani M, de Kerchove L, Watremez C, Glineur D, Vanoverschelde JL, Noirhomme P, et al. Assessment and repair of aortic valve cusp prolapse: implications for valve-sparing procedures. J Thorac Cardiovasc Surg. 2011;141(4):917–25.

15. Boodhwani M, de Kerchove L, Glineur D, El Khoury G. A simple method for the quantification and correction of aortic cusp prolapse by means of free margin plication. J Thorac Cardiovasc Surg. 2010;139(4):1075–7. Available from https://www.ncbi.nlm.nih.gov/pubmed/19660418

16. Schäfers HJ, Bierbach B, Aicher D. A new approach to the assessment of aortic cusp geometry. J Thorac Cardiovasc Surg. 2006;132(2):436–8.

17. Schäfers HJ, Schmied W, Marom G, Aicher D. Cusp height in aortic valves. J Thorac Cardiovasc Surg. 2013;146(2):269–74.

18. Pethig K, Milz A, Hagl C, Harringer W, Haverich A. Aortic valve reimplantation in ascending aortic aneurysm: risk factors for early valve failure. Ann Thorac Surg. 2002;73(1):29–33. Available from http://ovidsp.ovid.com/ovidweb.cgi?T=JS&PAGE=reference&D=med4&NEWS=N&AN=11834030

19. Stephens EH, Liang DH, Kvitting JPE, Kari FA, Fischbein MP, Mitchell RS, et al. Incidence and progression of mild aortic regurgitation after Tirone David reimplantation valve-sparing aortic root replacement. J Thorac Cardiovasc Surg. 2014;147(1):169–178.e3. https://doi.org/10.1016/j.jtcvs.2013.09.009.

20. le Polain de Waroux JB, Pouleur AC, Robert A, Pasquet A, Gerber BL, Noirhomme P, et al. Mechanisms of recurrent aortic regurgitation after aortic valve repair. Predictive value of intraoperative transesophageal echocardiography. JACC Cardiovasc Imaging. 2009;2(8):931–9. https://doi.org/10.1016/j.jcmg.2009.04.013.

21. Underwood MJ, El Khoury G, Deronck D, Glineur D, Dion R. The aortic root: structure, function, and surgical reconstruction. Heart. 2000;83(4):376–80.

22. Franke UFW, Isecke A, Nagib R, Breuer M, Wippermann J, Tigges-Limmer K, et al. Quality of life after aortic root surgery: reimplantation technique versus composite replacement. Ann Thorac Surg. 2010;90(6):1869–75.

23. Hughes GC, Zhao Y, Rankin JS, Scarborough JE, O'Brien S, Bavaria JE, et al. Effects of institutional volumes on operative outcomes for aortic root replacement in North America. J Thorac Cardiovasc Surg. 2013;145(1):166–70. Available from http://ovidsp.ovid.com/ovidweb.cgi?T=JS&PAGE=reference&D=emed15&NEWS=N&AN=51846122

24. Mosbahi S, Stak D, Gravestock I, Burgstaller JM, Steurer J, Eckstein F, et al. A systemic review and meta-analysis: Bentall versus David procedure in acute type A aortic dissection. Eur J Cardiothorac Surg. 2019;55(2):201–9. Available from https://www.ncbi.nlm.nih.gov/pubmed/30084969

25. Sievers HH, Richardt D, Diwoky M, Auer C, Bucsky B, Nasseri B, et al. Survival and reoperation after valve-sparing root replacement and root repair in acute type A dissection. J Thorac Cardiovasc Surg. 2018;156(6):2076–2082.e2. Available from https://www.ncbi.nlm.nih.gov/pubmed/30454910

26. Subramanian S, Leontyev S, Borger MA, Trommer C, Misfeld M, Mohr FW. Valve-sparing root reconstruction does not compromise survival in acute type a aortic dissection. Ann Thorac Surg. 2012;94(4):1230–4.

27. Fila P, Ondrasek J, Bedanova H, Nemec P. Aortic valve sparing operations versus composite graft implantation in acute aortic dissections. Cor Vasa. 2012;54(5–6):224–9.

28. Mastrobuoni S, De Kerchove L, Navarra E, Astarci P, Noirhomme P, El Khoury G. Valve sparing-aortic root replacement with the reimplantation technique in acute type A aortic dissection. Ann Cardiothorac Surg. 2016;5(4):397–400.

29. Rosenblum JM, Leshnower BG, Moon RC, Lasanajak Y, Binongo J, McPherson L, et al. Durability and safety of David V valve-sparing root replacement in acute type A aortic dissection. J Thorac Cardiovasc Surg. 2019;157(1):14–23.e1. Available from https://www.ncbi.nlm.nih.gov/pubmed/30557940

30. Bavaria JE, Desai N, Szeto WY, Komlo C, Rhode T, Wallen T, et al. Valve-sparing root reimplantation and leaflet repair in a bicuspid aortic valve: comparison with the 3-cusp David procedure. J Thorac Cardiovasc Surg. 2015;149(2 Suppl):S22–8. Available from https://www.ncbi.nlm.nih.gov/pubmed/25500099

31. Ouzounian M, Feindel CM, Manlhiot C, David C, David TE. Valve-sparing root replacement in patients with bicuspid versus tricuspid aortic valves. J Thorac Cardiovasc Surg. 2019;158(1):1–9. https://doi.org/10.1016/j.jtcvs.2018.10.151.

32. Svensson LG, Pillai ST, Rajeswaran J, Desai MY, Griffin B, Grimm R, et al. Long-term survival, valve durability, and reoperation for 4 aortic root procedures combined with ascending aorta replacement. J Thorac Cardiovasc Surg. 2016;151(3):764.

33. Semaan E, Markl M, Malaisrie SC, Barker A, Allen B, McCarthy P, et al. Haemodynamic outcome at four-dimensional flow magnetic resonance imaging following valve-sparing aortic root replacement with tricuspid and bicuspid valve morphology. Eur J Cardiothorac Surg. 2014;45(5):818–25. Available from http://ovidsp.ovid.com/ovidweb.cgi?T=JS&PAGE=reference&D=medl&NEWS=N&AN=24317086

34. Collins JD, Semaan E, Barker A, McCarthy PM, Carr JC, Markl M, et al. Comparison of hemodynamics after aortic root replacement using valve-sparing or bioprosthetic valved conduit. Ann Thorac Surg. 2015;100(5):1556–62. Available from http://www.elsevier.com/locate/athoracsur

35. Oechtering TH, Hons CF, Sieren M, Hunold P, Hennemuth A, Huellebrand M, et al. Time-resolved 3-dimensional magnetic resonance phase contrast imaging (4D Flow MRI) analysis of hemodynamics in valve-sparing aortic root repair with an anatomically shaped sinus prosthesis. J Thorac Cardiovasc Surg. 2016;152(2):418–427.e1.

36. Markl M, Draney MT, Miller DC, Levin JM, Williamson EE, Pelc NJ, et al. Time-resolved three-dimensional magnetic resonance velocity mapping of aortic flow in healthy volunteers and patients after valve-sparing aortic root replacement. J Thorac Cardiovasc Surg. 2005;130(2):456–63.

37. Oechtering TH, Frydrychowicz A, Sievers HH. Malrotated sinus vortices in straight graft valve-sparing aortic root treatment: a matter of concern? J Thorac Cardiovasc Surg. 2017;154(3):794–7. https://doi.org/10.1016/j.jtcvs.2017.02.024.

38. David TE. On sinuses and vortices. J Thorac Cardiovasc Surg. 2017;154(3):791–3. https://doi.org/10.1016/j.jtcvs.2017.05.056.

Coronary Artery Bypass Graft vs. Percutaneous Intervention

18

Donna Kimmaliardjuk and David Glineur

Introduction

This chapter reviews the current evidence in support of percutaneous coronary intervention (PCI) and coronary artery bypass grafting (CABG) for coronary revascularization. The first section of the chapter reviews important criteria to consider when deciding upon revascularization strategy. The second section of the chapter reviews current evidence supporting revascularization strategy based on anatomical lesions, such as: the left main, proximal left anterior descending artery, and multivessel disease. After reading this chapter, the reader will: identify and understand the important criteria to assess to guide revascularization strategy, will have a basic understanding of the findings of major PCI and CABG revascularization trials, and how those results have influenced the current European Society of Cardiology (ESC) and European Association of Cardio-Thoracic Surgery (EACTS) Guidelines on revascularization.

Criteria for Decision-Making

The three main criteria that should be considered when deciding upon revascularization strategy are:

1. Predicted surgical mortality
2. Anatomical complexity of coronary artery disease (CAD)
3. Completeness of revascularization

Whether PCI vs. CABG is performed should depend on the risk-benefit ratios of the treatments, evaluating the risks of procedural complications against the improvements in quality of life, and long-term freedom from death, MI, or repeat revascularization. The following recommendations are based on the 2018 ESC/EACTS Guidelines on myocardial revascularization [1].

Predicted Surgical Mortality

The European System for Cardiac Operative Risk Evaluation (EuroSCORE II) (www.euroscore. org/calc.html) and the Society of Thoracic Surgeons (STS) score (http://riskcalc.sts.org) were both developed to estimate the surgical in-hospital or 30-day mortality risk. These scores are useful; however, there is not a single risk model that provides perfect risk assessment. The scores are limited by: (1) the definitions used or the methodology applied, (2) lacking important variables (such as frailty), (3) the practicability of

D. Kimmaliardjuk · D. Glineur (✉)
Division of Cardiac Surgery, The University of
Ottawa Heart Institute, Ottawa, ON, Canada
e-mail: dkimmaliardjuk@ottawaheart.ca;
dglineur@ottawaheart.ca

© Springer Nature Switzerland AG 2022
P. P. Punjabi, P. G. Kyriazis (eds.), *Essentials of Operative Cardiac Surgery*,
https://doi.org/10.1007/978-3-031-14557-5_18

calculation, (4) a failure to reflect all relevant mortality and morbidity endpoints, and (5) limited external validation. Therefore, these scores should be used as a guide within the multidisciplinary Heart Team discussion.

Anatomical Complexity of Coronary Artery Disease

The SYNTAX score was prospectively developed for the SYNTAX trial to grade the anatomical complexity of coronary lesions in patients with left main (LM) or three-vessel disease [2]. In the SYNTAX trial, and in external validation studies of this score, the SYNTAX score was found to be an independent predictor of long-term major adverse cardiac and cerebrovascular events (MACCE) and death in patients treated with PCI but not CABG [3–6]. In the SYNTAX trial, patients with low and intermediate SYNTAX scores had similar outcomes with PCI and CABG, but patients with high SYNTAX scores had improved outcomes with CABG [7–9]. In subsequent RCTs, the interaction of SYNTAX score with the effect of the randomized treatment was less pronounced and did not reach statistical significance [10–12]. However, in a collaborative individual patient pooled analysis of randomized trials of 11,518 patients, the test for trend across the ordered terciles of the SYNTAX score (low, intermediate, and high) was positive at P = 0.0011 [13]. Thus, the SYNTAX score should be considered as an effect modifier.

Completeness of Revascularization

The aim of myocardial revascularization is to minimize residual ischemia. The sub study of the COURAGE (Clinical Outcomes Utilizing Revascularization and Aggressive Drug Evaluation) trial demonstrated a decreased risk of death and MI by decreasing residual stress-induced ischemia from >10% of the myocardium to 5% or less [14]. In the SYNTAX trial, anatomical complete revascularization was defined as PCI or bypass of all epicardial vessels with a diameter of 1.5 mm or greater, and a luminal reduction of ≥50% in at least one angiographic view. In a post hoc analysis of the SYNTAX trial, anatomical incomplete revascularization was

associated with inferior long-term outcomes after both CABG and PCI [15]. A residual SYNTAX score >8 after PCI was associated with a significantly higher risk of death at 5 years and of the composite of death, myocardial infarction (MI), and stroke. In fact, any residual SYNTAX score >0 was associated with a risk of repeat intervention [16]. A meta-analysis of 89,883 patients in RCTs and observational studies demonstrated lower long-term mortality (RR 0.71, 95% CI 0.65–0.77), MI (RR 0.78, 95% CI 0.68–0.90), and repeat revascularization (RR 0.74, 95% CI 0.65–0.83) with complete revascularization compared to incomplete revascularization [17]. There were consistent findings in a pooled analysis of 3212 patients of the SYNTAX, BEST (Randomised Comparison of Coronary Artery Bypass Surgery and Everolimus-Eluting Stent Implantation in the Treatment of Patients with Multivessel Coronary Artery Disease), and PRECOMBAT (Premier of Randomized Comparison of Bypass Surgery versus Angioplasty Using Sirolimus-Eluting Stent in Patients with Left Main Coronary Artery Disease) trials. In a propensity matched analysis, mortality and the composite risk of death, MI, and stroke were significantly lower in PCI patients that had complete vs. incomplete revascularization [18]. After PCI with complete revascularization, the risk of death or of the composite of death, MI, or stroke was not significantly different from that after CABG with complete revascularization (adjusted HR 1.16, 95% CI 0.83–1.63, P = 0.39, and 1.14, 95% CI 0.87–1.48, P = 0.35, respectively). However, these risks were significantly elevated after PCI with incomplete revascularization.

Functional complete revascularization means that all lesions causing resting or stress-induced ischemia are revascularized. These lesions are identified by fractional flow reserve (FFR) or instantaneous wave-free ratio (iwFR) during angiography. The FAME study demonstrated that using the guidance of functionally-significant lesions for PCI resulted in superior long-term outcomes compared with anatomically-guided lesions for PCI [19]. In contrast, FAME 2 demonstrated that leaving functionally significant lesions untreated resulted in a high rate of reintervention [20]. Based on the results of FAME and FAME 2, achieving complete revascularization based on the functional definition is the preferred strategy for PCI. The role of functional guidance for CABG however is not as clear [21, 22]. One of the potential benefits of CABG is protection against disease progression in proximal segments; if a surgeon limits bypassing to only functionally relevant lesions, the benefit of proximal protection is lessened. This has to be weighed against the risk of competitive flow causing bypass closure when there is high native vessel flow. Thus, for indeterminate lesions by visual estimation, functional testing may help guide surgical revascularization strategy, with respect to which conduit to use, and where.

Results Per Coronary Territory

Various trials have assessed outcomes post-PCI and post-CABG depending on anatomical lesions. This next section discusses the three major anatomical lesions, isolated proximal left anterior descending (LAD), left main coronary artery disease, and multivessel CAD, and major trials' outcomes for PCI and CABG for each territory.

Isolated Proximal LAD Coronary Artery Disease

Current evidence suggests similar outcomes of death, MI, and stroke in patients with isolated proximal LAD disease among CABG and PCI patients. Be that as it may, there is a higher risk of repeat revascularization with PCI [23–32].

Left Main Coronary Artery Disease

The available evidence from RCTs and meta-analyses comparing CABG with PCI using DES among patients with LM disease suggests equivalent results for the safety composite of death, MI, and stroke up to 5 years of follow-up [33]. There is a significant interaction with time: PCI provides early benefit in terms of MI and peri-interventional stroke, which is then offset by a higher risk of MI during long-term follow-up. Repeat revascularization is higher with PCI than

with CABG. The EXCEL (Everolimus-Eluting Stents or Bypass Surgery for Left Main Coronary Artery Disease) trial compared CABG with PCI using new-generation DES, EES, among 1905 patients with significant LM disease [12]. At 3 years of follow-up, the primary endpoint of death, stroke, or MI was similar in the CABG and PCI groups (14.7 vs. 15.4%; HR 1.00, 95% CI 0.79–1.26, P = 0.98). The pre-planned landmark analysis from 30 days to 3 years showed a significant benefit in CABG patients with respect to the primary endpoint (7.9 vs. 11.5%, P = 0.02). The 5-year primary endpoint was also similar between the two groups (19.2% in CABG vs. 22.0% in PCI group, P = 0.13). However, the composite of death, stroke, MI, or ischemia-driven revascularization was higher in the PCI group (31.1 vs. 24.9%, 95% CI 2.4–10.6) [34]. The explanation of the absence primary endpoint difference between the two groups is mainly related to the definition of periprocedural MI. Indeed, when looking at the results of an observational cohort study from a Korean center using serial creatine kinase–(CK-MB) measurements from more than 7600 patients who had undergone PCI or CABG showed widely disparate rates of MI depending on the definition used [35]. They ranged from 19% for PCI vs. 3% for CABG with use of the second universal definition of MI to 5.5% for PCI vs. 18.3% for CABG if the Society for Cardiovascular Angiography and Interventions (SCAI) definition was used. EXCEL used the SCAI definition of MI. This is crucial because the 37% higher rate of peri-procedural MI in the CABG arm of EXCEL likely drove the comparative event rates. The Kaplan-Meier curves in the EXCEL paper show that rates of MI are higher in the PCI group as the trial progresses. Compared with PCI, there were 22 more MIs in the CABG arm in the first 30 days, but 29 fewer MIs after 30 days [34]. Notably, death from any cause at 5 years was 13.0% in the PCI group, and 9.9% in the CABG group, which is only a 3.1-percentage-point difference, however the odds ratio was 1.38 (95% CI 1.03–1.85). These results differ slightly from those in the NOBLE (Nordic-Baltic-British Left Main Revascularization Study) trial.

The NOBLE trial compared CABG with PCI using new-generation DES [biolimus-eluting stents (BES)] among 1201 patients with significant LM disease (mean SYNTAX score of 23) [11]. At a median follow-up of 3.1 years, the primary endpoint of death, MI, stroke, and repeat revascularization occurred more frequently in the PCI group (29 vs. 19%; HR 1.48, 95% CI 1.11–1.96, P = 0.007). The 5-year primary endpoint occurred in 28% of PCI patients, compared to 19% of CABG patients (HR 1.58; 95% CI 1.24–2.01, P = 0.0002) [36]. The 5-year all-cause mortality was 9% in the PCI group and 9% in the CABG group (HR 1.08, 0.74–1.59, P = 0.68). PCI patients had a higher occurrence of non-procedural MI (8 vs. 3%; HR 2.99, 95% CI 1.66–5.39, P = 0.0002), and repeat revascularization (17 vs. 10%; HR 1.73, 95% CI 1.25–2.40, P = 0.0009).

A recent collaborative individual patient pooled analysis of randomized trials including 11,518 patients comparing CABG with PCI for LM or multivessel disease demonstrated that CABG was associated with a significant survival benefit during a mean follow-up of 3.8 ± 1.4 years (5-year all-cause mortality 11.2% after PCI vs. 9.2% after CABG; HR 1.20, 95% CI 1.06–1.37, P = 0.0038) [13]. There was a linear trend for increasing hazard ratios of death with increasing SYNTAX terciles. However, among 4478 patients with LM disease, patients randomly assigned to CABG or PCI with a mean follow-up of 3.4 ± 1.4 years had similar risks for the primary outcome of all-cause mortality (PCI 10.7 vs. CABG 10.5%; HR 1.07, 95% CI 0.87–1.33, P = 0.52). In patients with a high SYNTAX score, there was a trend towards better survival with CABG. Overall, there were no significant differences in mortality between PCI and CABG in subgroup analyses according to SYNTAX scores [13]. However, the number of patients with a high SYNTAX score was limited due to the inclusion criteria of the studies. Based on current evidence, PCI is appropriate in LM disease and low-to-intermediate anatomical complexity. In patients with LM disease and low anatomical complexity, there is evidence that the outcomes are similar for PCI and CABG. For PCI in LM with intermedi-ate anatomical complexity, it is a class IIa recommendation in the ESC/EACTS revascularization guidelines. Among patients with LM disease and high anatomical complexity, the number of patients studied in RCTs is low due to exclusion criteria. The risk estimates and confidence intervals are imprecise, but suggest a trend towards better survival with CABG. Therefore, PCI is not recommended in the ESC/EACTS revascularization guidelines for LM disease with high anatomical complexity.

Multivessel Coronary Artery Disease

The survival advantage of CABG over PCI has been consistent among patients with intermediate to high SYNTAX scores, and has been attributed at least partly due to the protection that bypass grafts provide against new proximal disease that may develop. The BEST trial, comparing CABG with PCI using new-generation DES, in patients with multivessel CAD (77% three-vessel CAD and 23% two-vessel disease, mean SYNTAX score 24), demonstrated that PCI had a higher incidence of the primary endpoint of death, MI, and target vessel revascularization (TVR) than CABG at a median follow-up of 4.6 years (15.3 vs. 10.6%; HR 1.47, 95% CI 1.01–2.13, P = 0.04) [10]. The risk of death, MI, and stroke was not statistically different between the two groups (11.9 vs. 9.5%; HR 1.26, 95% CI 0.84–1.89, P = 0.26). However, repeat revascularization of any vessel (11.0 vs. 5.4%; HR 2.1, 95% CI 1.28–3.41, P = 0.003) but not TVR (5.7 vs. 3.8%; HR 1.51, 95% CI 0.82–2.80, P = 0.19) was higher in the PCI group. CABG resulted in more complete revascularization (71.5 vs. 50.9%; P < 0.001) and a lower incidence of revascularization for new lesions (5.5 vs. 2.3%; HR 2.47, 95% CI 1.18–5.17, P = 0.01). The collaborative individual patient pooled analysis found that in 7040 patients with multivessel disease, CABG patients had significantly lower 5-year all-cause mortality than PCI patients (PCI 11.5 vs. CABG 8.9%; HR 1.28, 95% CI 1.09–1.49, P = 0.0019) [13]. Two variables that affected all-cause mortality were: diabetes and disease complexity, as defined by the SYNTAX score. Mortality was higher after PCI than CABG in patients with diabetes compared to patients without diabetes (15.5 vs. 10.0%; HR 1.48,95% CI 1.19–1.84, P = 0.0004, P interaction = 0.045). There was also a linear increase in risk of mortality for PCI according to SYNTAX score tercile (low SYNTAX score: 10.5 vs. 8.4%; HR 1.11, 95% CI 0.77–1.62, P = 0.57; intermediate SYNTAX score: 14.0 vs. 9.5%; HR 1.50, 95% CI 1.09–2.08, P = 0.0129; high SYNTAX score: 19.2 vs. 11.2%; HR 1.70, 95% CI 1.13–2.55, P = 0.0094). The 10-year outcomes of all-cause death in the SYNTAX trial occurred more frequently in the PCI group compared to the CABG group (27 vs. 24%, HR 1.17, 95% CI 0.97–1.41, P = 0.092) [37]. In the subgroup analyses of LM and triple vessel disease cohorts, the rate of all-cause death was lower in CABG patients with triple vessel disease compared to PCI patients (21 vs. 28%, HR 1.41, 95% CI 1.10–1.80). The rate of all-cause death in LM CABG patients was 28% compared to 26% in LM PCI patients (HR 0.90, 95% CI 0.68–1.20). In patients with a high SYNTAX score and triple vessel disease, PCI resulted in higher 10-year all-cause death than CABG (HR 1.83, 95% CI 1.20–2.81).

An individual patient data pooled analysis of SYNTAX and BEST, comparing CABG with PCI using DES among 1275 non-diabetic patients with multivessel disease, demonstrated a lower risk of death (6.0 vs. 9.3%; HR 0.65, 95% CI 0.43–0.98, P = 0.04) and MI (3.3 vs. 8.3%; HR 0.40, 95% CI 0.24–0.65, P < 0.001) in CABG patients at a median follow-up of 61 months [38]. For patients with a low SYNTAX score, the risk of death was not significantly different (6.0 vs. 7.5%, P = 0.66). The benefit of CABG over PCI was greater in patients with intermediate-to-high SYNTAX scores (7.1 vs. 11.6%, P = 0.02). Another individual patient data pooled analysis of SYNTAX and BEST patients with multivessel disease involving the proximal LAD (88% three-vessel CAD, mean SYNTAX score 28), reported that the PCI group had a higher risk of the composite of death, MI, and stroke (16.3 vs. 11.5%; HR 1.43, 95% CI 1.05–1.96, P = 0.02), cardiac death, MI, and repeat revascularization at 5 years of follow-up [39]. Current evidence suggests that in non-diabetic patients with multivessel CAD

and low anatomical complexity, PCI and CABG result in similar long-term outcomes of survival, and the composite of death, MI, and stroke.

However, in non-diabetic patients with multivessel CAD and intermediate-to-high anatomical complexity, two large trials using DES, SYNTAX and BEST, found a significantly higher mortality and a higher incidence of death, MI, and stroke with PCI [10, 37]. In a recent meta-analysis, these results were consistently obtained for patients with multivessel CAD [13]. Therefore, PCI is not recommended for multivessel CAD with intermediate-to-high complexity.

Conclusion

This chapter reviewed the current evidence supporting methods of myocardial revascularization. The first section reviewed the important criteria to assess when deciding upon revascularization strategy, including: predicted surgical mortality, anatomical complexity of CAD, and the ability of achieving complete revascularization. Using risk scores, such as the EuroSCORE II and STS score will help predict surgical mortality, and anatomical complexity can be assessed using the SYNTAX score. Tools such as FFR and iwFR can help ensure complete revascularization. Achieving complete revascularization is one of the most important determinants of long-term outcomes post-revascularization and should be the primary goal regardless of method of revascularization. The second section of the chapter reviewed the major trials that have compared PCI to CABG for revascularizing isolated proximal LAD CAD, LM CAD, and multivessel CAD and their respective outcomes. Reviewing these results should clarify why a certain revascularization strategy is recommended based on anatomical lesions, and current evidence.

Key Pearls and Pitfalls

- Aortic valve sparing (AVS) operations were developed to treat aortic root aneurysms while preserving the native aortic valve and have become established alternatives to composite valve graft (CVG) procedures for patients with favourable cusp morphology

- Although AVS operations have undergone several technical modifications, all developed with a common objective of avoiding the thromboembolic complications associated with mechanical valves and structural valve deterioration associated with biological prostheses
- Understanding the mechanism of AI, as assessed by Transthoracic or Transesophageal Echocardiography (TTE or TEE), is a crucial step in deciding candidacy for reimplantation or any AVS procedure
- Optimal root management in the context of acute type A dissection remains controversial
- The larger the root aneurysm, the more likely that the cusps have been damaged by chronic AI and are not appropriate substrates for a durable repair

References

1. Neumann FJ, Sousa-Uva M, Ahlsson A, Alfonso F, Banning AP, Benedetto U, et al. 2018 ESC/EACTS Guidelines on myocardial revascularization. Eur Heart J. 2019;40(2):87–165.
2. Sianos G, Morel MA, Kappetein AP, Morice MC, Colombo A, Dawkins KD, et al. The SYNTAX Score: an angiographic tool grading the complexity of coronary artery disease. EuroIntervention. 2005;1(2):219–27.
3. Wykrzykowska JJ, Garg S, Girasis C, de Vries T, Morel MA, van Es GA, et al. Value of the SYNTAX score for risk assessment in the all-comers population of the randomized multicenter LEADERS (Limus Eluted from A Durable versus ERodable Stent coating) trial. J Am Coll Cardiol. 2010;56(4):272–7.
4. Garg S, Serruys PW, Silber S, Wykrzykowska J, van Geuns RJ, Richardt G, et al. The prognostic utility of the SYNTAX score on 1-year outcomes after revascularization with zotarolimus- and everolimus-eluting stents: a substudy of the RESOLUTE All Comers Trial. JACC Cardiovasc Interv. 2011;4(4):432–41.
5. Zhao M, Stampf S, Valina C, Kienzle RP, Ferenc M, Gick M, et al. Role of euroSCORE II in predicting long-term outcome after percutaneous catheter intervention for coronary triple vessel disease or left main stenosis. Int J Cardiol. 2013;168(4):3273–9.
6. Cavalcante R, Sotomi Y, Mancone M, Whan Lee C, Ahn JM, Onuma Y, et al. Impact of the SYNTAX

scores I and II in patients with diabetes and multivessel coronary disease: a pooled analysis of patient level data from the SYNTAX, PRECOMBAT, and BEST trials. Eur Heart J. 2017;38(25):1969–77.
7. Mohr FW, Morice M-C, Kappetein AP, Feldman TE, Ståhle E, Colombo A, et al. Coronary artery bypass graft surgery versus percutaneous coronary intervention in patients with three-vessel disease and left main coronary disease: 5-year follow-up of the randomised, clinical SYNTAX trial. Lancet. 2013;381(9867):629–38.
8. Morice MC, Serruys PW, Kappetein AP, Feldman TE, Stahle E, Colombo A, et al. Five-year outcomes in patients with left main disease treated with either percutaneous coronary intervention or coronary artery bypass grafting in the synergy between percutaneous coronary intervention with taxus and cardiac surgery trial. Circulation. 2014;129(23):2388–94.
9. Head SJ, Davierwala PM, Serruys PW, Redwood SR, Colombo A, Mack MJ, et al. Coronary artery bypass grafting vs. percutaneous coronary intervention for patients with three-vessel disease: final five-year follow-up of the SYNTAX trial. Eur Heart J. 2014;35(40):2821–30.
10. Park SJ, Ahn JM, Kim YH, Park DW, Yun SC, Lee JY, et al. Trial of everolimus-eluting stents or bypass surgery for coronary disease. N Engl J Med. 2015;372(13):1204–12.
11. Mäkikallio T, Holm NR, Lindsay M, Spence MS, Erglis A, Menown IBA, et al. Percutaneous coronary angioplasty versus coronary artery bypass grafting in treatment of unprotected left main stenosis (NOBLE): a prospective, randomised, open-label, non-inferiority trial. Lancet. 2016;388(10061):2743–52.
12. Stone GW, Sabik JF, Serruys PW, Simonton CA, Genereux P, Puskas J, et al. Everolimus-Eluting Stents or Bypass Surgery for Left Main Coronary Artery Disease. N Engl J Med. 2016;375(23):2223–35.
13. Head SJ, Milojevic M, Daemen J, Ahn J-M, Boersma E, Christiansen EH, et al. Mortality after coronary artery bypass grafting versus percutaneous coronary intervention with stenting for coronary artery disease: a pooled analysis of individual patient data. Lancet. 2018;391(10124):939–48.
14. Shaw LJ, Berman DS, Maron DJ, Mancini GB, Hayes SW, Hartigan PM, et al. Optimal medical therapy with or without percutaneous coronary intervention to reduce ischemic burden: results from the Clinical Outcomes Utilizing Revascularization and Aggressive Drug Evaluation (COURAGE) trial nuclear substudy. Circulation. 2008;117(10):1283–91.
15. Farooq V, Serruys PW, Garcia-Garcia HM, Zhang Y, Bourantas CV, Holmes DR, et al. The negative impact of incomplete angiographic revascularization on clinical outcomes and its association with total occlusions: the SYNTAX (Synergy Between Percutaneous Coronary Intervention with Taxus and Cardiac Surgery) trial. J Am Coll Cardiol. 2013;61(3):282–94.
16. Farooq V, Serruys PW, Bourantas CV, Zhang Y, Muramatsu T, Feldman T, et al. Quantification of

incomplete revascularization and its association with five-year mortality in the synergy between percutaneous coronary intervention with taxus and cardiac surgery (SYNTAX) trial validation of the residual SYNTAX score. Circulation. 2013;128(2):141–51.

17. Garcia S, Sandoval Y, Roukoz H, Adabag S, Canoniero M, Yannopoulos D, et al. Outcomes after complete versus incomplete revascularization of patients with multivessel coronary artery disease: a meta-analysis of 89,883 patients enrolled in randomized clinical trials and observational studies. J Am Coll Cardiol. 2013;62(16):1421–31.

18. Ahn JM, Park DW, Lee CW, Chang M, Cavalcante R, Sotomi Y, et al. Comparison of stenting versus bypass surgery according to the completeness of revascularization in severe coronary artery disease: patient-level pooled analysis of the SYNTAX, PRECOMBAT, and BEST trials. JACC Cardiovasc Interv. 2017;10(14):1415–24.

19. van Nunen LX, Zimmermann FM, Tonino PAL, Barbato E, Baumbach A, Engstrøm T, et al. Fractional flow reserve versus angiography for guidance of PCI in patients with multivessel coronary artery disease (FAME): 5-year follow-up of a randomised controlled trial. Lancet. 2015;386(10006):1853–60.

20. Fearon WF, Nishi T, De Bruyne B, Boothroyd DB, Barbato E, Tonino P, et al. Clinical outcomes and cost-effectiveness of fractional flow reserve-guided percutaneous coronary intervention in patients with stable coronary artery disease: three-year follow-up of the FAME 2 trial (Fractional flow reserve versus angiography for multivessel evaluation). Circulation. 2018;137(5):480–7.

21. Toth G, De Bruyne B, Casselman F, De Vroey F, Pyxaras S, Di Serafino L, et al. Fractional flow reserve-guided versus angiography-guided coronary artery bypass graft surgery. Circulation. 2013;128(13):1405–11.

22. Layland J, Oldroyd KG, Curzen N, Sood A, Balachandran K, Das R, et al. Fractional flow reserve vs. angiography in guiding management to optimize outcomes in non-ST-segment elevation myocardial infarction: the British Heart Foundation FAMOUS-NSTEMI randomized trial. Eur Heart J. 2015;36(2):100–11.

23. Yusuf SZD, Peduzzi P, Fisher LD, Takaro T, Kennedy JW, Davis K, Killip T, Passamani E, Norris R, Morris C, Mathur V, Varnauskas E, Chalmers TC. Effect of coronary artery bypass graft surgery on survival: overview of 10-year results from randomised trials by the Coronary Artery Bypass Graft Surgery Trialists Collaboration. Lancet. 1994;344(8922):563–70.

24. Dzavik V, Ghali WA, Norris C, Mitchell LB, Koshal A, Saunders LD, et al. Long-term survival in 11,661 patients with multivessel coronary artery disease in the era of stenting: a report from the Alberta Provincial Project for Outcome Assessment in Coronary Heart Disease (APPROACH) Investigators. Am Heart J. 2001;142(1):119–26.

25. Hannan EL WC, Walfrod G, Culliford AT, Gold JP, Smith CR, Higgins RS, Carlson RE, Jones RH. Drug-eluting stents vs. coronary-artery bypass grafting in multivessel coronary disease. N Engl J Med. 2008;358(4):331–41.

26. Jeremias A, Kaul S, Rosengart TK, Gruberg L, Brown DL. The impact of revascularization on mortality in patients with nonacute coronary artery disease. Am J Med. 2009;122(2):152–61.

27. Aziz O, Rao C, Panesar SS, Jones C, Morris S, Darzi A, et al. Meta-analysis of minimally invasive internal thoracic artery bypass versus percutaneous revascularisation for isolated lesions of the left anterior descending artery. BMJ. 2007;334(7594):617.

28. Kapoor JR, Gienger AL, Ardehali R, Varghese R, Perez MV, Sundaram V, et al. Isolated disease of the proximal left anterior descending artery comparing the effectiveness of percutaneous coronary interventions and coronary artery bypass surgery. JACC Cardiovasc Interv. 2008;1(5):483–91.

29. Blazek S, Holzhey D, Jungert C, Borger MA, Fuernau G, Desch S, et al. Comparison of bare-metal stenting with minimally invasive bypass surgery for stenosis of the left anterior descending coronary artery: 10-year follow-up of a randomized trial. JACC Cardiovasc Interv. 2013;6(1):20–6.

30. Hannan EL, Zhong Y, Walford G, Holmes DR Jr, Venditti FJ, Berger PB, et al. Coronary artery bypass graft surgery versus drug-eluting stents for patients with isolated proximal left anterior descending disease. J Am Coll Cardiol. 2014;64(25):2717–26.

31. Blazek S, Rossbach C, Borger MA, Fuernau G, Desch S, Eitel I, et al. Comparison of sirolimus-eluting stenting with minimally invasive bypass surgery for stenosis of the left anterior descending coronary artery: 7-year follow-up of a randomized trial. JACC Cardiovasc Interv. 2015;8(1 Pt A):30–8.

32. Thiele H, Neumann-Schniedewind P, Jacobs S, Boudriot E, Walther T, Mohr FW, et al. Randomized comparison of minimally invasive direct coronary artery bypass surgery versus sirolimus-eluting stenting in isolated proximal left anterior descending coronary artery stenosis. J Am Coll Cardiol. 2009;53(25):2324–31.

33. Giacoppo DCR, Cassese S, Frangieh AH, Wiebe J, Joner M, Schunkert H, Kastrati A, Byrne RA. Percutaneous coronary intervention vs coronary artery bypass grafting in patients with left main coronary artery stenosis: a systematic review and meta-analysis. JAMA Cardiol. 2017;2(10):1079–88.

34. Stone GW, Kappetein AP, Sabik JF, Pocock SJ, Morice MC, Puskas J, et al. Five-year outcomes after PCI or CABG for left main coronary disease. N Engl J Med. 2019;381(19):1820–30.

35. Cho MS, Ahn JM, Lee CH, Kang DY, Lee JB, Lee PH, et al. Differential rates and clinical significance of periprocedural myocardial infarction after stenting or bypass surgery for multivessel coronary disease according to various definitions. JACC Cardiovasc Interv. 2017;10(15):1498–507.

36. Holm NR, Mäkikallio T, Lindsay MM, Spence MS, Erglis A, Menown IBA, et al. Percutaneous coronary

angioplasty versus coronary artery bypass grafting in the treatment of unprotected left main stenosis: updated 5-year outcomes from the randomised, non-inferiority NOBLE trial. Lancet. 2019;395(10219):191–9.

37. Thuijs DJFM, Kappetein AP, Serruys PW, Mohr F-W, Morice M-C, Mack MJ, et al. Percutaneous coronary intervention versus coronary artery bypass grafting in patients with three-vessel or left main coronary artery disease: 10-year follow-up of the multicentre randomised controlled SYNTAX trial. Lancet. 2019;394(10206):1325–34.

38. Chang M, Ahn JM, Lee CW, Cavalcante R, Sotomi Y, Onuma Y, et al. Long-term mortality after coronary revascularization in nondiabetic patients with multivessel disease. J Am Coll Cardiol. 2016;68(1):29–36.

39. Cavalcante R, Sotomi Y, Lee CW, Ahn JM, Farooq V, Tateishi H, et al. Outcomes after percutaneous coronary intervention or bypass surgery in patients with unprotected left main disease. J Am Coll Cardiol. 2016;68(10):999–1009.

Index

© Springer Nature Switzerland AG 2022
P. P. Punjabi, P. G. Kyriazis (eds.), *Essentials of Operative Cardiac Surgery*,
https://doi.org/10.1007/978-3-031-14557-5